Ophthalmology: A Collection of Cases

Ophthalmology: A Collection of Cases

Editor: Jaxon Gray

AMERICAN
MEDICAL PUBLISHERS
www.americanmedicalpublishers.com

AMERICAN
MEDICAL PUBLISHERS
www.americanmedicalpublishers.com

Cataloging-in-Publication Data

Ophthalmology: a collection of cases / edited by Jaxon Gray.
p. cm.
Includes bibliographical references and index.
ISBN 979-8-88740-650-3
1. Ophthalmology. 2. Eye--Diseases. I. Gray, Jaxon.
RE46 .C55 2023
617.7--dc23

American Medical Publishers,
41 Flatbush Avenue,
1st Floor, New York,
NY 11217, USA

ISBN 979-8-88740-650-3 (Hardback)

Contents

Preface

This book aims to highlight the current researches and provides a platform to further the scope of innovations in this area. This book is a product of the combined efforts of many researchers and scientists, after going through thorough studies and analysis from different parts of the world. The objective of this book is to provide the readers with the latest information of the field.

Ophthalmology is a medical specialty focused on the diagnosis and treatment of diseases and disorders related to the eyes and visual system. It seeks to provide medical and surgical care for a wide range of eye conditions such as glaucoma, age-related macular degeneration and retinal detachment. Glaucoma refers to a group of eye conditions which are characterized by damage to the optic nerve, and it is often associated with increased intraocular pressure. It can be treated through medications, laser therapy and surgical interventions. Age-related macular degeneration is a progressive degenerative disease which affects the central portion of the retina. It can lead to central vision loss and can be treated through injections, medications and laser therapy, depending on the type and stage of the disease. Different approaches, evaluations and advanced studies on ophthalmology have been included in this book. Researchers and students in this field will be assisted by it.

I would like to express my sincere thanks to the authors for their dedicated efforts in the completion of this book. I acknowledge the efforts of the publisher for providing constant support. Lastly, I would like to thank my family for their support in all academic endeavors.

Editor

1

A Rare Presentation of Orbital Castleman's Disease

Ruchi Goel,[1] Akash Raut,[1] Ayushi Agarwal,[1] Shweta Raghav,[1] Sumit Kumar,[1] Simmy Chaudhary,[2] Priyanka Golhait,[1] Sushil Kumar,[1] and Ravindra Saran[3]

[1]*Guru Nanak Eye Centre, Maulana Azad Medical College, New Delhi 110002, India*
[2]*Kallam Anji Reddy Campus, L V Prasad Marg, Banjara Hills, Hyderabad 500034, India*
[3]*Department of Pathology, Govind Ballabh Pant Post Graduate Institute of Education and Medical Research, New Delhi 110002, India*

Correspondence should be addressed to Ayushi Agarwal; ayushiagarwal.2110@gmail.com

Academic Editor: Alexander A. Bialasiewicz

Castleman's disease (CD) is an uncommon group of atypical lymphoproliferative disorders. Extranodal involvement such as the orbit is extremely rare. We aim to report a case of a 62-year-old male who presented with left painless proptosis for the past three years. Examination revealed a firm, lobulated mass in the left superotemporal orbit, displacing the globe inferomedially. A well-defined extraconal orbital lesion encasing the left lateral rectus muscle with intraconal extension was seen on Magnetic Resonance Imaging (MRI) that led to the provisional diagnosis of left solitary encapsulated venous malformation. Excision of the mass via lateral orbitotomy was performed. However, on histopathology, the features were consistent with a mixed-cell variant of Castleman's disease. A detailed systemic workup was unremarkable. Proptosis resolved after surgery and no recurrence was noted in the three-year follow-up. To the best of our knowledge, this is the first case report of a mixed-cell variant of unicentric orbital CD without any systemic features. This case highlights the importance of including CD in the differential diagnosis of well-defined orbital lesions so as to enable its early detection and timely management.

1. Introduction

Castleman's disease (CD), a rare entity first described in 1956 by Dr. Benjamin Castleman, is a group of atypical lymphoproliferative disorders [1, 2]. Also called as angiofollicular lymphoid hyperplasia, it can present as either a unicentric (one site involvement) or a multicentric disease (more than one site involvement) [3]. On the basis of histopathology, four subtypes are found, namely, the hyaline-vascular variant, plasma cell variant, mixed-cell type, and plasmablastic type (plasmablasts expressing Human Herpes Virus-(HHV-) 8 antigen) [4]. Extranodal involvement such as the orbit is extremely uncommon, and so far, very few cases of orbital CD have been reported in the literature [5]. The most common histopathological type of orbital CD is the hyaline-vascular variant (approximately 90% of cases) which is usually unicentric, clinically presenting as a gradually progressive orbital mass. We describe a rare case of unicentric mixed-cell variant orbital CD that was initially misdiagnosed as a solitary encapsulated venous malformation.

2. Case

A 62-year-old man presented with protrusion of the left eye for the past three years. It was insidious in onset, painless, and gradually progressive. There was no history of trauma, systemic illness, previous surgery, or diplopia. The best corrected visual acuity (BCVA) in the right eye was 20/200 and in the left eye 20/50. On examination, a nontender, nonpulsatile, lobulated, firm mass was palpated in the left superotemporal region, not associated with a change in size on valsalva. A horizontal dystopia of 2 mm and a vertical dystopia of 4 mm were observed displacing the eyeball inferomedially (Figure 1). The extraocular movement of the left eye was limited in levoelevation. Pupillary reaction and fundoscopy were unremarkable. No associated ocular involvement

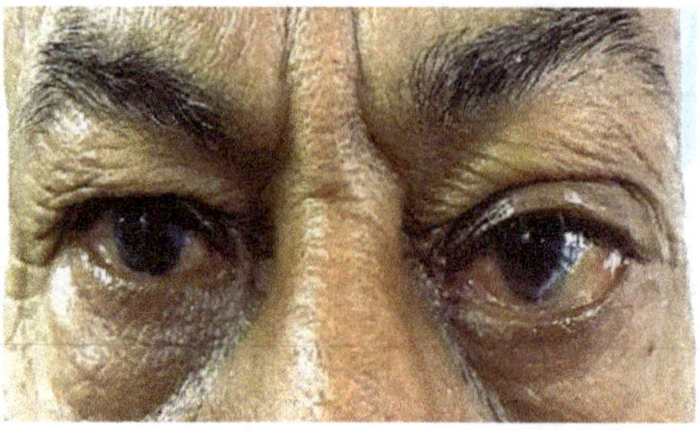

Figure 1: Clinical photograph showing left superior orbital fullness displacing the eyeball inferomedially.

was detected. The systemic examination was within normal limits with no lymphadenopathy or organomegaly. A complete blood workup, including immunological profile, showed a relatively increased Erythrocytic Sedimentation Rate (ESR) of $25\,mm/1^{st}$ hour. The rest of the parameters were within normal limits. Immunocompromised status was ruled out. The ultrasound B-scan of the left orbit revealed a mass lesion of low internal reflectivity in the lacrimal gland region.

A Contrast-Enhanced Magnetic Resonance Imaging (CE-MRI) of the orbit revealed a well-defined soft tissue lesion predominantly in the superolateral aspect of the extraconal compartment of the left orbit with intraconal extension, abutting the left lateral rectus muscle (Figure 2). The lesion measured $3.2\,cm\,(anteroposterior) \times 1.6\,cm\,(transverse) \times 2.4\,cm\,(craniocaudal)$. It appeared isointense on T1 and hyperintense on T2-Weighted Image (T2WI) with tiny hypointense foci on T1 as well as T2WI. Dynamic contrast-enhanced scans revealed progressive accumulation of contrast with persistence on delayed sequences with the lesion showing diffuse restriction. The lesion reached up to the lateral orbital wall laterally and the roof of the orbit superiorly. Since a provisional diagnosis of left solitary encapsulated venous malformation with bilateral immature senile cataract $(right > left)$ was made, the patient was planned for mass excision via lateral orbitotomy.

Macroscopically, a $3.5 \times 3 \times 2\,cm$ well-defined, greyish-red lobulated, firm mass was excised (Figure 3). Histopathological examination revealed sheets of mature-looking lymphoid tissue with attempted pseudofollicle formation and interfollicular hyalinized thick-walled blood vessels. Focal eccentric layering of the mantle zone ("onion skinning") was present. There was increased reticulin framework in the interfollicular area. On immunohistochemistry, an intermixed population of CD5 and CD20 with numerous plasma cells highlighted by CD138 was noted. Polyclonal expression of both kappa and lambda was seen (Figure 4). These findings were consistent with extranodal Castleman's disease of mixed-cell variant. Systemic involvement was ruled out as serum Interleukin-6 levels, gamma globulins, and Computed Tomography (CT) of the chest, abdomen, brain, and pelvis were unremarkable. A confirmatory diagnosis of unicentric, mixed-cell type of orbital CD was made. Surgical excision resulted in complete resolution of proptosis.

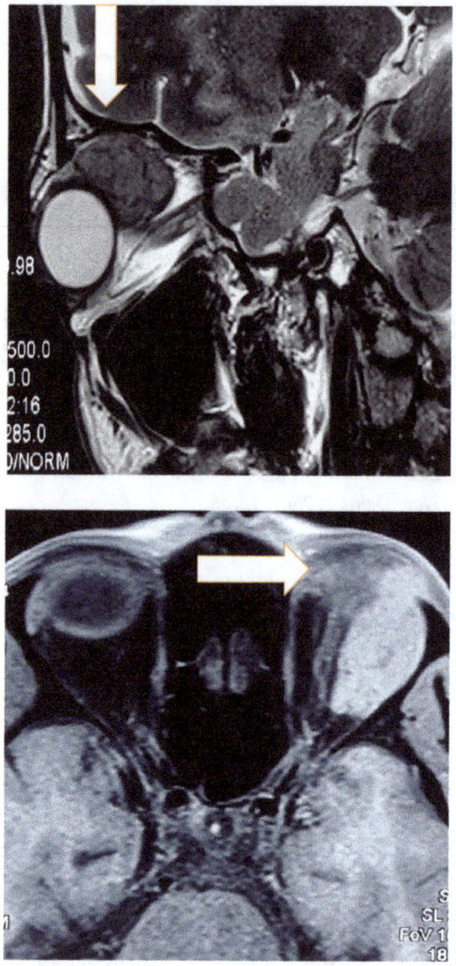

Figure 2: CE-MRI (Contrast-Enhanced Magnetic Resonance Imaging) showing left well-defined orbital lesion in the extraconal compartment abutting the left lateral rectus muscle with intraconal extension.

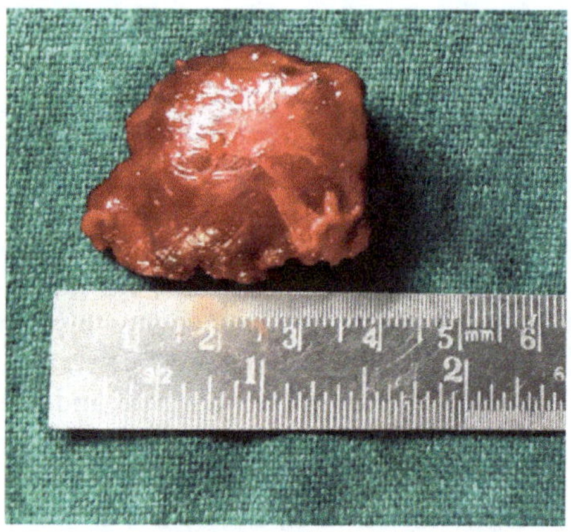

Figure 3: Gross examination showing a 3.5 × 3 × 2 cm well-defined, greyish-red, lobulated, and firm mass.

3. Discussion

Orbital CD, an extremely rare entity, most commonly presents as a progressive painless swelling resulting in proptosis or as B symptoms, i.e., weight loss, fever, and night sweats in

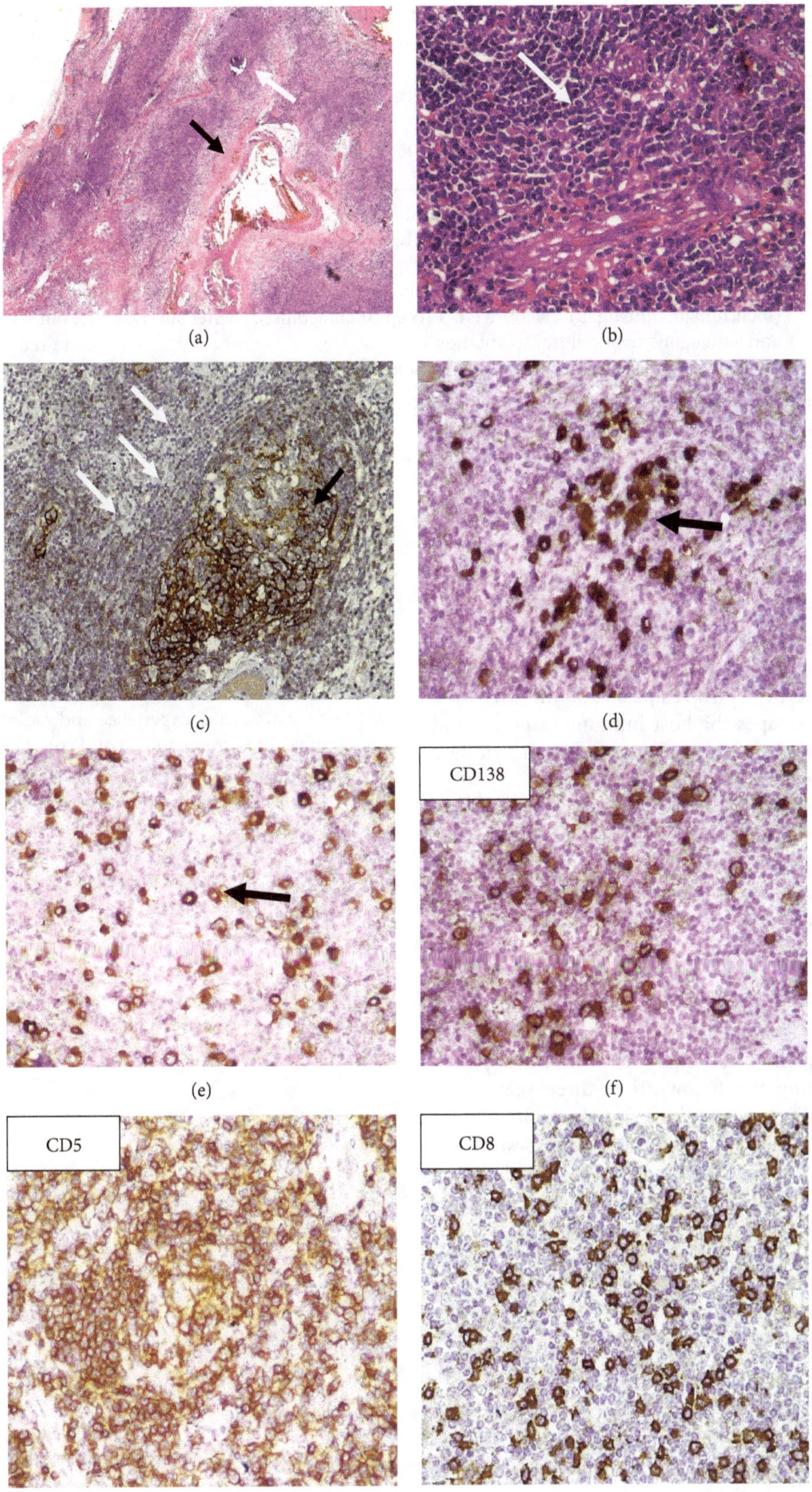

Figure 4: Histopathology suggestive of extranodal CD revealed (a) extranodal tissue showing a dilated blood vessel (black arrow) with multiple sheaths of lymphoid cells with attempted ill-formed follicles (white arrow) (HES2X), (b) mature looking lymphocytes (white arrow) (HES40X), (c) follicular dendritic cells positive for CD23 (black arrow) with garlanding ("onion skinning") of lymphocytes around it (white arrow), (d) polyclonal expression of kappa and (e) lambda, and (f) CD138-positive for plasma cells (g) CD5-positive T cells and (h) cytotoxic CD8 cells.

TABLE 1: Management of CD: an overview.

	Treatment	Prognosis
Unicentric (orbital) CD	Surgery (cornerstone)±neoadjuvant chemotherapy alternative: radiotherapy (i) If associated ocular involvement—trial of steroids (unless contraindicated) followed by radiotherapy	Surgery: excellent prognosis with 10-year survival rate > 95% Radiotherapy alone: 2- year survival rate—approximately 80% [7]
Multicentric CD	(i) Cytotoxic chemotherapy (CHOP/etoposide/CVAD/COP) (ii) Monoclonal antibody—rituximab (+CHOP) (iii) Corticosteroids (limited role) (iv) Emergent therapies: IL-6 receptor antagonist (tocilizumab, siltuximab), anakinra (IL-1 receptor antagonist), and autologous stem cell transplantation (v) Antiviral agents (in combination/maintenance therapy)	Multicentric CD has a long-term poor prognosis (worst in idiopathic MCD) Emergent therapies including rituximab show a better survival rate, but larger multicenter studies are required

CHOP: cyclophosphamide, doxorubicin, vincristine, and prednisolone; CVAD: cyclophosphamide, vincristine, doxorubicin, dexamethasone; COP: cyclophosphamide, vincristine, prednisolone.

presence of systemic involvement. The aetiology is multifactorial. Viral, neoplastic, and inflammatory mechanisms play an important role in the pathogenesis of unicentric CD (UCD). Of all these, the primary driving force is believed to be Neoplastic Follicular Dendritic Cells (FDCs). Aberrant production of interleukin-6 (IL-6) has also been implicated in unicentric CD [6]. In immunocompromised conditions, HHV-8 (Human Herpes Virus/Kaposi-sarcoma virus), a lymphotropic virus, escapes the host immune response and replicates in the tissues, resulting in uncontrolled cytokine production mainly seen in multicentric CD [6].

Associated posterior segment or intracranial involvement must always be ruled out [2]. CD-like clinicopathological findings can be seen in lymphomas, Ig-G4-related disease, autoimmune disorders (rheumatoid arthritis, systemic lupus erythematosus), Idiopathic Orbital Inflammatory Disease (IOID), and metastatic lesions. Histopathological examination with IHC remains the gold standard for confirmatory diagnosis. Various management options are available depending upon the location (Table 1). A complete surgical excision in this case was curative, with no signs of recurrence seen during the follow-up of three years.

To conclude, CD must be included as a differential diagnosis of a well-defined orbital lesion. To the best of our knowledge, this is the first case report of a unicentric, mixed-cell variant of orbital CD in the absence of systemic features. A step-wise multidisciplinary approach is crucial for an early diagnosis and appropriate treatment.

References

[1] D. L. Choi, K. Brannock, and A. L. Tang, "Castleman disease presenting as a parapharyngeal mass: a case report and review of the literature," *Clinical Medicine Insights: Case Reports*, vol. 12, 2019.

[2] J. W. Gittinger Jr., "Ocular involvement in Castleman's disease: response to radiotherapy," *Ophthalmology*, vol. 96, no. 11, pp. 1646–1649, 1989.

[3] N. W. Jones, T. R. Fountain, B. Thakral, and M. Eldibany, "Castleman's disease in the orbit of a 17-year-old girl: a case report," *Ophthalmic Plastic and Reconstructive Surgery*, vol. 30, no. 1, pp. e17–e20, 2014.

[4] D. C. Fajgenbaum, F. van Rhee, and C. S. Nabel, "HHV-8-negative, idiopathic multicentric Castleman disease: novel insights into biology, pathogenesis, and therapy," *Blood*, vol. 123, no. 19, pp. 2924–2933, 2014.

[5] H. Alkatan, A. Galindo-Ferreiro, S. Elkhamary, A. Maktabi, A. Galvez-Ruiz, and S. Schellini, "Orbital Castleman's disease: tertiary eye center experience and radiological characteristics," *Archives of Inflammation*, vol. 1, pp. 1–4, 2016.

[6] D. C. Fajgenbaum and D. Shilling, "Castleman disease pathogenesis," *Hematology/Oncology Clinics of North America*, vol. 32, no. 1, pp. 11–21, 2018.

[7] K.-L. Chan, S. Lade, H. M. Prince, and S. J. Harrison, "Update and new approaches in the treatment of Castleman disease," *Journal of Blood Medicine*, vol. 7, pp. 145–158, 2016.

2

Eales' Disease: When the Rare Sounds Frequent

Beatriz Oliveira Lopes[1], **Margarida Sena Brízido**[1], **Ana Isabel Reis**[2], **Margarida Maria Miranda**[1], and **Susana Morais Pina**[1]

[1]*Department of Ophthalmology, Beatriz Ângelo Hospital, Loures, Portugal*
[2]*Department of Medicine, Beatriz Ângelo Hospital, Loures, Portugal*

Correspondence should be addressed to Beatriz Oliveira Lopes; bibas.oliveiralopes@gmail.com

Academic Editor: Takaaki Hayashi

Eales' disease is a peripheral occlusive retinal phlebitis, with an unclear pathogenesis. The classic association with hypersensitivity to *Mycobacterium tuberculosis* protein infers that immunologic disturbance may be involved. Here, we described three cases of Eales' disease. All patients are Caucasian men aged 27-58 years and presented with vitreous hemorrhage and/or peripheral venous vasculitis. Tuberculin skin sensitive test (*Mantoux* screening test) and interferon-gamma release assay (IGRA) were positive in all patients. Therapeutic approach included antituberculosis therapy and systemic steroids, associated or not to immunosuppressive therapy, and retinal scatter photocoagulation in all cases. Antivascular endothelial grow factor (*VEGF*) intravitreal injections were also required in two cases. Since various retinal diseases can resemble this presentation, Eales' disease is considered a diagnosis of exclusion. Early diagnosis and appropriate therapeutic approach are both essential to accomplish disease control and reduce ophthalmologic complications.

1. Introduction

Eales' disease is a primary idiopathic peripheral obstructive retinal vasculopathy, reported in 1880 by Henry Eales for the first time [1]. A relation to ocular inflammation was described few years later [2, 3]. Healthy young men are the most affected by this disease, which is more prevalent in India and the Middle East [1]. In recent years, more cases affecting older adults have been described.

The clinical findings of Eales' disease include perivascular phlebitis and secondary proliferative retinopathy with neovascularization, recurrent vitreous hemorrhages, and possible tractional retinal detachment [1, 2]. Other signs of ocular inflammation as vitritis and anterior chamber cell reaction may also be present. The clinical course of Eales' disease is highly variable, presenting itself with gradual progression in few cases and temporary or even permanent remission in others [4].

Although the pathophysiology is poorly clarified, literature suggests that there is a clear association between Eales disease and *Mycobacterium tuberculosis* [2, 4, 5].

Different therapeutic approaches are suggested for Eales' disease, depending on its clinical stage [3, 5]. The typical retinal vasculitis usually requires treatment with systemic steroids in combination with complete antituberculosis therapy for a minimal period of 9 months. Steroid- paring immunosuppressive agents, like methotrexate, cyclosporine, and azathioprine, are usually reserved for cases which corticosteroids are not sufficient, need to be discontinued, or are contraindicated. Peripheral retinal scatter photocoagulation and anti-*VEGF* intravitreal injections are also essential therapeutic approaches in cases of proliferative disease and important retinal ischemia [2, 5]. In case of secondary ocular complications such as tractional retinal detachment and/or persistent vitreous hemorrhage, pars plana vitrectomy surgery may improve visual prognosis [2].

Table 1: Description of the presented cases. Abbreviations: OD: right eye; OS: left eye; FA: fluorescein angiography; *SD-OCT*: spectral domain optical coherence tomography; ERM: epiretinal membrane; CME: cystoid macular edema; CT: computed tomography; IGRA: interferon-gamma release assay; VEGF: antivascular endothelial grow factor.

	Case 1	Case 2	Case 3
Sex	Male	Male	Male
Age (years)	27	49	58
Laterality	Unilateral	Bilateral	Bilateral
Clinical presentation	Progressive blurred vision in the right eye	Acute bilateral decrease visual acuity and floaters	Floaters in the left eye over the previous 6 months
Anterior segment evaluation	Low-grade iridocyclitis	Unremarkable	Unremarkable
Fundus features	Vitritis, optic disc edema, venous vasculitis, and perivascular haemorrhages in nasal quadrants (OD)	Bilateral vitritis, vitreous hemorrhage, retinal vasculitis, hemorrhages in all retinal quadrants, and macular edema	Bilateral peripheral hemorrhages, vascular remodeling, neovascularization, vitreous hemorrhage, and macular edema (OS)
Ophthalmology multimodal evaluation	FA: venous vasculitis with retinal ischemia	FA: bilateral occlusive venous vasculitis with retinal ischemia SD-OCT: bilateral CME	FA: bilateral venous vasculitis with peripheral ischemia, neovascularization *SD-OCT*: ERM+ CME (OS)
Tuberculin skin sensitive and *IGRA* test	Positive	Positive	Positive
Thorax TC	Cisural micronodule with a 4 mm ganglion	Unspecific small bilateral hilar ganglia	Apical reticular pattern, residual fibrotic, and retracted changes
Systemic evaluation	Negative	Negative	Negative
Systemic treatment	Quadruple antitubercular treatment, prednisolone (1 mg/kg/day) with progressive withdrawal, and methotrexate (20 mg/week)	Quadruple antitubercular treatment, prednisolone (1 mg/kg/day) with progressive withdrawal, and methotrexate (20 mg/week)	Quadruple antitubercular treatment and prednisolone (1 mg/kg/day) with progressive withdrawal
Ocular treatment	Topical prednisolone and bromofenac Sectorial laser photocoagulation	Scatter laser photocoagulation and intravitreal anti-*VEGF* in both eyes	Scatter laser photocoagulation and intravitreal anti-VEGF in both eyes
Time on follow-up	2 years	2 years	4 years
Follow-up	Clinically stable with no need for therapy Complete visual acuity recovery	Clinically stable, under methotrexate (20 mg/week) and prednisolone (2.5 mg/day) Significant visual acuity recovery, restriction of visual field	Clinically stable with no need for therapy Significant visual acuity recovery

2. Clinical Cases

2.1. Patient 1. A healthy 27-year-old Caucasian male presented with progressive blurred vision in the right eye (OD) (Table 1). He denied ocular pain, headaches, and other ocular or systemic symptoms. Best corrected visual acuity (BCVA) was 10/10 in both eyes. Anterior segment evaluation showed low-grade iridocyclitis in the OD. Dilated ocular fundus examination revealed moderate vitritis, optic disc edema, vascular tortuosity, and venous vasculitis with perivascular hemorrhages mainly in the nasal quadrants of the OD (Figure 1). Fluorescein angiography showed severe venous vasculitis with important retinal ischemia in the correspondent quadrants of the same eye (Figure 1 and Table 1). Unilateral panuveitis with retinal vasculitis, prompted for the search of an etiology study while topical therapy with prednisolone and bromofenac, was implemented.

Initial investigation included hemogram, platelet count, hepatic and renal function, erythrocyte sedimentation rate, human leukocyte antigen (HLA) B51, antinuclear antibody, lysozyme, angiotensin-converting enzyme (ACE), and infectious serologic analysis. No suspicious lesions indicating active tuberculosis or sarcoidosis were found in the computed tomography (CT) of the thorax; although, it showed a cisural micronodule with a 4 mm ganglion (Table 1). A further systematic review was unremarkable. Tuberculin skin sensitive test and *IGRA test* (5.59) were positive, and Eales' disease was considered the likely diagnosis.

Besides topical therapy, corticoid therapy (1 mg/Kg/day oral prednisolone) with slow progressive withdrawal was started, associated with quadruple antituberculosis therapy (ethambutol, rifampicin, pyrazinamide and isoniazid). Oral methotrexate (15 mg/week) was introduced two months later, keeping slow progressive corticosteroids withdrawal

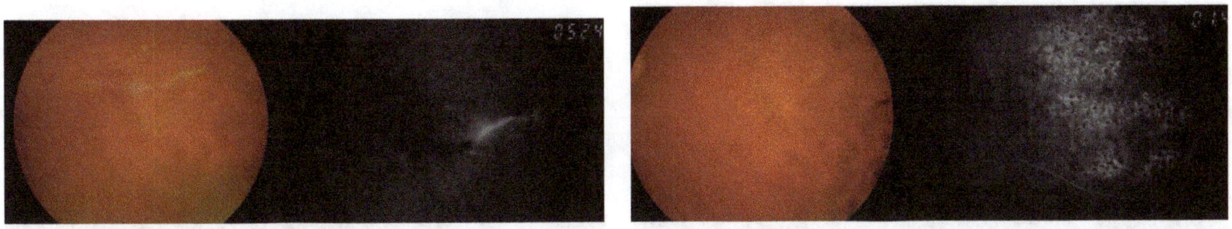

(a) (b)

Figure 1: Retinography and fluorescein angiography evidencing (a) active venous vasculitis with perivascular hemorrhages and retinal ischemia in the nasal quadrants OD in patient 1and (b) after medical treatment and scatter laser photocoagulation.

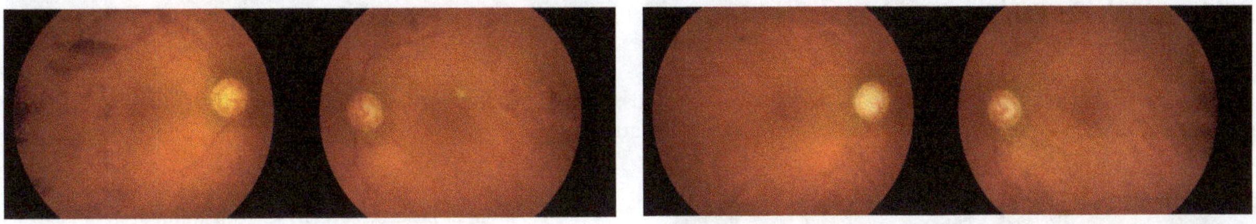

(a) (b)

Figure 2: Image of ocular fundus showing (a) active venous vasculitis with hemorrhages in all retinal quadrants in both eyes in patient 2 and (b) after treatment, including scatter laser photocoagulation and intravitreal anti-VEGF therapy.

with clinical improvement (Table 1). Sectorial laser photocoagulation of the ischemic nasal quadrants of the retina was performed after vasculitis remission (Figure 1).

Two years after diagnosis, having completed one year of antitubercular and two years of immunosuppressive treatment, the patient remains clinically stable, with no signs of active vasculitis and no need for further therapy.

2.2. Patient 2. A healthy 48-year-old Caucasian male came to the emergency room with acute bilateral decrease visual acuity and floaters (Table 1). He denied ocular pain, fever, anorexia, and other systemic symptoms. BCVA in OD was 6/10 and in OS was 5/10. Biomicroscopic examination was unremarkable in both eyes. Dilated ocular fundus examination showed vitritis, vitreous haemorrhage, and extensive retinal venous vasculitis with haemorrhages in all retinal quadrants and macular edema (Figure 2). Fluorescein angiography showed bilateral severe occlusive venous vasculitis associated with paramacular, midperipheral, and peripheral retinal ischemia (Figure 3), and spectral domain optical coherence tomography (*SD-OCT*) revealed cystoid macular edema (CME) in both eyes (Table 1).

Investigation of the etiology included hemogram, inflammatory markers (C-reactive protein and erythrocyte sedimentation rate), human leukocyte antigen (HLA) B51, lysozyme, angiotensin-converting enzyme (ACE), infectious serologic testing and hemoglobin electrophoresis, coagulation, and prothrombotic evaluation that were all unremarkable, except for tuberculin skin sensitive test (20 mm) and IGRA (>10) which were positive. X-ray and CT scan of the thorax also revealed unspecific small bilateral hilar ganglia (Table 1).

Eales' disease was suspected, and patient started complete quadruple antituberculosis treatment, which was maintained for nine months, associated with oral corticoid therapy (prednisolone 1 mg/Kg/day) with slow progressive withdrawal and subsequent introduction of oral methotrexate (20 mg/week) in order to achieve control of the disease. Serial treatment regime with anti-*VEGF* vitreous injections was also performed in both eyes (in a total of 11 in each eye). Laser photocoagulation was also required in both eyes over four sessions (Figure 2 and Table 1). This therapeutic approach allowed progressive clinical improvement.

After two years of follow-up, the patient maintains immunosuppression with oral methotrexate (20 mg/week) associated with prednisolone (2.5 mg/day) and achieved almost complete visual acuity recovery for 10/10 in both eyes, although with significant restriction of visual field, induced by both severe retinal ischemia and photocoagulation (Table 1).

2.3. Patient 3. A 58-year-old Caucasian male with known medical history of dyslipidemia, diabetes mellitus type 2 for 15 years, and ischemic stroke 15 years before presented to the emergency room with complaints of floaters in his left eye over the previous 6 months (Table 1). At presentation, BCVA was 8/10 OD and 5/10 OS. Anterior segment evaluation was unremarkable. Fundoscopy revealed peripheral retinal hemorrhages in both eyes and irregular macular reflex, inferior vitreous hemorrhage, vascular remodeling, and neovascularization in OS (Table 1). Fluorescein angiography showed retinal venous vasculitis with peripheral ischemia and neovascularization in both eyes, with no suggestive appearance of diabetic retinopathy (Figure 4). Patient also performed *SD-OCT* which revealed epiretinal membrane (ERM) with CME in the OS (Table 1).

Detailed clinical history and thorough systemic examination including serologic analysis, hemogram, inflammatory

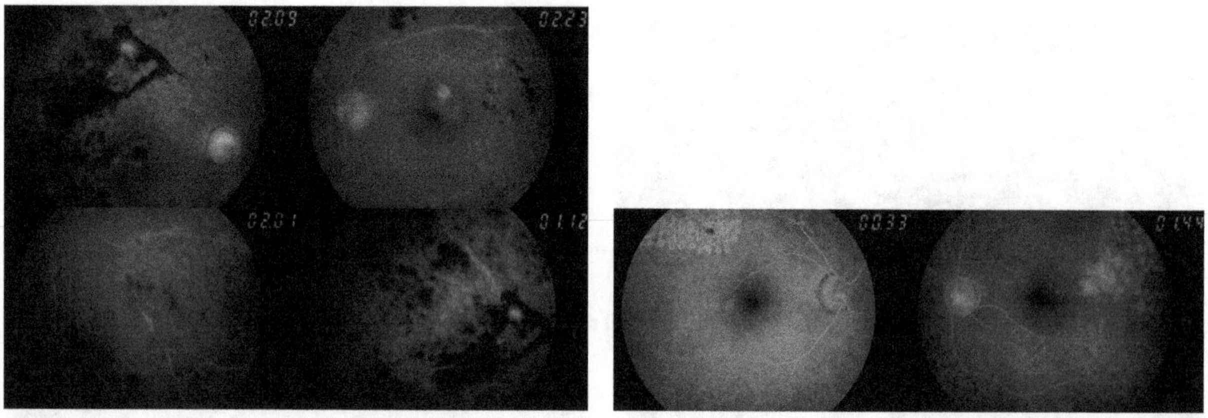

(a) (b)

FIGURE 3: Fluorescein angiography showing (a) retinal venous vasculitis, perivascular hemorrhages, and severe retinal ischemia in both eyes in patient 2 and (b) after treatment, including scatter laser photocoagulation.

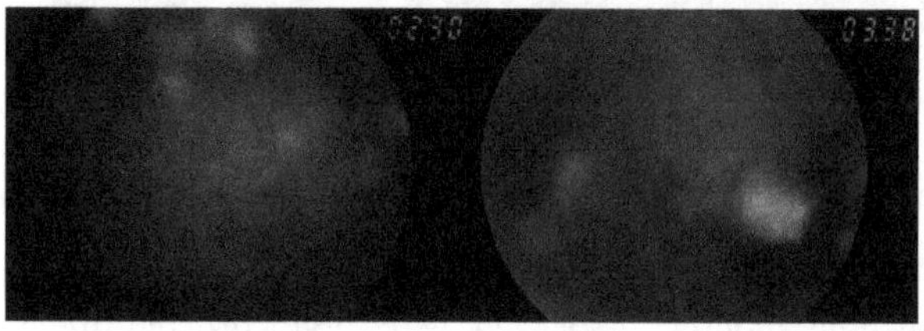

FIGURE 4: Fluorescein angiography showing significant occlusive vasculitis associated with peripheral ischemia, hemorrhages, and neovascularization in both eyes in patient 3.

markers, protein, and hemoglobin electrophoresis were unremarkable. X-ray and CT scan of the thorax evidenced pulmonary parenchyma with apical reticular pattern and residual fibrotic and retracted changes (Table 1). Once other causes of vasculitis and infections have been ruled out and tuberculin skin sensitive test (41 mm) and *IGRA* (2.77) were positive, Eales' disease was considered.

Patient started a complete quadruple antituberculosis treatment associated with oral corticoid therapy (prednisolone 1 mg/Kg/day) with progressive withdrawal. Scatter laser photocoagulation and three anti-VEGF vitreous injections were also performed in both eyes (Table 1). Although poor patient's compliance, clinical improvement with complete regression of vasculitis and neovascularization was achieved.

Almost 4 years after diagnosis, patient remains clinically stable and had significant visual acuity recovery (BCVA was 10/10 OD and 8/10 OS), maintaining close follow-up and no need for treatment.

3. Discussion

Defined as a primary idiopathic disorder of peripheral retinal vessel, Eales' disease pathophysiology is still poorly understood. This disease classically progresses in sequential stages involving retinal inflammation, occlusion, and neovascularization [2, 5]. Early inflammatory stage presents with retinal periphlebitis, which manifests as sheathing of blood vessels, primarily venous. This vasculitis leads to capillary occlusion

TABLE 2: Disease severity classification system [13].

Stage	Description
Ia	Periphlebitis of small caliber vessels with superficial retinal hemorrhages
Ib	Periphlebitis of large caliber vessels with superficial retinal hemorrhages
IIa	Capillary nonperfusion
IIb	Neovascularization elsewhere/of the disc
IIIa	Fibrovascular proliferation
IIIb	Vitreous hemorrhage
IVa	Traction/rhegmatogenous retinal detachment
IVb	Rubeosis iridis, neovascular glaucoma, complicated cataratac, and optic atrophy

in the middle stage which contributes to retinal ischemia with increased vascular endothelial growth factor [2]. Neovascularization seen at the boundaries between perfused and nonperfused zones of the retina is observed consequently in the late proliferative stage. It can happen up to 80% of the cases [1, 2], unlike disc neovascularization, which is rare [2]. Recently, it has been created a new 4 stage-grading classification in order to facilitate assess severity and functional prognosis of the disease [1, 2] (Table 2).

Eales is a bilateral condition in approximately 90% of patients. However, due to the inherent asymmetry, it can manifest itself unilaterally, as observed in patient 1, as sudden blurring of vision or floaters, caused by vitreous hemorrhage [1]. Sometimes, this presentation may difficult the correct diagnosis. In our case series, neovascularization associated with vitreous hemorrhages was present in patients 2 and 3. We speculated that in the first patient, the diagnosis was made sooner at an earlier stage, which allowed preventing this serious complication.

Immunologic mechanisms, mainly cell-mediated, have been proposed for Eales' etiology [3, 5]. From the various causes suggested, *Mycobacterium tuberculosis* is the most common reported. Although the role of this antigen is not completely determined, several studies propose that Eales disease is strongly related to both tuberculin protein hypersensitivity and previous exposure to tuberculosis [2, 5]. Indeed, the *Mycobacterium tuberculosis* genome had been detected through polymerase chain reaction studies in epiretinal membranes and vitreous samples of several Eales patients with tuberculin skin test positivity [6, 7].

In our case series, tuberculin skin sensitive test as well as *IGRA* test was positive in all patients, supporting the possible etiologic role of *Mycobacterium tuberculosis* in the pathogenesis of this entity and contributing to the diagnosis as well. However, the diagnosis of Eales' disease requires exclusion of several other ocular or systemic inflammatory and noninflammatory diseases which can easily resemble its features [5]. Branch retinal vein occlusion, proliferative diabetic retinopathy, Coats disease, and sickle cell disease are all retinal entities which manifest with similar peripheral retinal nonperfusion that must be ruled out [1, 5]. It is also important to exclude systemic infections and noninfectious diseases such as syphilis, sarcoidosis, toxoplasmosis, systemic lupus erythematosus, or Behçet disease [5, 8]. As we reported with our case series a detailed clinical history, ocular and systemic examination with appropriate diagnostic testing, including serologic analysis, hemoglobin electrophoresis, tuberculin skin sensitive test, and/or *IGRA* is usually required and essential for a complete diagnosis approach.

Treatment approach is defined in accordance with the clinical stage of the disease. Systemic corticosteroids are the mainstay of treatment for active vasculitis, especially in severe bilateral cases [2]. Although the role of antituberculosis therapy in Eales disease remains some point controversial, authors believe that its association with corticosteroids is extremely important in the disease control when IGRA and/or tuberculin sensitivity test are positive, or patients present with a presumably lung tubercular lesion [2, 8, 9]. In this way, all presented cases have been treated with the association of systemic corticosteroids and antituberculosis therapy, and two of them required immunosuppressive therapy with oral methotrexate as well, to achieve disease control and to prevent the adverse effects of corticosteroid treatment complications. In the proliferative stage, retinal photocoagulation combined with anti-*VEGF* intravitreal injections is the treatment of choice [10]. In cases of macular edema, anti-*VEGF* intravitreal injections are also indicated [9, 11]. Retinal photocoagulation was performed in all cases, and anti-*VEGF* intravitreal injections required in patients 2 and 3 for macular edema and/or associated neovascularization treatment. Photocoagulation is not recommended in case of active vasculitis, as it may release more angiogenic factors, with potential worsening of neovascularization [5]. Previous treatment with corticosteroid or immunosuppressive therapy may avoid demand of subsequent photocoagulation [5]. The major indication for pars plana vitrectomy is persistent vitreous hemorrhage and less commonly, tractional retinal detachment or ERM [5, 12]. Patient 3 developed ERM, although with no need for surgical treatment yet.

Although the progressive nature of this disease and the possible associated ocular complications such as tractional retinal detachment, neovascular glaucoma, rubeosis iridis, and cataract, visual prognosis is generally good. Recurrent vitreous hemorrhages are the most frequent cause of visual loss, which is transitory most of the time, as observed in our patients. Therefore, patients with Eales' disease can have a hopeful prognosis, being mainly affected by early diagnosis, prompt treatment, and regular long-term follow-up.

Our case series intend to draw attention to this rare entity which has become more frequent in the western world and between older adults. In this way, clinical suspicious and knowledge of the appropriate therapeutic management of the disease are essential to prevent clinical progression and the onset of ocular complications, as we accomplished with our patients.

Consent

Consent for publication was obtained from patients.

References

[1] J. Davis, S. H. Schecter, and J. Sowka, "Eales' disease: the great masquerader," *Optometry*, vol. 80, no. 7, pp. 354–359, 2009.

[2] J. Biswas, R. K. Ravi, A. Naryanasamy, L. T. Kulandai, and H. N. Madhavan, "Eales' disease - current concepts in diagnosis and management," *Journal of Ophthalmic Inflammation and Infection*, vol. 3, no. 1, p. 11, 2013.

[3] M. H. Errera, A. Pratas, P. Goldschmidt, N. Sedira, J. A. Sahel, and J. Benesty, "Eales' disease," *Journal Français d'Ophtalmologie*, vol. 39, no. 5, pp. 474–482, 2016.

[4] J. Biswas, T. Sharma, L. Gopal, H. N. Madhavan, K. N. Sulochana, and S. Ramakrishnan, "Eales disease–an update," *Survey of Ophthalmology*, vol. 47, no. 3, pp. 197–214, 2002.

[5] P. Namperumalsamy and D. Shukla, *Retina*, Elsevier, 5th edition, 2013.

[6] J. Biswas, L. Therese, and H. N. Madhavan, "Use of polymerase chain reaction in detection of Mycobacterium tuberculosis complex DNA from vitreous sample of Eales' disease," *British Journal of Ophthalmology*, vol. 83, no. 8, p. 994, 1999.

[7] H. N. Madhavan, K. L. Therese, P. Gunisha, U. Jayanthi, and L. Biswas, "Polymerase chain reaction for detection of Mycobacterium tuberculosis in epiretinal membrane in Eales' disease," *Investigative Ophthalmology and Visual Science*, vol. 41, no. 3, pp. 822–825, 2000.

[8] D. Călugăru, M. Călugăru, and C. el Ghali, "Eales disease in a young adult man Case report," *Romanian Journal of Ophthalmology*, vol. 61, no. 4, pp. 306–309, 2017.

[9] T. Das, A. Pathengay, N. Hussain, and J. Biswas, "Eales' disease: diagnosis and management," *Eye*, vol. 24, no. 3, pp. 472–482, 2010.

[10] S. D. Patwardhan, R. Azad, B. M. Shah, and Y. Sharma, "Role of intravitreal bevacizumab in Eales disease with dense vitreous hemorrhage: a prospective randomized control study," *Retina*, vol. 31, no. 5, pp. 866–870, 2011.

[11] S. R. Gupta and C. J. Flaxel, "The use of a vascular endothelial growth factor inhibitor (ranibizumab) in macular edema due to eales disease," *Retinal Cases & Brief Reports*, vol. 6, no. 1, pp. 122–124, 2012.

[12] A. M. A. el-Asrar and S. A. al-Kharashi, "Full panretinal photocoagulation and early vitrectomy improve prognosis of retinal vasculitis associated with tuberculoprotein hypersensitivity (Eales' disease)," *The British Journal of Ophthalmology*, vol. 86, no. 11, pp. 1248–1251, 2002.

[13] S. Saxena and D. Kumar, "A new staging system for idiopathic retinal periphlebitis," *European Journal of Ophthalmology*, vol. 14, no. 3, pp. 236–239, 2004.

3

Unilateral Toxic Anterior Segment Syndrome Resulting in Cataract and Urrets-Zavalia Syndrome after Sequential Uneventful Implantation of a Posterior Chamber Phakic Toric Intraocular Lens at Two Different Surgical Facilities: A Series of Unfortunate Events

Kepa Balparda,[1] Claudia Marcela Vanegas-Ramirez,[2] Johny Márquez-Tróchez,[2] and Tatiana Herrera-Chalarca[3]

[1]*Department of Cornea and Refractive Surgery, Black Mammoth Surgical, Medellín, Colombia*
[2]*Department of Ophthalmology, Universidad Pontificia Bolivariana, Medellín, Colombia*
[3]*Department of Clinical Research, Black Mammoth Surgical, Medellín, Colombia*

Correspondence should be addressed to Kepa Balparda; kb@kepabalparda.com

Academic Editor: Nicola Rosa

Background. Phakic Intraocular Lens (P-IOL) implantation is a safe, easy, predictable intervention designed to manage moderate to high refractive errors. Complications are relatively uncommon and include mainly cataract and intraocular pressure spikes. Toxic Anterior Segment Syndrome (TASS) is a rather unusual sterile anterior segment inflammation after uneventful intraocular surgery, extremely rarely reported after P-IOL implantation. Urrets-Zavalia Syndrome (UZS) is also very rarely described after P-IOL. To date, to the best of the authors' knowledge, no article has ever described the simultaneous occurrence of TASS and UZS in a patient after P-IOL implantation. *Objective.* In this article, the authors present the case of a female patient with moderate myopic astigmatism, who underwent sequential P-IOL implantation at two different facilities. The postoperative course of the first eye was uneventful, but she developed complications associated to the intervention in the second eye. *Materials.* The article describes the case of a young patient who underwent a sequential Phakic Intraocular Lens (P-IOL) implantation at two different institutions. The postoperative course of the first eye (left eye) was uneventful; however, the second eye (right eye) initially developed Toxic Anterior Segment Syndrome (TASS). Although timely and correct management was instituted, upon resolution of TASS, the patient developed Urrets-Zavalia Syndrome, anterior subcapsular cataract, and significant endothelial damage in the same eye. *Results.* The patient was followed closely and managed accordingly; corneal edema and anterior segment inflammation of the right eye eventually resolved. Nevertheless, an anterior subcapsular cataract and a fixed dilated pupil remained; with normal intraocular pressure (IOP). Specular microscopy confirmed an endothelial cell loss in the TASS eye (right eye). Pupil size showed no reaction to repeated doses of Pilocarpine 2%. A month after surgery, refraction on her right eye was $+0.25 + 0.75 \times 93$, which resulted in a 20/50 vision. *Conclusions.* TASS and UZS are both extremely rare complications after uneventful P-IOL implantation, with only a handful of cases having been reported of each of them. To date, this is the very first case where UZS ensued after and potentially as a consequence of TASS in a patient who had undergone P-IOL implantation. Although a direct causative element could not be pinpointed, the fact that the complication ensued after being operated in one surgical institution and not the other, could suggest some role of different sterilization and handling procedures, but no direct conclusion can be made on this case.

1. Introduction

Phakic Intraocular Lens (P-IOL) implantation is a safe, easy, predictable intervention to manage moderate to high refractive errors. Complications are relatively uncommon and include mainly subcapsular anterior cataracts, most of which are not visually significant. Toxic Anterior Segment Syndrome (TASS) is a rather unusual sterile anterior segment inflammation after uneventful intraocular surgery, very rarely reported after P-IOL implantation. Urrets-Zavalia Syndrome (UZS) is defined as a fixed dilated pupil, initially described after penetrating keratoplasty in keratoconus patients who had received atropine. Nowadays, it has been related to many other anterior segment surgeries. To date, no article has ever described the simultaneous occurrence of TASS and UZS in a patient after P-IOL implantation.

In this article, the authors present the case of a female patient with moderate myopic astigmatism, who underwent sequential P-IOL implantation at two different facilities. The postoperative course of the first eye was uneventful, but she developed TASS in the second eye. Although timely and correct management was instituted, upon resolution of TASS, the patient developed UZS, anterior subcapsular cataract, and significant endothelial damage.

2. Case Report

A female, 26-year-old patient, lawyer by profession, concurred to the main author's (K. B.) private practice in the search for surgical correction of her refractive error. She had a history of soft contact lens use for most of the day, with some mild foreign body sensation at the end of the day. She had no prior ocular surgeries. Otherwise, her clinical history was unremarkable.

Upon clinical evaluation, her uncorrected distance visual acuity (UDVA) was 20/1600 on both eyes. Her subjective refraction was $-6.50 + 2.00 \times 90$ and $-7.75 + 1.75 \times 80$ on her right and left eyes, respectively, and she achieved a 20/20 vision in both eyes with refraction. Anterior segment evaluation was utterly unremarkable. Her posterior segment was evaluated by a Retina Specialist who determined there were no predisposing peripheral lesions.

Preoperatory Pentacam, endothelial cell count, and biometry were all normal. The patient and the main author discussed different refractive options and jointly decided to perform EyeCryl Phakic Toric IOL (Biotech Vision Care; Ahmedabad, India) implantation in order to better preserve corneal biomechanical stability and avoid potential ectatic risks associated with laser surgery. Lenses were calculated using Biotech's proprietary calculator, with a planned refractive target of +0.50 in both eyes. White-to-white distance was measured both by Pentacam and with a caliper at the slit lamp.

The patient was first operated on her left eye at a big multispecialty hospital located in Rionegro (Colombia), and a $-9.50 + 2.00 \times 90$ was implanted uneventfully; the lens was left at 80 degrees following calculation. Surgical implantation was performed under peribulbar anesthesia by the main author (K. B.) as follows: the patient was draped and the eye cleaned; then, a 1.2 mm paracentesis and a 2.8 mm main incision were created, and the anterior chamber was filled with 2.4% Sodium Hyaluronate Ophthalmic Viscosurgical Device (Bio-Hyalur HV; Biotech Vision Care; Ahmedabad, India). The P-IOL was mounted and injected inside the anterior chamber. Afterward, the lens was positioned in the correct toric markings, and all four haptics were positioned behind the iris over the ciliary sulcus. Then, the Ophthalmic Viscosurgical Device was removed, and 1% Acetylcholine was injected intracamerally to achieve proper pupillary miosis. The postsurgical regimen for the left eye was Gatifloxacin 0.3% and Prednisolone 1.0% (Zypred; Allergan; Dublin, Ireland). In the first week after surgery, the operated eye was calm, with no pain, a UDVA of 20/15, and refraction of $+0.25 + 0.25 \times 85$ (Figure 1).

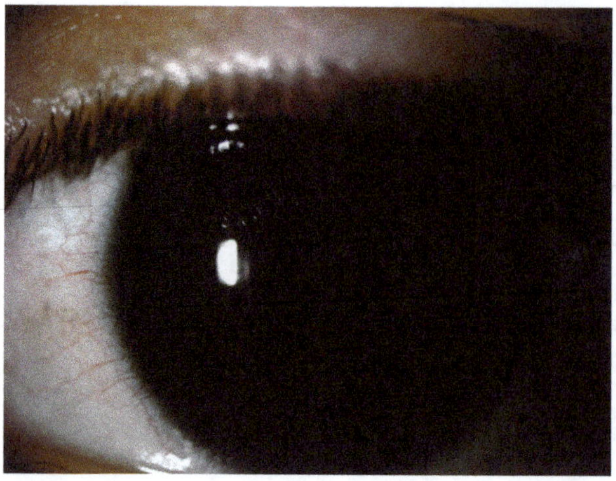

Figure 1: Left eye one week after surgery, with an uneventful clinical course.

The right eye was operated on a month later at a smaller, Ophthalmology-only surgical facility in Medellín (Colombia). The reason for the change was due to the patient's direct preference due to a shorter waiting list in the second facility. The surgical process was exactly the same as with the other eye, using the same brands of fluids and medicines. A $-8.00 + 2.50 \times 90$ EyeCryl Phakic Toric IOL was implanted without complications in a comfortable, uneventful surgery. The lens was left at the 90° meridian. The postsurgical regimen was started with Ciprofloxacin 0.3% and Dexamethasone 0.1% (Flobact-D; Ophtha; Bogotá, Colombia).

The patient requested for an urgent evaluation about 10 hours after surgery, because of exacerbated, uncontrolled pain in her just-operated eye. On clinical evaluation, a grade I corneal edema was found, with a mildly dilated, poorly-reactive pupil and an intraocular pressure of 30 mmHg. She was started on preservative-free Dorzolamide 2%, Timolol Maleate 0.5%, and Brimonidine 0.2% (Krytantek Ofteno PF; Sophia, Mexico) and oral Acetazolamide at a dose of 250 mg every 8 hours. The next day, corneal edema had increased to grade III (Figure 2), with a wider unreactive pupil, with an IOP of 20 mmHg and no pain. A TASS was suspected, so she was instructed to use Prednisolone 1% every hour and keep on using the other medicines.

During the course of four days, she was seen daily, finding a normal, stable IOP of 10 mmHg, but with a constantly

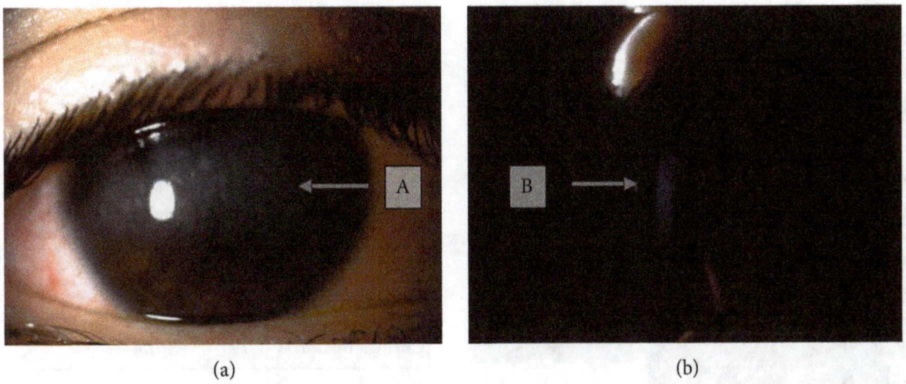

FIGURE 2: Corneal edema in the right eye during TASS, as seeing both with diffuse (a) and laminar (b) lighting.

edematous cornea and a widely mydriatic, fixed pupil. Pentacam confirmed an edematous cornea, and an anterior segment OCT discarded Descemet's membrane detachment. Due to nonresponsiveness, she was started on oral Prednisolone at a dose of 0.8/mg/kg/day. Infectious endophthalmitis was discarded.

During two weeks, she was followed closely. Corneal edema and anterior segment inflammation eventually resolved, and topical and systemic steroids were eventually tapered. Nevertheless, an anterior subcapsular cataract (Figure 3) and a fixed dilated pupil remained. A month after surgery, refraction on her right eye was $+0.25 + 0.75 \times 93$, which gave her a 20/50 vision. Her IOP has remained normal. Specular microscopy confirmed an endothelial cell loss in the TASS eye, with a normal cell count in the contralateral eye (Figure 4). Pentacam has confirmed the resolution of edema (Figure 5). Pupil size showed absolutely no reaction to repeated doses of Pilocarpine 2% (IsoptoCarpina; Laboratorios Alcon, Colombia) (Figure 6).

Her left eye has remained uneventful, with a stable $+ 0.25 + 0.25 \times 82$ refraction and a UDVA of 20/15.

We attach the corneal thickness before surgery, during and after TASS of the right eye; and the contralateral eye thickness (Figure 7).

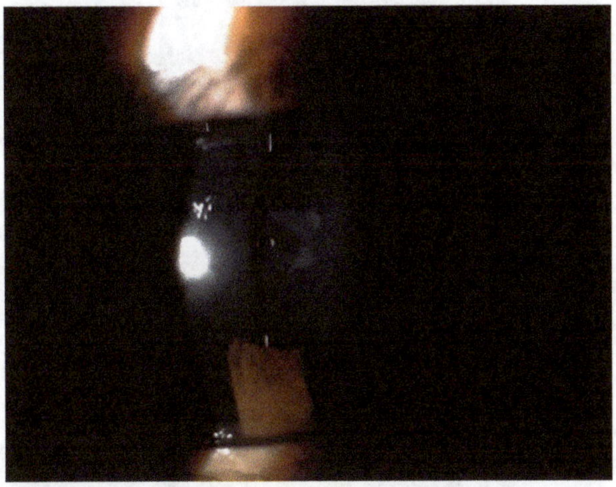

FIGURE 3: Anterior subcapsular cataract after TASS resolved.

3. Discussion

A myriad of data has confirmed P-IOL to be an effective option for surgical correction of moderate to high myopia and astigmatism, with an excellent safety profile. [1] Yasa et al. [2] published their experience in 58 eyes of 29 patients implanted with the EyeCryl Phakic IOL, finding a great increase in UDVA with stable postoperative refraction after 12 months of following. The group did not find any "significant cataract formation, significant endothelial cell loss, glaucoma, uveitis, or any other vision-threatening complication." [2] A recent paper by Bianchi also found Implantable Phakic Contact Lens (IPCL V2.0; Care Group, India) implantation to be safe and effective, with stable endothelial cell count and no cases of cataract after 6 months of following. [3]

Long-term following studies have also confirmed these findings. Nakamura et al. [4] retrospectively evaluated results of 114 eyes from 61 patients who underwent Implantable Collamer Lens (ICL; STAAR Surgical; Monrovia, California, United States) implantation at least 10 years before, finding an endothelial cell loss of 5.3% over the years, with only four eyes (3.5%) requiring IOL extraction due to subcapsular cataract. It is to be mentioned that the models of ICL included in this study lacked the central hole currently used, which could theoretically decrease the incidence of symptomatic cataract due to improved aqueous flow in the anterior capsular area [5].

TASS is a very uncommon, but potentially devastating, [6] complication of intraocular surgery, characterized by a severe, sterile postoperative inflammation generally occurring within days of surgery; although, delayed cases have also been reported [7]. Overall, between 3 and 20 cases of TASS occur in the United States of America every year [8]. Sengupta et al. [9] have suggested the incidence of TASS to be around 0.22% in cataract surgeries. Although clusters of TASS have been demonstrated to occur [10], half of the cases are sporadic [9]. By far, most cases of TASS are related to cataract surgery, but some authors have reported its occurrence after keratoplasty [11] and other surgeries.

TASS after P-IOL implantation is considered to be an extremely rare complication, [12] with only a handful of

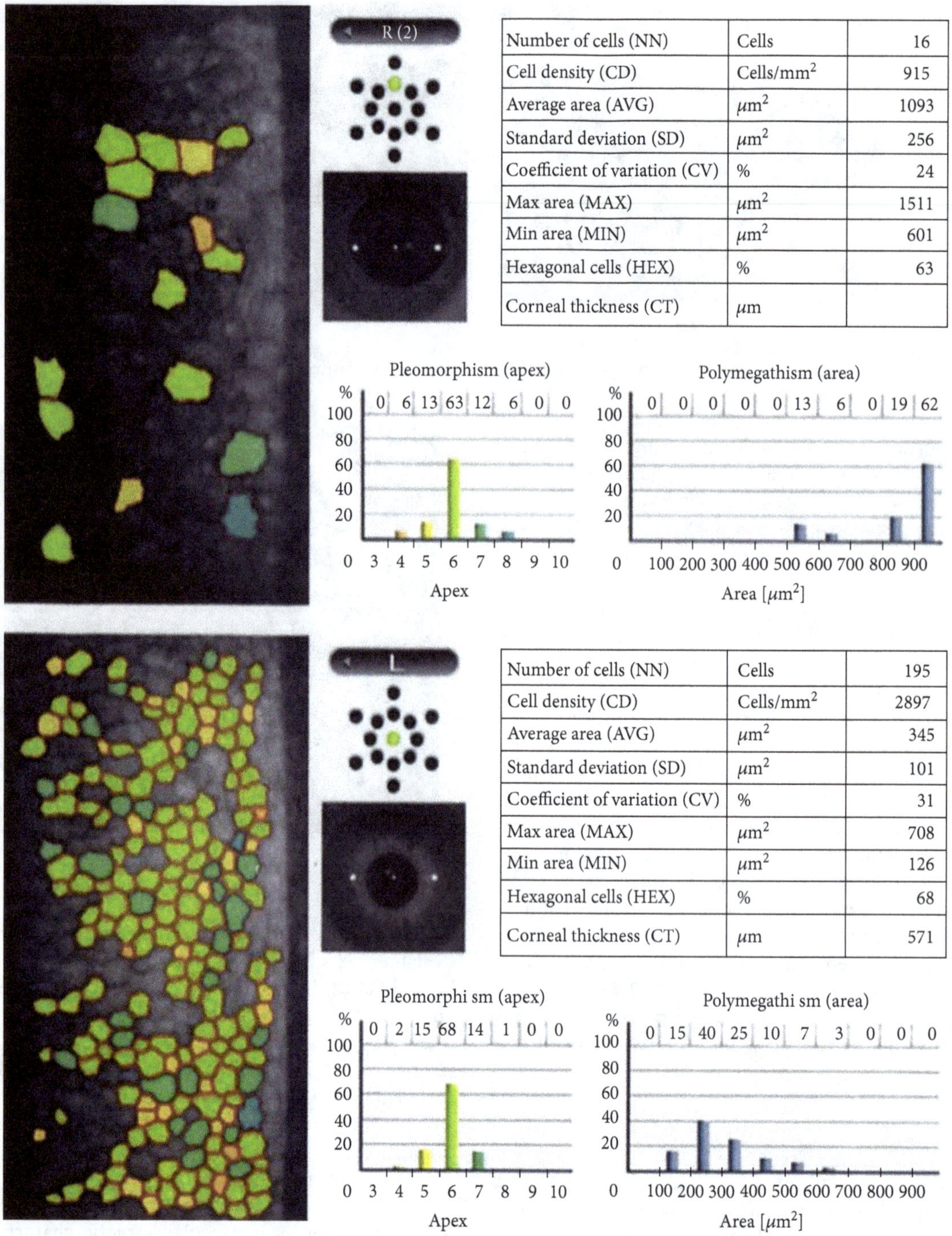

FIGURE 4: Specular microscopy of both eyes, showing a significant decrease in cell count and a clear increase in cell area in the right eye, while values remain normal in the left eye. Please also note the difference in pupil size between the right (UZS) and left (normal) eyes.

cases being reported so far worldwide [6, 12–14]. Singh et al. [12] reported a case of unilateral TASS in a young patient implanted with ICL, which responded to both oral and topical steroids [12]. Van Philips [6] has published four cases of TASS (two occurring sequentially in one patient) after uneventful implantation of an iris-fixated foldable P-IOL (Artiflex; Ophtec Inc; Groningen, The Netherlands). So far, the biggest case series of TASS after P-IOL implantation is the article published by Hernández-Bogantes et al. [15] that presented the occurrence of six cases of TASS in three patients after same day implantation of ICL. Although no direct causative element could be demonstrated, the authors suggested "the most probable cause [to be] the handling of the ICLs or instrument tips with powdered-gloves as reported by the surgeon" [15].

UZS is another rare complication occurring after uneventful intraocular surgery, initially described after penetrating keratoplasty, but reported after multiple surgeries. It

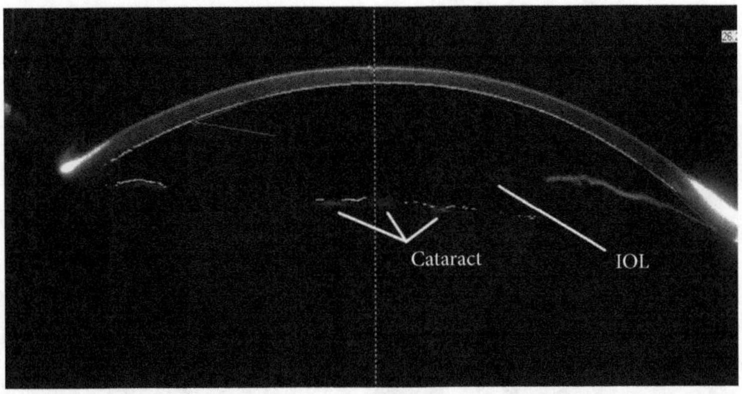

FIGURE 5: Anterior segment densitometry (Pentacam) demonstrating a correctly implanted intraocular lens (IOL) with a proper vault over the crystalline lens. Anterior subcapsular cataract can also be seen.

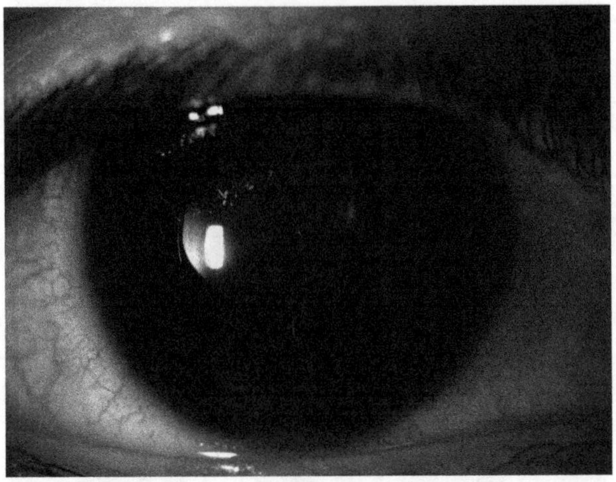

FIGURE 6: Fixed dilated asymmetric pupil in the right eye, consistent with UZS.

is characterized by a fixed, dilated pupil, with no responsiveness to topical Pilocarpine [16]. Although the exact mechanism for the occurrence of UZS has not been elucidated, [17] "an acute increase in intraocular pressure and ischemia of the iris most probably play a major role" [16]. UZS after P-IOL is extremely rare and has only been reported a couple of times [18, 19]. Arendt and Gerding [20] reported the occurrence of UZS after Artiflex implantation, which developed a pupillary block (IOP 50 mmHg) due to a malfunctioning iridectomy and had to undergo another surgical iridectomy. After the second surgery, the patient developed an unresponsive, fixed, dilated pupil. UZS has also been reported in two patients undergoing uneventful ICL implantation [19].

So far, to the best of the authors' knowledge, no case of associated UZS and TASS secondary to P-IOL has ever been reported in the literature before. In our patient, TASS coursed with an increase in intraocular pressure (30 mmHg) for two days, which may explain the later occurrence of UZS in concordance to the main etiologic theory of iris ischemia secondary to elevated intraocular pressure. Although transient increases in intraocular pressure may be secondary to other causes after P-IOL implantation (such as retained OVD), TASS is directly related to increases in intraocular pressure and seems to be the most plausible culprit in the case presented. After intensive local and systemic steroids, TASS resolved completely, leaving a fixed dilated pupil and other permanent damages, such as anterior subcapsular cataract and endothelial damage. All these changes can be explained by the intense sterile anterior segment inflammation that characterizes TASS.

Although an exact causative agent for the occurrence of TASS cannot be pinpointed in many cases, there is a myriad of potential culprits, including residues of enzymatic detergents in the tip of the instruments, idiopathic response to certain medications, stabilizing agents, and bacterial contamination in the solutions used. It is interesting that the patient developed TASS after being operated in a determined surgical facility, after having had an unremarkable postoperative course when the first eye was operated at another hospital. It may be feasible that different sterilization and handling protocols at the different facilities, as well as the use of different brands of fluids and medications, may have played a role in the appearance of this complication [21]. Nevertheless, the facility where the TASS ensued is an Ophthalmology-only center, with no known outbreaks or previously reported cases of TASS, so it may be reasonable to assume that current sterilization and handling protocols are mainly correct. The change of medication brands may have played a role, and potentially, the patient had an idiopathic response to one of the stabilizing elements used by one brand and not the other.

After a judicious evaluation of the case by the whole surgical and administrative team, no exact, demonstrable causative element for TASS could be determined.

4. Conclusion

Literature has demonstrated P-IOL implantation to be "predictable and safe option for refractive correction in highly myopic eyes" [22], with a very low incidence of adverse events. TASS and UZS are both extremely rare complications after uneventful P-IOL implantation, with only a handful of cases having been reported of each of them. To date, this is

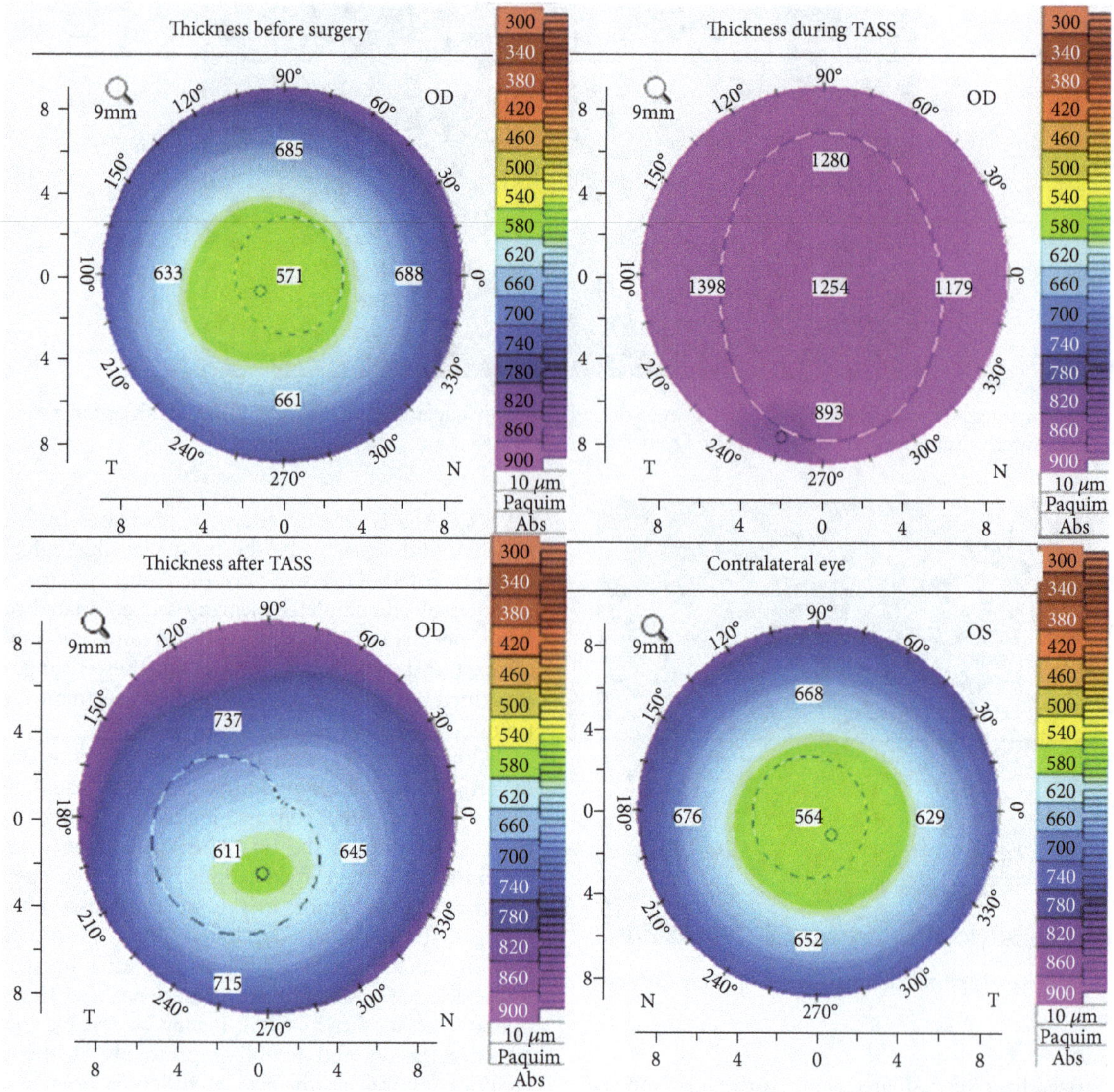

Figure 7: Corneal thickness before surgery, during and after TASS of the right eye. Thickness of contralateral eye.

the very first case where UZS ensued after and potentially as a consequence of TASS in a patient who had undergone P-IOL implantation. Although a direct causative element could not be pinpointed, the fact that the complication ensued after being operated in one surgical facility and not the other could suggest some role of different sterilization and handling procedures, but no direct conclusion can be made on this case.

Acknowledgments

The authors wish to thank the help of Dr. Hernán Arboleda (Retina Specialist) and Dr. Martha Luz Zuluaga (Cornea Specialist) for their kind help in the management of this patient.

References

[1] S. K. Pandey and V. Sharma, "Commentary: expanding indications of newer and economically viable phakic posterior chamber intraocular lens designs," *Indian Journal of Ophthalmology*, vol. 67, no. 7, pp. 1066-1067, 2019.

[2] D. Yaşa, U. Ürdem, A. Ağca et al., "Early results with a new posterior chamber phakic intraocular lens in patients with high myopia," *Journal of Ophthalmology*, vol. 2018, Article ID 1329874, 8 pages, 2018.

[3] G. R. Bianchi, "Initial results from a new model of posterior chamber implantable phakic contact lens: IPCL V2.0," *Medical Hypothesis, Discovery and Innovation in Ophthalmology*, vol. 8, no. 2, pp. 57–63, 2019.

[4] T. Nakamura, N. Isogai, T. Kojima, Y. Yoshida, and

Y. Sugiyama, "Posterior chamber phakic intraocular lens implantation for the correction of myopia and myopic astigmatism: a retrospective 10-year follow-up study," *American Journal of Ophthalmology*, vol. 206, pp. 1–10, 2019.

[5] T. Kawamorita, K. Shimizu, and N. Shoji, "Effect of hole size on fluid dynamics of a posterior-chamber phakic intraocular lens with a central perforation by using computational fluid dynamics," *Graefe's Archive for Clinical and Experimental Ophthalmology*, vol. 254, no. 4, pp. 739–744, 2016.

[6] L. A. M. van Philips, "Toxic anterior segment syndrome after foldable artiflex iris-fixated phakic intraocular lens implantation," *Journal of Ophthalmology*, vol. 2011, Article ID 982410, 5 pages, 2011.

[7] C. Y. Park, J. K. Lee, and R. S. Chuck, "Toxic anterior segment syndrome-an updated review," *BMC Ophthalmology*, vol. 18, no. 1, p. 276, 2018.

[8] M. B. Eydelman, M. E. Tarver, D. Calogero, S. Y. Buchen, and K. Y. Alexander, "The Food and Drug Administration's proactive toxic anterior segment syndrome program," *Ophthalmology*, vol. 119, no. 7, pp. 1297–1302, 2012.

[9] S. Sengupta, D. F. Chang, R. Gandhi, H. Kenia, and R. Venkatesh, "Incidence and long-term outcomes of toxic anterior segment syndrome at Aravind Eye Hospital," *Journal of Cataract and Refractive Surgery*, vol. 37, no. 9, pp. 1673–1678, 2011.

[10] A. Matsou, A. Tzamalis, N. Chalvatzis, A. Mataftsi, I. Tsinopoulos, and P. Brazitikos, "Generic trypan blue as possible cause of a cluster of toxic anterior segment syndrome cases after uneventful cataract surgery," *Journal of Cataract and Refractive Surgery*, vol. 43, no. 6, pp. 848–852, 2017.

[11] N. Sevimli, R. Karadag, O. Cakici, H. Bayramlar, S. Okumus, and U. Sari, "Toxic anterior segment syndrome following deep anterior lamellar keratoplasty," *Arquivos Brasileiros de Oftalmologia*, vol. 79, no. 5, pp. 330–332, 2016.

[12] A. Singh, N. Gupta, V. Kumar, and R. Tandon, "Toxic anterior segment syndrome following phakic posterior chamber IOL: a rarity," *BML Case Reports*, vol. 11, no. 1, 2018.

[13] M. Moshirfar, G. Whitehead, B. C. Beutler, and N. Mamalis, "Toxic anterior segment syndrome after Verisyse iris-supported phakic intraocular lens implantation," *Journal of Cataract and Refractive Surgery*, vol. 32, no. 7, pp. 1233–1237, 2006.

[14] I. Kremer, E. Levinger, and S. Levinger, "Toxic anterior segment syndrome following iris-supported phakic IOL implantation with viscoelastic Multivisc BD," *European Journal of Ophthalmology*, vol. 20, no. 2, pp. 451–453, 2018.

[15] E. Hernandez-Bogantes, A. Ramirez-Miranda, A. Olivo-Payne, A. Abdala-Figuerola, A. Navas, and E. O. Graue-Hernandez, "Toxic anterior segment syndrome after implantation of phakic implantable collamer lens," *International Journal of Ophthalmology*, vol. 12, no. 1, pp. 175–177, 2019.

[16] O. Spierer and M. Lazar, "Urrets-Zavalia syndrome (fixed and dilated pupil following penetrating keratoplasty for keratoconus) and its variants," *Survey of Ophthalmology*, vol. 59, no. 3, pp. 304–310, 2014.

[17] O. A. Magalhaes, C. L. Kronbauer, E. G. Muller, and C. T. Sanvicente, "Update and review of Urrets-Zavalia syndrome," *Arquivos Brasileiros de Oftalmologia*, vol. 79, no. 3, pp. 202–204, 2016.

[18] R. J. Perez-Cambrodi, D. P. Pinero-Llorens, J. P. Ruiz-Fortes, F. J. Blanes-Mompo, and A. Cervino-Exposito, "Fixed mydriatic pupil associated with an intraocular pressure rise as a complication of the implant of a phakic refractive lens (PRL)," *Seminars in Ophthalmology*, vol. 29, no. 4, pp. 205–209, 2014.

[19] A. Al Habash, K. Al Arfaj, and O. Al Abdulsalam, "Urrets-Zavalia syndrome after implantable Collamer lens placement," *Digital Journal of Ophthalmology*, vol. 21, no. 3, 2016.

[20] P. Arendt and H. Gerding, "Urrets-Zavalia syndrome after iris-claw-lens implantation, inadequate iridectomy and acute glaucoma," *Klinische Monatsblätter für Augenheilkunde*, vol. 233, no. 4, pp. 373-374, 2016.

[21] S. Cetinkaya, Z. Dadaci, H. Aksoy, N. O. Acir, H. I. Yener, and E. Kadioglu, "Toxic anterior-segment syndrome (TASS)," *Clinical Ophthalmology*, vol. 8, pp. 2065–2069, 2014.

[22] K. Balparda, C. M. Vanegas-Ramírez, L. Segura-Muñoz, and M. Gómez-Londoño, "Contralateral posterior chamber phakic intraocular lens implantation as rehabilitation of refractive lens exchange with a monofocal intraocular lens in a young, nonpresbyopic, bilateral highly-myopic patient," *Case Reports in Ophthalmological Medicine*, vol. 2019, Article ID 8791071, 5 pages, 2019.

4

Paracentral Acute Middle Maculopathy and Nonischemic Central Retinal Vein Obstruction in a Young Patient with Protein C Deficiency

Mojtaba Abrishami, Seyedeh Maryam Hosseini, Nasser Shoeibi, and Hamid Reza Heidarzadeh

Eye Research Center, Mashhad University of Medical Sciences, Mashhad, Iran

Correspondence should be addressed to Hamid Reza Heidarzadeh; dr.hamidreza.heidarzade@gmail.com

Academic Editor: Cristiano Giusti

Purpose. To report a case of protein C deficiency with paracentral acute middle maculopathy (PAMM) and nonischemic central retinal vein obstruction (NI-CRVO). *Case Report.* A previously healthy twenty-one-year-old male was referred with sudden-onset, painless, unilateral paracentral scotomata in the right eye for a week. His uncorrected visual acuity was 20/20 in both eyes. In fundus examination of the right eye, mild venous tortuosity, retinal hemorrhages, and a gray-white opacity in the papillomacular bundle were observed. In the macular spectral-domain optical coherence tomography images, a hyperreflective band was noticed at the level of the inner nuclear layer, indicating PAMM. Fundus appearance and fluorescein angiography findings indicated NI-CRVO diagnosis made. The systemic and laboratory evaluations disclosed a protein C deficiency. *Conclusion.* In this report, in a healthy young male, combined PAMM and NI-CRVO showed to be the cause of blurred vision in the setting of protein C deficiency.

1. Introduction

Paracentral acute middle maculopathy (PAMM) is an ischemic retinal lesion of the inner nuclear layer (INL). It is the result of global hypoperfusion at the level of the retinal capillary plexuses (RCP), especially the deep vascular complex (DVC) [1]. The most common associated conditions with PAMM are retinal vascular diseases like central retinal vein occlusion (CRVO) and central retinal artery occlusion [2]. The majority of CRVO cases are older than 50 years, and it is a rare condition in younger patients [3]. Primary thrombophilia like protein C deficiency is found rarely among patients with CRVO, and its association with this condition is unclear [4].

In this report, we present a young man without any remarkable past medical history who developed PAMM and nonischemic CRVO (NI-CRVO) in the setting of protein C deficiency.

2. Case Report

A twenty-one-year-old male without significant past medical history presented with sudden onset, painless, unilateral blurred vision in the right eye since one week before. Uncorrected visual acuity (UCVA) for both eyes was 20/20. The relative afferent pupillary defect was negative. The slit-lamp examination had no pathologic finding, and intraocular pressure was in the normal range. The fundus examination of the right eye showed disc swelling, multiple diffuse spot-like retinal hemorrhages, venous tortuosity, and a gray-white opacity retinal patch in the papillomacular bundle. The left eye was entirely normal (Figure 1(a)). In macular spectral-domain optical coherence tomography (SD-OCT), a hyperreflective band in the level of INL was noticed (Figure 1(b)). In fundus autofluorescence, the white opacity in the fundus examination was revealed as a hypoautofluorescence lesion (Figure 1(c)). Fluorescein angiography disclosed a slight

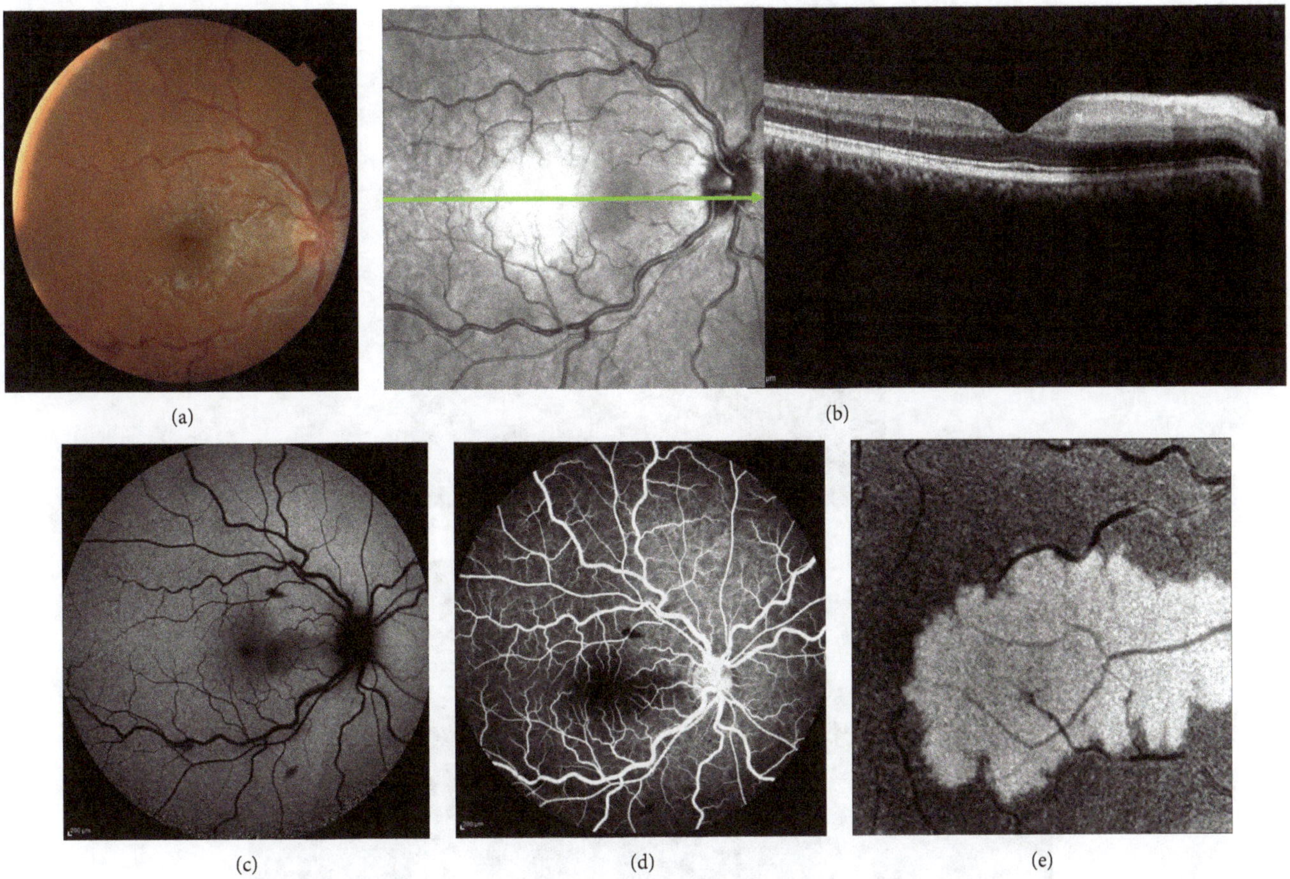

Figure 1: (a) The fundus photograph of the right eye shows disc swelling, multiple dot-like retinal hemorrhages, venous tortuosity, and a gray-white opacity in the papillomacular bundle. (b) Spectral-domain optical coherence tomography illustrates a hyperreflective band in the level of INL, and in infrared reflectance image, a grayish lesion with sharp borders in the papillomacular bundle can be observed. (c) Fundus autofluorescence shows the lesion as a hypoautofluorescence lesion. (d) The late phase of fluorescein angiography ($3':1''$) discloses no significant nonperfusion area. (e) $3 * 3$ mm en face optical coherence tomography angiography image of the right eye lesion revealed edema in the level of deep capillary plexus.

delay in the venous phase without any significant nonperfusion area in the late phase (Figure 1(d)). Optical coherence tomography angiography images of the retinal lesion area showed flow deficit in the level of the choriocapillaris and a hyperreflective area in the level of the deep capillary plexus (Figure 1(e)).

With a diagnosis of PAMM and NI-CRVO in the right eye, evaluation for systemic diseases and the hypercoagulopathy states was performed. Complete blood count and biochemistry tests, including fasting blood sugar and hemoglobin A1C, were in the normal ranges. He had normal values for prothrombin time (PT), partial thromboplastin time (PTT), international normalized ratio (INR), protein S, factor 5 Leiden, antiphospholipid, and anti-cardiolipin immunoglobulin G. The only significant abnormality in systemic evaluations was a low level of protein C (66.5%). Consultation with a hematologist for further evaluation was done, and the diagnosis of protein C deficiency was confirmed. Regarding the coronavirus 2019 (COVID-19) pandemic, we evaluated COVID-19 infection. Neither nasopharyngeal swab sample for reverse transcriptase polymerase chain reaction test nor antibodies against severe acute respiratory syndrome coronavirus 2 was conclusive for COVID-19.

Besides the hematology consult, the patient was followed, and after one month, he had a stable vision with no decreased visual acuity. Macular SD-OCT demonstrates decreased thickness and attenuation of the hyperreflective band in INL (Figure 2).

3. Discussion

Herein, we report PAMM and NI-CRVO in a young patient with protein C deficiency. CRVO is mainly associated with age, and nearly 90% of cases are older than 50 [3]. The association of systemic disease with CRVO is less prominent in young patients; on the other hand, thrombophilia is more associated with CRVO [5]. Regarding the young age of our patient, evaluation for coagulopathy disorders was performed and resulted in the diagnosis of protein C deficiency.

CRVO is the most common cause of PAMM. A retrospective, observational case-series of 484 American patients with NI-CRVO reported that the prevalence of PAMM development was approximately 5.17% [6]. In a case series of patients with PAMM and retinal vascular disease in Chinese patients, the prevalence of PAMM was 5.23% in 555

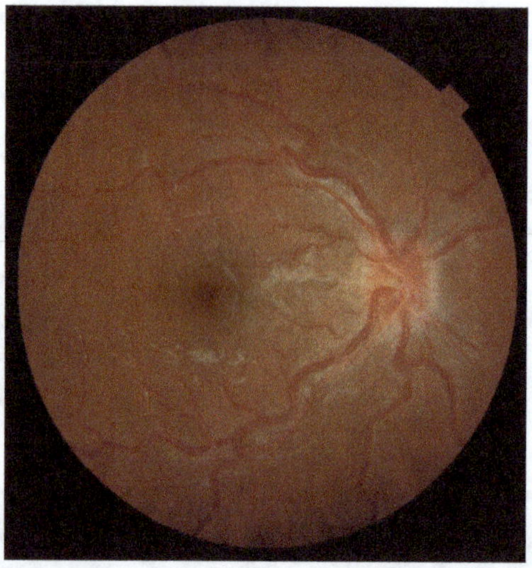

(a)

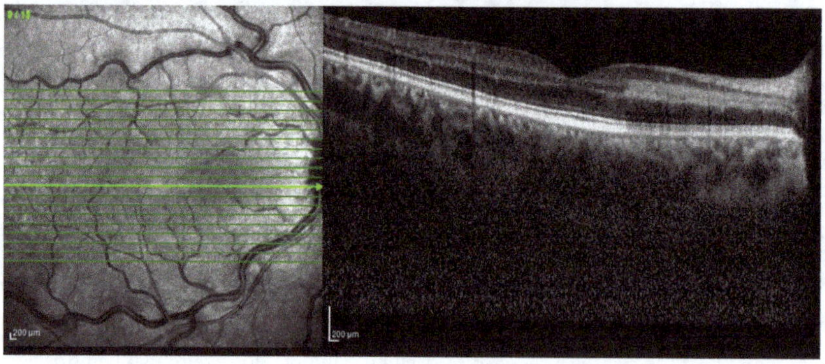

(b)

FIGURE 2: Fundus imaging following one month. (a) Fundus photograph of the right eye shows the vanishing of dot-like retinal hemorrhages and decrease in the opacity of papillomacular bundle lesion. (b) SD-OCT of the right eye revealed diminution in the thickness and edema of the hyperreflective retinal lesion.

patients with retinal vein occlusion. They also reported its prevalence was 19.44% in patients with retinal artery occlusion [7].

Clinical manifestation of PAMM can be unilateral or bilateral and typically presents with one or multiple paracentral scotomata, blurred central vision, and difficulty in focusing. The visual acuity can be normal, like in our case, or slightly decreased. Fundus examination can be normal or associated with deep, smooth grayish lesions [2]. SD-OCT shows PAMM lesions as a hyperreflective band in the INL that progress to atrophy with INL thinning over time, and OCTA shows the extent of ischemia in the inner and deep capillary plexus [8].

PAMM has been reported being associated with systemic diseases like idiopathic intracranial hypertension, meningitis, leptomeningeal infiltration by tumors, carotid arterial disease, vascular surgeries, antiphospholipid syndrome, giant cell arteritis, and some drugs [2]. Ocular disease associations are reported as inflammatory chorioretinopathy, congenital glaucoma, and foveal hypoplasia. Also, it was reported in the otherwise healthy patients following viral flu-like disease, H1N1 vaccination, and pregnancy [2].

Protein C is a critical vitamin K-dependent protease in the regulation of thrombin. It also has some cytoprotective functions in the regulation of inflammation and sepsis. The mild protein C deficiency incident is about 1 in 200 to 1 in 500, but the severe deficit incident is about 1 in 20000 people [9].

Protein C deficiency has been reported in patients with CRVO, but in a large series with control groups, there was no significant association [4]. To the best of our knowledge, there is no report on PAMM association with protein C deficiency; however, in the review of its pathogenesis, it is identified secondary to DVC flow failure, and it could be secondary to thrombosis in the setting of protein C deficiency [10].

Here, we report a previously healthy young male who developed PAMM and NI-CRVO in the setting of protein C deficiency, and it is the first time that a case of protein C deficiency with PAMM has been reported. In conclusion, PAMM and NI-CRVO could develop in young patients. However, the association between primary thrombophilia disorders, like protein C deficiency, and the retinal vessel occlusive disorders is unclear.

Consent

Consent for publication was acquired from the patient.

Authors' Contributions

All the authors contributed significantly to this report, and all authors agree to be accountable for all aspects of the work. All authors read and approved the final manuscript.

References

[1] D. Sarraf, E. Rahimy, A. A. Fawzi et al., "Paracentral acute middle maculopathy," *JAMA Ophthalmology*, vol. 131, no. 10, pp. 1275–1287, 2013.

[2] N. Moura-Coelho, T. Gaspar, J. T. Ferreira, M. Dutra-Medeiros, and J. P. Cunha, "Paracentral acute middle maculopathy-review of the literature," *Graefe's Archive for Clinical and Experimental Ophthalmology*, vol. 258, no. 12, pp. 2583–2596, 2020.

[3] L. L. Lim, N. Cheung, J. J. Wang et al., "Prevalence and risk factors of retinal vein occlusion in an Asian population," *The British Journal of Ophthalmology*, vol. 92, no. 10, pp. 1316–1319, 2008.

[4] J. M. Lahey, J. J. Kearney, and M. Tunc, "Hypercoagulable states and central retinal vein occlusion," *Current Opinion in Pulmonary Medicine*, vol. 9, no. 5, pp. 385–392, 2003.

[5] A. C. Fong, H. Schatz, H. R. McDonald et al., "Central retinal vein occlusion in young adults (papillophlebitis)," *Retina*, vol. 12, no. 1, pp. 3–11, 1992.

[6] E. Rahimy, D. Sarraf, M. L. Dollin, J. D. Pitcher, and A. C. Ho, "Paracentral acute middle maculopathy in nonischemic central retinal vein occlusion," *American Journal of Ophthalmology*, vol. 158, no. 2, pp. 372–380.e1, 2014.

[7] Z. Zhang, Y. Jiang, X. Huang, Z. Wu, and B. Ke, "Clinical characteristics of paracentral acute middle maculopathy in eyes with retinal vascular occlusion diseases in Chinese patients," *Journal of Ophthalmology*, vol. 2021, Article ID 8867570, 8 pages, 2021.

[8] E. Rahimy, L. Kuehlewein, S. R. Sadda, and D. Sarraf, "Paracentral acute middle maculopathy," *Retina*, vol. 35, no. 10, pp. 1921–1930, 2015.

[9] A. Gupta and S. Patibandla, "Protein C deficiency," in *StatPearls*, StatPearls Publishing, Treasure Island (FL), 2021.

[10] J. Scharf, K. B. Freund, S. Sadda, and D. Sarraf, "Paracentral acute middle maculopathy and the organization of the retinal capillary plexuses," *Progress in Retinal and Eye Research*, vol. 81, p. 100884, 2021.

5

Ophthalmic Diagnosis and Novel Management of Infantile Refsum Disease with Combination Docosahexaenoic Acid and Cholic Acid

Omar Elghawy,[1] Alice Y. Zhang,[2] Ryan Duong,[1] William G. Wilson,[3] and Eugene Y. Shildkrot[2]

[1]*University of Virginia School of Medicine, Charlottesville, Virginia, USA*
[2]*UVA Health Department of Ophthalmology, Charlottesville, Virginia, USA*
[3]*UVA Health Department of Pediatrics, Charlottesville, Virginia, USA*

Correspondence should be addressed to Eugene Y. Shildkrot; ys8q@hscmail.mcc.virginia.edu

Academic Editor: Takaaki Hayashi

Infantile Refsum disease is a rare peroxisomal biogenesis disorder characterized by impaired alpha-oxidation and accumulation of phytanic acid in the tissues. Patients often present with fundus changes resembling retinitis pigmentosa, developmental delay, sensorineural hearing loss, ataxia, and hepatomegaly. Traditionally, mainstay treatment for this condition has been a phytanic acid-restricted diet, although supplementation with either docosahexaenoic acid or cholic acid has rarely been described in the literature. We present a case of infantile Refsum disease in a child with retinitis pigmentosa-like ocular findings, sensorineural hearing loss, and self-resolving hepatic disease, who developed novel findings of macular edema refractory to carbonic anhydrase inhibitors. We describe management with a phytanic acid-restricted diet and combination docosahexaenoic acid, and cholic acid therapy, which helped to limit progression of her disease.

1. Introduction

Heredopathia Atactica Polyneuritiformis (Refsum disease) is a rare autosomal recessive disorder characterized by the accumulation of phytanic acid in the blood and tissues. A variant of this disease that occurs in children is infantile Refsum disease (IRD) which is biochemically, genetically, and clinically distinct from the adult form [1]. IRD is a mild Zellweger spectrum disorder characterized by retinitis pigmentosa-like fundi, developmental delay, sensorineural hearing loss, ataxia, and hepatomegaly [2]. The pathophysiology of IRD is driven by pathogenic variations in one of the 12 different genetic PEX genes that code for the biogenesis of peroxisomes [3]. This peroxisomal biogenesis abnormality leads to defective alpha-oxidation of dietary phytanic acid, a branched chain fatty acid present in meat, fish oils, and dairy products [3, 4]. The disorder is rare, although no exact estimates of IRD prevalence are available [5]. Low incidence and relatively nonspecific presentation may lead to a delay in diagnosis of the disease. We present the case of a five-year-old girl in whom the diagnosis of IRD was prompted by retinal pigmentary changes atypical for retinitis pigmentosa. Multimodal imaging of the retinal fundus is presented, documenting a novel finding of bilateral cystic macular edema (CME) in a patient with IRD. Early detection allowed systemic management of this patient with a phytanic acid-restricted diet and novel combination management with docosahexaenoic acid (DHA) and cholic acid.

2. Case Presentation

A 5-year-old girl with a clinical diagnosis of Usher syndrome was referred for initial retinal evaluation in our clinic. Her past ocular history was significant for left-sided esotropia treated with patching and atropine penalization of the dominant eye. She had a history of developmental delay, seizures, and significant hearing impairment. At the age of four months, she presented with severe hepatic dysfunction, with elevated serum levels of transaminases, and liver biopsy results were consistent with Alagille syndrome or a peroxisomal storage disorder. Previous workup included negative skin biopsy and no evidence of TORCH infection or renal dysfunction. Her enzyme levels improved spontaneously. The mother had a history of fetal demise at about 16 weeks of gestation secondary to cystic hygroma. The family history was otherwise unremarkable for congenital anomalies or known genetic disorders.

Her physical exam upon our initial evaluation at age 5 years revealed the presence of epicanthal folds, upper lid ptosis, and bilateral single transverse palmar creases. She had approximately 15 degrees of residual left esotropia at presentation. Snellen visual acuity and intraocular pressure could not be obtained during the initial visit due to poor cooperation. The patient was able to fix and follow with each eye. Fundoscopic examination revealed bilateral "salt and pepper" changes, a hypopigmented patch in the macula of both eyes, and bilateral nummular patches of hyperpigmentation in the periphery, without significant ocular nerve pallor or vascular attenuation. OCT revealed few cystic changes in the macula with loss of foveal depression and ellipsoid zone in the right eye (Figure 1(a)).

Given the involvement of both the central and peripheral retinas with atypical hypopigmented nummular patches, the absence of disc pallor or significant vascular attenuation, and the absence of typical bone spicules, the previous diagnosis of Usher syndrome was questioned. Measurement of serum very long chain fatty acids showed elevation of C26:0 and C22:0 puritanic acid and phytanic acid, suggestive of a possible peroxisomal biogenesis disorder. Review of an electroretinogram (ERG) obtained under anesthesia at an outside facility revealed complete extinction of scotopic and photopic responses. Chromosomal microarray testing and Usher syndrome mutation panel were unremarkable. Genetic evaluation revealed that she was homozygous for a PEX1 mutation (c.2528 G>A, p. GLY843ASB) consistent with infantile Refsum disease.

Following the diagnosis, the patient was started on a phytanic acid-restricted diet and underwent audiology evaluation with subsequent hearing aid prescription for severe sensorineural hearing loss. At 6 years of age, she was noted to develop new bilateral cystoid macular edema, a finding not previously reported in this syndrome (Figure 1(b)). At the age of 9, she began therapy with 200 mg daily docosahexaenoic acid and 350 mg daily cholic acid (Cholbam). The patient's developmental delay improved on this treatment regimen, and the patient began excelling in schoolwork. However, despite long-term therapy with topical dorzolamide for 5 years, her macular edema persisted (Figure 1(c)) through her most recent follow-up at 13 years of age. At this time, 8 years after initial presentation, her Snellen visual acuity was 20/100 in the right eye and 1/200 E in the left. No cataracts were noted. Retinal autofluorescence revealed a diffuse spotted pattern of hyperautofluorescence in the midperiphery (Figure 1(d)). Fundus photos demonstrated stable bilateral salt and pepper changes, with bilateral nummular patches of hyperpigmentation with a hypopigmented patch in the macula of each eye (Figures 1(e) and 1(f)). The patient has some dental enamel irregularities but is currently doing well with no further complications due to her condition.

3. Discussion

This case highlights the unique clinical features that should prompt an investigation for systemic conditions in a pediatric patient with retinal findings mimicking retinitis pigmentosa. The diagnosis of IRD is challenging but can be life-changing, if made early, by preventing progression of the disease, developmental delay, and subsequent clinical sequelae. The diagnosis is complicated by the paucity of literature on IRD and confusion between the adult and infantile forms. The findings that prompted further testing and eventual diagnosis in this patient included her young age and atypical nummular pigmented patches without significant optic nerve pallor or vascular attenuation. It is interesting that the patient's earlier liver abnormalities had stabilized without specific treatments following a genetic diagnosis in infancy. Successful diagnosis allowed our patient to receive treatment with phytanic acid diet restriction, docosahexaenoic acid, and cholic acid and has allowed for normal cognitive development, thus far no additional systemic manifestations of the disease.

IRD is rare, and its clinical characteristics have not been fully elucidated [5]. In contrast to classic Refsum disease, the infantile form is associated with minor dysmorphism, mental retardation, hepatomegaly, and sensorineural hearing loss [2]. Within the limited literature, retinal pigmentary degeneration and accompanying night blindness are commonly reported as earliest ocular clinical manifestations of IRD [6]. These ocular findings are similar to that of an inherited retinal dystrophy, which can be seen in a number of syndromes such as Bardet-Biedl [7]. However, the nummular patches of hyperpigmentation seen in our patient are not typical for an inherited dystrophy. Other nonspecific findings such as "salt and pepper" spots and nystagmus are also found in a variety of other conditions, but the patient's elevated phytanic acid is most suggestive of peroxisomal disease. As far as we are aware, this is the first report of a patient with IRD with cystoid macular edema. Furthermore, her CME was found to be refractory to treatment with topical carbonic anhydrase inhibitor.

The pathophysiology of IRD is driven by defective alpha oxidation of phytanic acid and other related structures derived from common dietary sources [8–10]. Clinical symptoms arise when excess phytanic acid accumulates in nervous tissues and liver [3–6, 11]. Consequently, detection and early management of IRD is critical in preventing irreversible long-term sensorineural degeneration [12]. Sequelae may include ataxia secondary to cerebellar degeneration, seizures, and even death from nerve fibrosis and fluid accumulation within the myelin sheath of critical nerves [13–15]. Vision loss also occurs secondary to deposition of excess phytanic acid within ocular tissue, manifesting as photoreceptor and ganglion cell death primarily in peripheral fields [16].

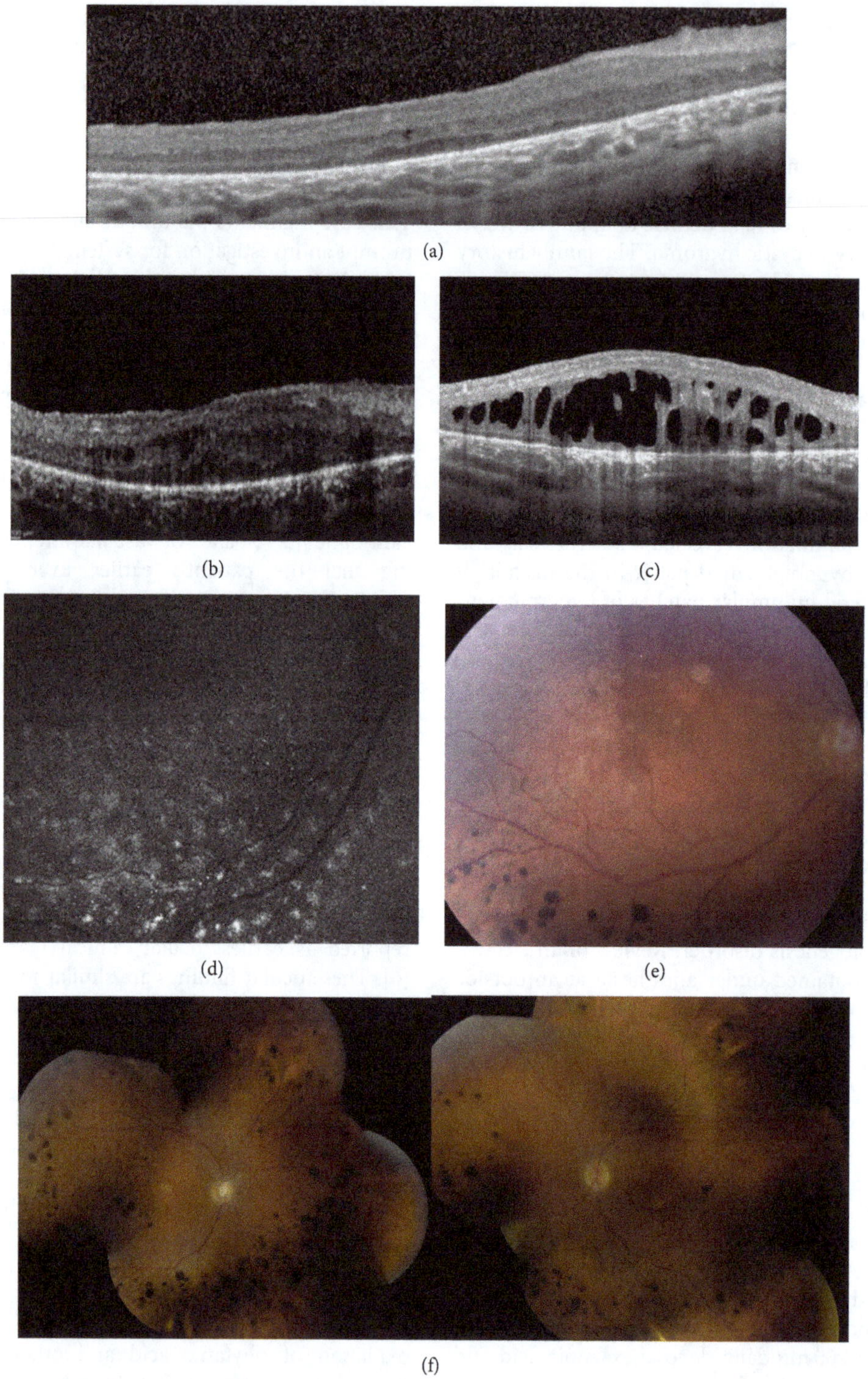

Figure 1: (a) OCT at age 5 on presentation of right eye showing minimal perifoveal cystic changes and extensive loss of IS/OS junction. (b) OCT of the right eye at 6 years of age demonstrating cystoid macular edema. Similar findings were noted in her left eye as well. (c) OCT of the right eye demonstrating persistent macular edema despite carbonic anhydrase inhibitors. Similar findings noted in the left eye. (d) Representative retinal autofluorescence revealed diffuse spotted pattern of hyperautofluorescence in midperiphery. (e) Central view of fundoscopic imaging revealing nummular patches. (f) Fundoscopic montage imaging at last follow-up revealing bilateral salt and pepper changes, a hypopigmented patch in the macula of both eyes, and bilateral nummular patches of hyperpigmentation in periphery. The optic nerve had no significant pallor, and the vessels were not attenuated.

The specific PEX1 pathogenic variation found in this patient (G843D) has previously been postulated in the literature to account for up to one-third of all pathogenic PEX1 gene alleles [16]. This variant has been shown to follow an autosomal recessive inheritance pattern though this was not confirmed with parental testing in our case. While functional studies analyzing the predicted effect on the PEX1 protein is lacking, it is believed to impact interactions with the PTS1 protein. However, one expression study assaying the G843D PEX1 allele's effect on PTS1 protein import demonstrated up to 15% residual catalase import activity compared to wild-type PEX1, suggesting that the G843D variant portends a more mild clinical phenotype compared other known PEX1 variants [16, 17].

Traditionally, the main treatment modality for patients with IRD has been centered around a phytanic acid-free diet. While it is possible for phytanic acid to be metabolized from adipose tissue, it predominantly comes from dietary sources [18]. Plasma exchange therapy has also been proposed to remove phytanic acid directly from the blood and has been demonstrated to improve patient outcomes when dietary restriction is insufficient in managing plasma phytanic acid. Though excluding phytanic acid from the diet has not been shown to reverse optic neuropathy [5], it can alleviate systemic complications and drastically improve quality of life [18]. However, phytanic acid-free foods are not palatable, leading to lower patient compliance with dietary regiments [19].

Our patient has benefitted from hearing aids, a switch to a vegan diet, and adjunctive treatment with a combination of docosahexaenoic acid and cholic acid, which appeared to slow progression of her IRD. To our knowledge, this is the first reported use of docosahexaenoic acid and cholic acid in combination for IRD. However, these drugs have been used individually in patients with Zellweger spectrum disorders with controversial efficacy. These drugs are aimed at increasing deficient polyunsaturated fatty acids in patients with Zellweger spectrum disorders and decreasing the concentrations of toxic bile acid intermediates [20, 21]. While some studies suggest a beneficial effect of DHA supplementation in patients with Zellweger spectrum disorders, a randomized double-blind placebo-controlled trial showed no improvement of visual function and growth [21, 22]. Similarly, despite FDA approval, studies surrounding cholic acid supplementation have not demonstrated improved growth and development or reduced urinary excretion of toxic intermediates in these patients [23, 24]. Additional research is needed to evaluate efficacy of DHA and cholic acid as combination therapy for IRD.

In summary, it is important to rule out the diagnosis of IRD or other inborn errors of metabolism in any young patient presenting with pigmentary retinopathy, as early detection is paramount for reducing morbidity and mortality of these conditions. Cystoid macular edema has not previously been reported but appears to be an important cause of visual decline in patients with IRD and may progress over time despite treatment with carbonic anhydrase inhibitors as seen in our patient. Combination therapy with docosahexaenoic acid (DHA), cholic acid, and dietary restriction when introduced at a young age may offer patients a chance at near normal development and life.

Abbreviations

DHAL: Docosahexaenoic acid
CME: Cystic macular edema
IRD: Infantile Refsum disease
OCT: Optical coherence tomography.

Acknowledgments

The authors would like to acknowledge the Genetics and Pediatrics Departments of the University of Virginia Medical Center for their technical assistance in the workup of this case.

References

[1] V. Choksi, E. Hoeffner, E. Karaarslan, C. Yalcinkaya, and S. Cakirer, "Infantile Refsum disease: case report," *American Journal of Neuroradiology*, vol. 24, no. 10, pp. 2082–2084, 2003.

[2] B. T. Poll-The, J. M. Saudubray, H. A. Ogier et al., "Infantile Refsum disease: an inherited peroxisomal disorder," *European Journal of Pediatrics*, vol. 146, no. 5, pp. 477–483, 1987.

[3] G. A. Jansen, H. R. Waterham, and R. J. A. Wanders, "Molecular basis of Refsum disease: sequence variations in phytanoyl-CoA hydroxylase (PHYH) and the PTS2 receptor (PEX7)," *Human Mutation*, vol. 23, no. 3, pp. 209–218, 2004.

[4] G. A. Jansen, R. Oftnan, S. Ferdinandusse et al., "Refsum disease is caused by mutations in the phytanoyl-CoA hydroxylase gene," *Nature Genetics*, vol. 17, no. 2, pp. 190–193, 1997.

[5] R. Kumar and O. De Jesus, *Refsum Disease*, StatPearls. StatPearls Publishing, 2021, February 2021, http://www.ncbi.nlm.nih.gov/books/NBK560618/.

[6] K. L. Pakzad-Vaezi and D. A. L. Maberley, "Infantile Refsum disease in a young ADULT," *Retinal Cases & Brief Reports*, vol. 8, no. 1, pp. 56–59, 2014.

[7] F. Parmeggiani, S. F. Sorrentino, D. Ponzin, V. Barbaro, S. Ferrari, and E. di Iorio, "Retinitis pigmentosa: genes and disease mechanisms," *Current Genomics*, vol. 12, no. 4, pp. 238–249, 2011.

[8] D. M. van den Brink, P. Brites, J. Haasjes et al., "Identification of *PEX7* as the Second Gene Involved in Refsum Disease," *The American Journal of Human Genetics*, vol. 72, no. 2, pp. 471–477, 2003.

[9] A. Kohlschütter, R. Santer, Z. Lukacs, C. Altenburg, M. J. Kemper, and K. Rüther, "A child with night Blindness," *Journal of Child Neurology*, vol. 27, no. 5, pp. 654–656, 2012.

[10] R. J. A. Wanders, G. A. Jansen, and O. H. Skjeldal, "Refsum disease, peroxisomes and phytanic acid oxidation: a review," *Journal of Neuropathology and Experimental Neurology*, vol. 60, no. 11, pp. 1021–1031, 2001.

[11] K. G. Claridge, F. B. Gibberd, and M. C. Sidey, "Refsum disease: The presentation and ophthalmic aspects of Refsum disease in a series of 23 patients," *Eye*, vol. 6, no. 4, pp. 371–375, 1992.

[12] V. P. Vandana, P. S. Bindu, M. Nagappa, S. Sinha, and A. B. Taly, "Audiological findings in infantile Refsum disease," *International Journal of Pediatric Otorhinolaryngology*, vol. 79, no. 8, pp. 1366–1369, 2015.

[13] E. Hansen, N. I. Bachen, and T. Flage, "Refsum's disease: eye manifestations in a patient treated with low phytol low phytanic acid diet," *Acta Ophthalmologica*, vol. 57, no. 5, pp. 899–913, 1979.

[14] A. J. Wills, N. J. Manning, and M. M. Reilly, "Refsum's's disease," *QJM*, vol. 94, no. 8, pp. 403–406, 2001.

[15] A. Abeshi, A. Zulian, T. Beccari, M. Dundar, F. D'Esposito, and M. Bertelli, "Genetic testing for Refsum disease," *The EuroBiotech Journal*, vol. 1, no. s1, pp. 89–91, 2017.

[16] J. Gärtner, N. Preuss, U. Brosius, and M. Biermanns, "Mutations in PEX1 in peroxisome biogenesis disorders: G843D and a mild clinical phenotype," *Journal of Inherited Metabolic Disease*, vol. 22, no. 3, pp. 311–313, 1999.

[17] B. E. Reuber, E. Germain-Lee, C. S. Collins et al., "Mutations in _PEX1_ are the most common cause of peroxisome biogenesis disorders," *Nature Genetics*, vol. 17, no. 4, pp. 445–448, 1997.

[18] F. C. C. Klouwer, K. Berendse, S. Ferdinandusse, R. J. A. Wanders, M. Engelen, and B. T. Poll-The, "Zellweger spectrum disorders: clinical overview and management approach," *Orphanet Journal of Rare Diseases*, vol. 10, no. 1, 2015.

[19] M. Martínez, E. Vázquez, M. T. García-Silva et al., "Therapeutic effects of docosahexaenoic acid ethyl ester in patients with generalized peroxisomal disorders," *The American Journal of Clinical Nutrition*, vol. 71, no. 1, pp. 376S–385S, 2000.

[20] M. T. Noguer and M. Martinez, "Visual follow-up in peroxisomal-disorder patients treated with docosahexaenoic acid ethyl ester," *Investigative Ophthalmology & Visual Science*, vol. 51, no. 4, pp. 2277–2285, 2010.

[21] M. Paker, J. S. Sunness, N. H. Brereton et al., "Docosahexaenoic acid therapy in peroxisomal diseases: results of a double-blind, randomized trial," *Neurology*, vol. 75, no. 9, pp. 826–830, 2010.

[22] K. D. R. Setchell, P. Bragetti, L. Zimmer-Nechemias et al., "Oral bile acid treatment and the patient with Zellweger syndrome," *Hepatology*, vol. 15, no. 2, pp. 198–207, 1992.

[23] F. C. C. Klouwer, B. G. P. Koot, K. Berendse et al., "The cholic acid extension study in Zellweger spectrum disorders: results and implications for therapy," *Journal of Inherited Metabolic Disease*, vol. 42, no. 2, pp. 303–312, 2019.

[24] K. Berendse, F. C. C. Klouwer, B. G. P. Koot et al., "Cholic acid therapy in Zellweger spectrum disorders," *Journal of Inherited Metabolic Disease*, vol. 39, no. 6, pp. 859–868, 2016.

6

Use of Autologous Platelets for Lamellar Macular Hole Repair

Andres Gonzalez,[1] Sarina Amin,[1] Omar Iqbal,[2] Stephen Myles Potter,[1] and Syed Gibran Khurshid[1]

[1] *University of Florida College of Medicine, Department of Ophthalmology, Gainesville, FL, USA*
[2] *University of Florida College of Medicine, Gainesville, FL, USA*

Correspondence should be addressed to Andres Gonzalez; 45.agonzalez@gmail.com

Academic Editor: Stephen G. Schwartz

The consensus of lamellar macular hole repair generally entails vitrectomy with internal limiting membrane with/without epiretinal membrane peeling with gas tamponade, although the risk of a full thickness macular hole remains. In this case report, we investigate the role of the regenerative properties of autologous platelets in the repair of a lamellar macular hole with pars plana vitrectomy, an autologous platelet plug, and 12% C3F8 without prone posturing. All three patients in this case report experienced visual improvement along with anatomic closure of the lamellar macular hole. Further randomized studies with larger sample sizes will contribute to the existing data regarding this procedure and its outcomes.

1. Introduction

A lamellar macular hole (LMH) is a term originally suggested by Gass in 1975 to encompass a macular lesion resulting from cystoid macular edema [1]. Today, a LMH refers to partial-thickness defects of the macula that present on optical coherence tomography (OCT) with an irregular foveal contour and with separation of the inner from the outer layers in the fovea [2]. The prognosis and visual acuity of patients with a LMH is usually good, and most cases have historically been managed conservatively. Vision can deteriorate in a certain subset of patients, in which intervention may be indicated [2]. The most frequently employed surgical standard technique for LMH repair is a pars plana vitrectomy (PPV) with internal limiting membrane (ILM) with/without epiretinal membrane (ERM) peeling with/without endotamponade and prone posturing [2–7]. Excellent anatomical and functional outcomes have been obtained with this surgical procedure. Although uncommon, the risk of a full thickness macular hole (FTHM) remains; the highest reported incidence of a FTHM in studies of at least 20 patients was three patients (27.7%) [8]. Prone posturing can also be difficult in some patients with previous neck or back injury, vertebral fusion surgery, large body habitus, or respiratory issues. Given the real risk of a FTMH, the call for alternative techniques has been advocated for [9].

Platelets play an active role in tissue repair and glial cell proliferation given its growth factor milieu [10]. PPV with autologous platelets has been reported to achieve high anatomic and visual success rates in full-thickness macular hole repair [11–13], although there are no reports of this surgical technique being applied to lamellar macular holes. The purpose of this study was to assess the outcomes of lamellar macular hole repair with PPV, an autologous platelet plug, and 12% C3F8 without prone posturing.

2. Case Report

Three patients presented to the University of Florida Eye Clinic between April 2015 and March 2016 with a central scotoma from a LMH found on OCT. All patients were pseudophakic, and there were no other significant eye diseases present. Patients 1 and 2 likely developed a LMH from a history of cystoid macular edema after cataract surgery. The etiology for LMH formation in Patient 3 was unclear, although the patient was noted to have a posterior vitreous

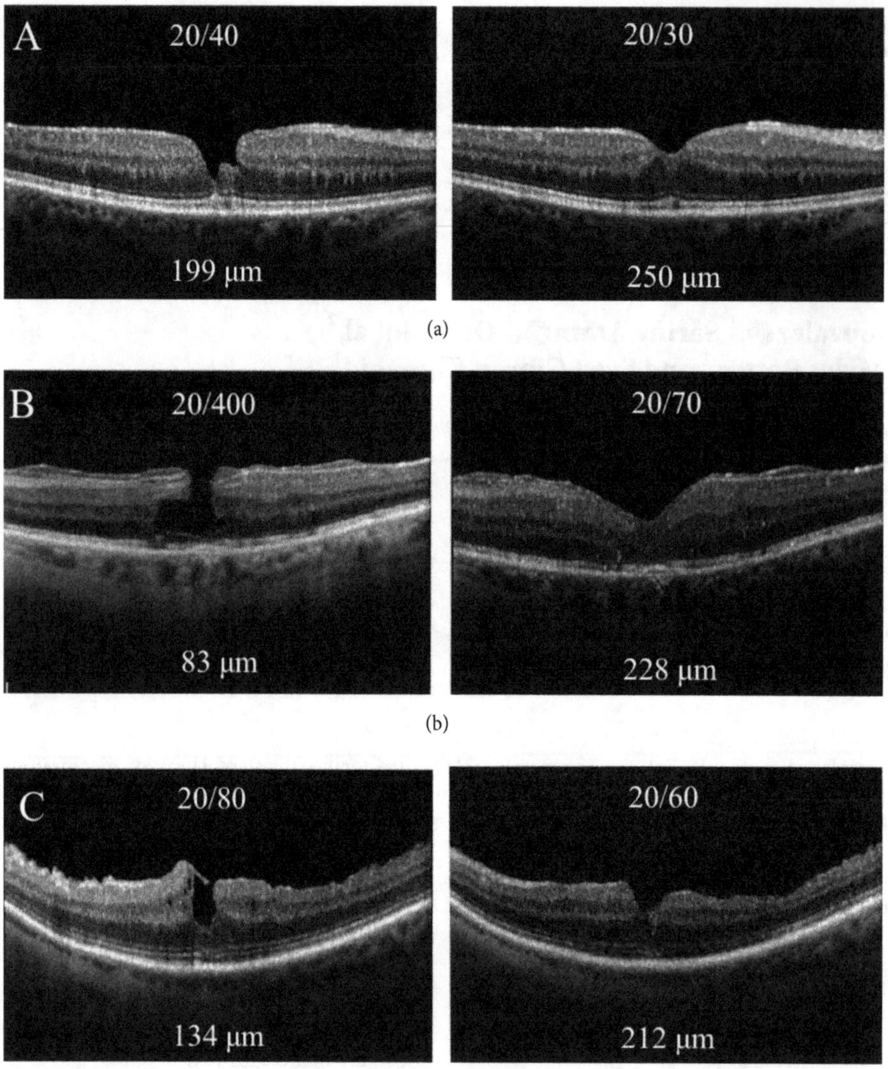

(a) (b) (c)

FIGURE 1: OCT images of Patients 1-3 (a-c) prior to surgery with respective visual acuities and CMT (left) and OCT images at last follow-up with respective visual acuities and CMT (right).

detachment on exam. No obvious operculum was seen in Patient 3 on exam. The OCT criteria defined by Witkin et al. were used as the reference for diagnosis of a LMH: (1) irregular foveal contour; (2) break in the inner fovea; (3) intraretinal split; and (4) intact foveal photoreceptors [14]. Using the 6-line radial pattern OCT, the LMH was differentiated from a macular pseudohole, a pseudocyst, and a full-thickness macular hole.

In all cases, a three-port 23-gauge PPV was performed by a single surgeon. Complete air-fluid exchange was performed. A 0.1mL autologous platelet plug was placed directly over the posterior pole at the macula. The air was then replaced with 12% octafluoropropane (C_3F_8). After surgery, patients were advised to remain in a supine position for one hour to allow the platelets to plug the LMH. No patients underwent ERM/ILM peeling. Patients were placed on a topical antibiotic-steroid drop for one month postoperatively. Follow-up examination occurred at one day, 1 month, 3 months, and 6 months.

The average patient age at the time of surgery was 72 years (range, 70–74 years). There were two female patients and one male patient. Postoperative OCT analysis revealed that all patients had LMH closure (Figure 1) with repopulation of foveal tissue and reformation of foveal architecture. All patients were followed up for at least 6 months. There were no recurrences of the LMH during this time. No surgical complications were observed.

Mean logMAR VA improved from 0.733 (Snellen equivalent 20/108; see [20/40 to 20/400]) preoperatively to 0.399 (Snellen equivalent 20/50; see [20/30 to 20/70]) at 6 months. All patients had functional visual improvement of their central scotoma and all patients had anatomic closure of the LMH on OCT. Central macular thickness improved in all patients, from an average of 138.7 μm preoperatively (range

TABLE 1: Patient characteristics.

Patient	1	2	3
Age (Gender)	70 (Female)	74 (Male)	72 (Female)
Lens status	Pseudophakic	Pseudophakic	Pseudophakic
Preoperative CMT (μm)	199	83	134
1-month CMT (μm)	230		
3-month CMT (μm)			
6-month CMT (μm)	250	228	212
Pre-treatment Snellen VA (logMAR)	20/40 (sc) 0.30	20/400 (sc) (NI PH) 1.3	20/80 (sc) 0.60
1-month Snellen VA (logMAR)	20/60 (sc) 0.48	20/200 (sc) (NI PH) 1	20/100 (sc) 0.70
3-month Snellen VA (logMAR)		20/50 (BCVA) 0.40	20/100 (sc) 0.70
6-month Snellen VA (logMAR)	20/30 (sc) 0.18	20/70 (BCVA) 0.54	20/60 (sc) 0.48
Observation Period (months)	6	12	6

∗ cc: with correction; ∗ sc: without correction.

83–199 microns) to 230 microns at 6 months (range 212–250 microns). See Table 1.

3. Discussion

Although excellent anatomic and functional results have been achieved with PPV with ILM with/without ERM peel with/without endotamponade [2–7], and the need for alternative surgical repairs has been advocated for given the uncommon but serious risk of a FTMH [9]. We present a case report of three patients that had a PPV, autologous platelet plug, and 12% C3F8 without prone posturing for LMH repair. Vitrectomy with autologous platelets has shown great success with macular holes [11–13]. There are no reports in the literature assessing this technique in LMH repair. Etiology of LMH was likely a history of cystoid macular edema after cataract surgery in Patient 1 and Patient 2 and possible hyaloidal traction from a posterior vitreous detachment in Patient 3. This case report showed an anatomical success rate of 100% along with visual improvement on Snellen and with respect to their central scotoma. No complications were noted after at least six months of follow-up for all patients. No patients received ERM/ILM peeling.

Müller cells are the principal glial cells of the retina and are integral for maintaining retinal architecture [15]. It is proposed that surgical decapitation of Müller cells' basement membrane stimulates glial cell proliferation and closure of a macular hole, hence the role of ILM peeling [10]. As an alternative, platelet suspensions have shown to achieve high anatomic success rates and good visual results for macular hole repairs [11–13]. The reason for this phenomenon is likely explained by the various growth factors present in platelets that have shown to stimulate Müller cells; these include platelet-derived growth factor (PDGF), epidermal growth factor (EGF), and fibroblast growth factor (FGF), among others [10]. Platelets become activated at the site of tissue injury, such as retinal tissue injury in a LMH. Activation releases these factors that support tissue repair by regulation of cell migration, mitosis, and differentiation [10]. We believe this is the pathophysiology as to why there was evidence of retinal glial cell proliferation, cellular repopulation of macular tissue, and reformation of normal foveal architecture in this case report. We believe that the regenerative properties of platelets reduce the risk of a FTMH. The disadvantage to using fresh autologous platelets is that intensive sterile preparation is needed.

We report another alternative treatment for LMH that involves PPV, autologous platelets, and endotamponade without postoperative prone posturing with good success in this pilot study. Further randomized studies with larger sample sizes will contribute to the existing data regarding this procedure and its outcomes.

Disclosure

This study is funded by an unrestricted grant from the foundation on Research to Prevent Blindness to the University of Florida Department of Ophthalmology, which had no role in the design/conduct of this work.

Authors' Contributions

Andres Gonzalez contributed to literature search, figures, data analysis, and writing. Sarina M. Amin contributed to literature search, figures, study design, data collection, data analysis, editing, and writing. Omar Iqbal contributed to literature search, figures, data collection, and writing. Stephen Myles Potter contributed to literature search, figures, study design, data collection, data analysis, editing, and writing. Gibran Syed Khurshid contributed to figures, study design, data collection, data analysis, editing, and writing.

References

[1] J. D. M. Gass, "Lamellar macular hole: a complication of cystoid macular edema after cataract extraction: a clinicopathologic case report," *Transactions of the American Ophthalmological Society*, vol. 73, pp. 231–250, 1975.

[2] Z. Michalewska, J. Michalewski, D. Odrobina et al., "Surgical treatment of lamellar macular holes," *Graefe's Archive for Clinical and Experimental Ophthalmology*, vol. 248, no. 10, pp. 1395–1400, 2010.

[3] S. J. Lee, S. Y. Jang, D. Moon, K. S. Choi, and G. Y. Jung, "Long-term surgical outcomes after vitrectomy for symptomatic lamellar macular holes," *Retina*, vol. 32, no. 9, pp. 1743–1748, 2012.

[4] H. Casparis and E. H. Bovey, "Surgical treatment of lamellar macular hole associated with epimacular membrane," *Retina*, vol. 31, no. 9, pp. 1783–1790, 2011.

[5] B. R. Garretson, J. S. Pollack, A. J. Ruby, K. A. Drenser, G. A. Williams, and R. Sarrafizadeh, "Vitrectomy for a symptomatic lamellar macular hole," *Ophthalmology*, vol. 115, no. 5, pp. 884.el–886.el, 2008.

[6] M. S. Figueroa, S. Noval, and I. Contreras, "Macular structure on optical coherence tomography after lamellar macular hole surgery and its correlation with visual outcome," *Canadian Journal of Ophthalmology*, vol. 46, no. 6, pp. 491–497, 2011.

[7] T. Sato, K. Emi, H. Bando, and T. Ikeda, "Retrospective comparisons of vitrectomy with and without air tamponade to repair lamellar macular hole," *Ophthalmic Surgery, Lasers and Imaging Retina*, vol. 46, no. 1, pp. 38–43, 2015.

[8] W. S. Choi, D. J. Merlau, and S. Chang, "Vitrectomy for macular disorders associated with lamellar macular hole epiretinal proliferation," *Retina*, vol. 38, no. 4, pp. 664–669, 2018.

[9] R. Frisina, E. Pilotto, and E. Midena, "Lamellar macular hole: state of the art," *Ophthalmic Research*, vol. 61, no. 2, pp. 73–82, 2019.

[10] S. L. Burmeister, D. Hartwig, G. Astrid Limb et al., "Effect of various platelet preparations on retinal Müller cells," *Investigative Ophthalmology & Visual Science*, vol. 50, no. 10, pp. 4881–4886, 2009.

[11] C. M. G. Cheung, V. Munshi, S. Mughal, J. Mann, and M. Hero, "Anatomical success rate of macular hole surgery with autologous platelet without internal-limiting membrane peeling," *Eye*, vol. 19, no. 11, pp. 1191–1193, 2005.

[12] M. Paques, C. Chastang, A. Mathis et al., "Effect of autologous platelet concentrate in surgery for idiopathic macular hole: results of a multicenter, double-masked, randomized trial," *Ophthalmology*, vol. 106, no. 5, pp. 932–938, 1999.

[13] B. J. Vote, W. L. Membrey, and A. G. Casswell, "Autologous platelets for macular hole surgery: the Sussex Eye Hospital experience," *Clinical & Experimental Ophthalmology*, vol. 32, no. 5, pp. 472–477, 2004.

[14] A. J. Witkin, T. H. Ko, J. G. Fujimoto et al., "Redefining lamellar holes and the vitreomacular interface: an ultrahigh-resolution optical coherence tomography study," *Ophthalmology*, vol. 113, no. 3, pp. 388–397, 2006.

[15] G. A. Limb, T. E. Salt, P. M. Munro, S. E. Moss, and P. T. Khaw, "In vitro characterization of a spontaneously immortalized human Müller cell line (MIO-M1)," *Investigative Ophthalmology & Visual Science*, vol. 43, no. 3, pp. 864–869, 2002.

7

A Case of Unilateral Coccidioidal Chorioretinitis in a Patient with HIV-Associated Meningoencephalitis

Christopher B. Toomey,[1] Andrew Gross,[2] Jeffrey Lee,[1] and Doran B. Spencer [1]

[1] *Viterbi Department of Ophthalmology, Shiley Eye Institute, University of California at San Diego, San Diego, CA, USA*
[2] *McGovern Medical School, University of Texas at Houston Health Science Center, Houston, TX, USA*

Correspondence should be addressed to Doran B. Spencer; dbspencer@ucsd.edu

Academic Editor: Claudio Campa

Intraocular coccidioidomycosis is a rare condition, with the most commonly reported presentation being an idiopathic iritis in patients who live in or have traveled thorough endemic areas. A paucity of reports exists describing the chorioretinal manifestations of coccidioidomycosis. Here we report a case of unilateral coccidioidal chorioretinitis and meningoencephalitis in an AIDS patient that led to near complete unilateral loss of vision. A 48-year-old Hispanic female with poorly controlled HIV/AIDS in southern California presented with a three-week history of headache, nausea, vomiting, right eye blurry vision, and a one-day history of subjective fever. Examination of the right eye revealed vitritis and several large chorioretinal lesions scattered throughout the periphery and macula with optic disc pallor. Serum coccidioidomycoses complement fixation (CF) was positive (titers of 1 : 256). Neuroimaging revealed a new area of enhancement in the left anterior frontal lobe consistent with meningoencephalitis. The patient was treated with intravenous fluconazole and intravitreal voriconazole with resolution of systemic symptoms and vitritis but persistence of unilateral, severe chorioretinal scarring and vision loss. In conclusion, in spite of the rarity of intraocular coccidioidomycosis, one must carry a degree of suspicion for this vision- and life-threatening condition as a potential etiology of chorioretinitis in individuals with pertinent risk factors.

1. Introduction

Coccidioidomycosis is a disease caused most frequently by *Coccidioides immitis*, a dimorphic fungus commonly found in the lower Sonoran Desert ecozone of the Western hemisphere [1]. The disease, which typically manifests as a self-limiting community-acquired pneumonia, was initially described in the late 1800s and thought to be of protozoan etiology (and hence the etymology of Coccidia) but was later identified as a dimorphic fungus [2]. Endemic areas include Arizona, New Mexico, West Texas, parts of Central America, Argentina, Northwest Mexico, and the San Joaquin Valley in California [1]. Populations at greater risk include pregnant women and those with immunosuppressed conditions [3]. Symptomatic patients usually present with 1–3 weeks after exposure with flu-like symptoms including night sweats, cough, myalgias, and rash [4].

Uveitis secondary to coccidioidomycosis is rare, and the few reports of it most frequently describe an idiopathic, bilateral iritis in patients who live or have traveled thorough endemic areas [5, 6]. A paucity of reports exists describing the chorioretinal manifestations of coccidioidomycosis. We report an unusual, unilateral case of coccidioidal chorioretinitis with panuveitis and meningoencephalitis in a patient with AIDS that led to near complete, unilateral loss of vision.

2. Case Presentation

A 48-year-old Hispanic female presented to a HIV clinic in southern California with a three-week history of headache, right eye blurry vision, dizziness, myalgia, nausea, and vomiting, and a one-day history of subjective fever. The past medical history was significant for human immunodeficiency virus (HIV) for 13 years (CD4 103, viral load 877 two weeks prior) with chronic associated cytomegalovirus (CMV) viremia, mycobacterium avium-intracellulare infection and toxoplasmosis encephalitis. The patient's medications included abacavir, dolutegravir, and lamivudine, as well as azithromycin, ethambutol, pyrimethamine, sulfadiazine, and valganciclovir

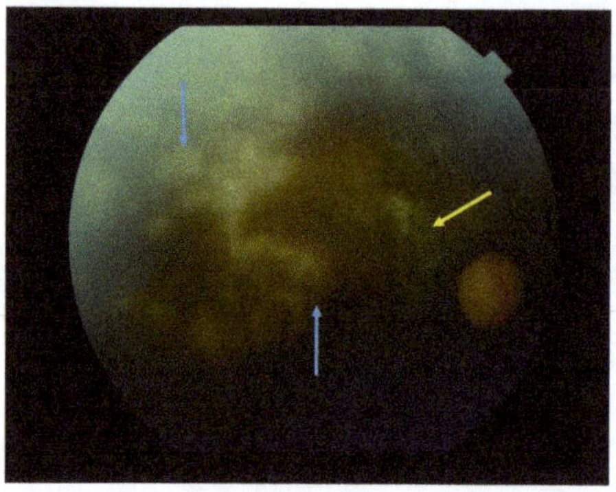

FIGURE 1: Fundus photograph with a yellow arrow marking an old, atrophic choroidal scar and blue lines delineating multiple white/off-yellow exudates around the macular and extending into the peripheral retina. Pallor of the optic disc is notable as well as minor vitreous haze.

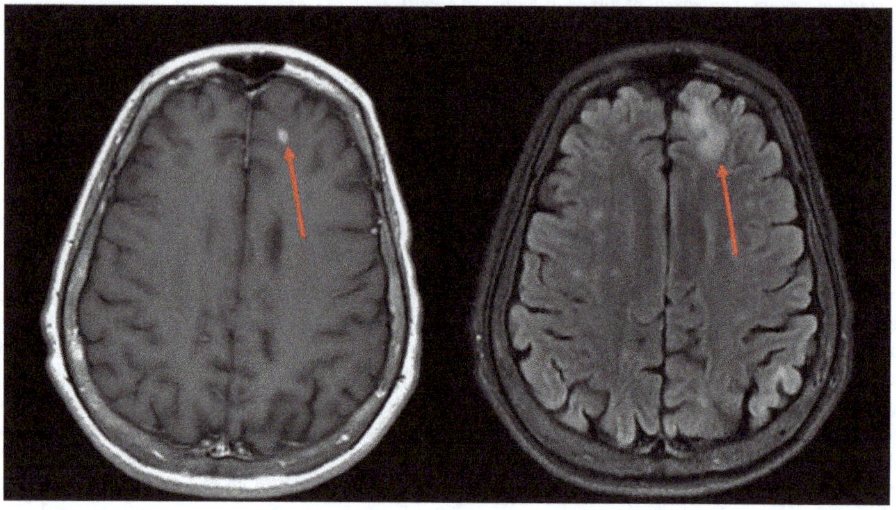

FIGURE 2: Axial T1 with contrast (left) and axial T2 FLAIR (right) magnetic resonance imaging (MRIs) demonstrating a peripherally enhancing 5 mm lesion in the left frontal lobe surrounded by moderate confluent vasogenic edema, marked by red arrows.

for opportunistic infections. Her temperature was 98.1°F, she had no abnormal vital signs, no recent weight change, no neurological symptoms and a normal systemic physical exam.

Ophthalmic examination revealed visual acuity of hand motion at 1 foot in the right eye (OD) and 20/20 in the left eye (OS), pupil constriction of 3 > 3 mm OD and 3 > 2 mm OS, and a positive right-sided relative afferent pupillary defect (RAPD). Intraocular pressures were within normal limits and extraocular movements were full in both eyes. Confrontational visual fields and color plates were unable to be obtained OD and within normal limits OS. Anterior segment examination was within normal limits on bedside exam. Dilated fundus exam OD revealed 1+ vitreous cell/haze, several large chorioretinal lesions scattered throughout the periphery and involving the macula with 2+ optic disc pallor. OS was within normal limits (Figure 1).

Due to the immunosuppressive state on presentation, as well as systemic symptoms, an extensive infectious work-up was performed as an inpatient with the Infectious Disease service and a vitreous tap was performed of the right eye. Serum coccidioidomycoses complement fixation (CF) was found to be positive (titers of 1 : 256). Serum syphilis enzyme immunoantibody, rapid plasma reagin, Borrelia burgdorferi antibody, CMV IgG/IgM, Varicella IgG, HSV type 1/2 IgM were negative. Gram stain showed polymorphonucleated white blood cells without organisms and cultures showed no growth. The encephalitis panel polymerase chain reaction was performed on the vitreous tap sample and was negative for Enterovirus, HSV1/2, Herpesvirus 6, Parechovirus, Varicella Zoster and *Cryptococcus neoformans/gatti*, E-coli K1, *Haemophilus influenza, Listeria monocytogenes, Neisseria meningitides, Strep. agalactiae, Strep. pneumoniae*. The vitreous PCR test was positive for Cytomegalovirus. CT head showed a new area of enhancement in the left anterior frontal lobe (Figure 2). Lumbar puncture (LP) with CSF gram stains, fungal cultures, and coccidioides CF were negative.

Based on the symptoms, positive serum coccidioidomycoses complement fixation and fundus appearance the patient was diagnosed with coccidioidal chorioretinitis with panuveitis. The vitreous PCR positive test was attributed to her long-standing CMV viremia secondary to sample contamination from the vitreous cells and trauma of the intravitreal biopsy and not deemed consistent with CMV retinitis given the absence of suspicious lesions. Additionally, her CD4 count of 103 places her outside of the highest risk strata of CMV retinitis, which occurs most commonly at a CD4 count of <50 [7]. The patient was treated with intravenous fluconazole and intravitreal voriconazole was preemptively given during the vitreous sampling. During her hospital course her systemic symptoms resolved. Follow-up examinations with serial fundus examinations showed progressive improvement in posterior vitritis, however, her visual acuity and retinal lesions remained stable throughout her hospital course. On follow-up examination at 3 and 5 months after discharge, her vision had decreased to light perception with no evidence of active lesions or vitritis and stable chorioretinal lesions.

3. Discussion

This case report describes the clinical manifestations of a patient with an unusual presentation of unilateral coccidioidal panuveitis with chorioretinitis; to our knowledge, this is unique in the literature. Few clinical reports exist describing the intraocular clinical manifestations of coccidioidomycosis [5, 6, 8–11]. Rodenbiker and Ganley reviewed a series of cases of ocular coccidioidomycoses with only 10 reported to have a posterior uveitis (retinitis, choroiditis, or chorioretinitis). The authors noted the anterior segment was often uninvolved and fundus findings included a range of lesions with yellow-white exudate ranging from <1 to 3 disc diameters [5]. Prevalence of asymptomatic chorioretinal scars in patients with coccidioidomycosis have been reported in 5 of 54 subjections (9.2%), suggesting the prevalence of coccidioidal chorioretinitis is higher than isolated reports suggest [12]. However, it is difficult to make assumptions on the prevalence of coccidioidal chorioretinitis in this manner given the difficulty of linking the chorioretinal scarring to the coccidioidomycosis.

The patient in this report presented with severe monocular vision loss with significant chorioretinal lesions and optic atrophy along with significant vitritis and a positive serum coccidioidomycoses CF. CSF coccidioidomycoses CF was negative, however, CSF testing has a low sensitivity in patients with coccidioidomycoses meningitis [13]. Our case report highlights the severity of coccidioidal chorioretinitis that can be associated with meningoencephalitis in a patient with HIV/AIDS, including in a unilateral fashion. Given the fundus appearance of old and new lesions, our clinical impression is that the chorioretinal involvement was on-going for many months and the patient presented for ophthalmologic evaluation once her central vision was affected. This supports the notion that ocular involvement of coccidioidomycosis may be an insidious process and highlights the essential role of routine ophthalmologic evaluation in AIDS patients in aiding in the diagnosis of systemic disease.

In spite of the rarity of intraocular coccidioidomycosis, recognizing the clinical appearance of this potentially vision and life-threatening condition is essential in individuals with pertinent risk factors including pregnancy and immunosuppression, along with a history of travel or living in endemic areas [1, 3].

Authors' Contributions

CBT, AG, JL, and DBS were responsible for data collection, analysis, and writing/preparation of the manuscript.

Acknowledgments

This work was supported by the NIH NEI P30 P30EY0225789 Vision Research Core.

References

[1] F. S Fisher, M. W Bultman, S. M Johnson, D. Pappagianis, and E. Zaborsky, "*Coccidioides* niches and habitat parameters in the Southwestern United States: a matter of scale," *Annals of the New York Academy of Sciences*, vol. 1111, no. 1, pp. 47–72, 2007.

[2] W. Ophuls, "Further observations on a pathogenic mould formerly described as a protozoon (*Coccidioides immitis, Coccidioides pyogenes*)," *Journal of Experimental Medicine*, vol. 6, no. 4–6, pp. 443–485, 1905.

[3] C. D. Odio, B. E. Marciano, J. N. Galgiani, and S. M. Holland, "Risk factors for disseminated coccidioidomycosis, United States," *Emerging Infectious Diseases*, vol. 23, no. 2, 2017.

[4] J. N. Galgiani, N. M. Ampel, J. E. Blair et al., "Coccidioidomycosis," *Clinical Infectious Diseases*, vol. 41, no. 9, pp. 1217–1223, 2005.

[5] H. T. Rodenbiker and J. P. Ganley, "Ocular coccidioidomycosis," *Survey of Ophthalmology*, vol. 24, no. 5, pp. 263–290, 1980.

[6] R. S. Moorthy, N. A. Rao, Y. Sidikaro, and R. Y. Foos, "Coccidioidomycosis Iridocyclitis," *Ophthalmology*, vol. 101, no. 12, pp. 1923–1928, 1994.

[7] R. D. Schrier, W. R. Freeman, C. A. Wiley, and J. A. McCutchan, "Immune predispositions for cytomegalovirus retinitis in AIDS. The HNRC group," *Journal of Clinical Investigation*, vol. 95, no. 4, pp. 1741–1746, 1995.

[8] K. A. Zakka, R. Y. Foos, and W J. Brown, "Intraocular coccidioidomycosis," *Survey of Ophthalmology*, vol. 22, no. 5, pp. 313–321, 1978.

[9] D. V. Vasconcelos-Santos, J. I. Lim, and N. A. Rao, "Chronic coccidioidomycosis endophthalmitis without concomitant systemic involvement: a clinicopathological case report," *Ophthalmology*, vol. 117, no. 9, pp. 1839–1842, 2010.

[10] E. T. Cunningham, "Intraocular coccidioidomycosis diagnosed by skin biopsy," *Archives of Ophthalmology*, vol. 116, no. 5, pp. 674–677, 1998.

[11] R. A. Shields, P. H. Tang, Z. M. Bodnar, S. J. Smith, and A. R. Silva, "Optical coherence tomography angiography highlights chorioretinal lesions in ocular coccidioidomycosis," *Ophthalmic Surgery, Lasers and Imaging Retina*, vol. 50, no. 3, pp. e71–e73, 2019.

[12] H. T. Rodenbiker, J. P. Ganley, J. N. Galgiani, and S. G. Axline, "Prevalence of chorioretinal scars associated with coccidioidomycosis," *Archives of Ophthalmology*, vol. 99, no. 1, pp. 71–75, 1981.

[13] G. Mathisen, A. Shelub, J. Truong, and C. Wigen, "Coccidioidal meningitis," *Medicine*, vol. 89, no. 5, pp. 251–284, 2010.

8

Brachybacterium paraconglomeratum Endophthalmitis Postcataract Operation

Kazuhiro Murata[1] **Kenji Ozawa,**[1] **Hideaki Kawakami**[2] **Kiyofumi Mochizuki,**[1] **and Kiyofumi Ohkusu**[3]

[1]*Department of Ophthalmology, Gifu University Graduate School of Medicine, 1-1 Yanagido, Gifu-shi, Gifu 501-1194, Japan*
[2]*Department of Ophthalmology, Gifu Municipal Hospital, 7-1 Kashima-cho, Gifu-shi, Gifu 500-8513, Japan*
[3]*Department of Microbiology, Tokyo Medical University, Japan*

Correspondence should be addressed to Kazuhiro Murata; kazoo88iya@yahoo.co.jp

Academic Editor: Nicola Rosa

Purpose. To present our findings in a case of delayed-onset postoperative endophthalmitis caused by *Brachybacterium paraconglomeratum*, a rare organism. *Observations.* A 57-year-old man presented with epiphora and photophobia 17 weeks after a routine cataract extraction with phacoemulsification and intraocular lens implantation. Because endophthalmitis was suspected to be caused by a low-grade pathogen or fungus, an anterior chamber tap was performed. However, both multiplex PCR and culturing were negative. The patient was treated with topical cefmenoxime, oral minocycline, and subconjunctival injection of vancomycin and ceftazidime, but the intraocular inflammation increased. Then, the anterior chamber was tapped again, and the second PCR amplification and direct sequencing which targeted *Actinomycetes* detected *Brachybacterium paraconglomeratum.* This pathogen is uncommon for human infections. He was treated with oral amoxicillin, and his intraocular condition slowly improved. *Conclusion.* This is the first reported case of an ocular disorder caused by *B. paraconglomeratum*. We recommend that *B. paraconglomeratum* be considered in cases of delayed-onset postcataract endophthalmitis.

1. Introduction

A rapid diagnosis is important for a fast recovery from ocular diseases and maintenance of ocular function. However, it is occasionally difficult to detect the causative pathogens from the collected samples by conventional examinations, microscopy, and culturing. The advances in the molecular techniques for detecting and identifying organisms by the polymerase chain reaction (PCR) method have enabled more accurate and faster identification of various pathogens which were unable to be detected earlier [1, 2].

We report our findings in a case of ocular infection caused by *B. paraconglomeratum* that was detected by PCR.

2. Case Report

A 57-year-old Japanese man underwent routine cataract surgery. He was examined in our hospital 17 weeks postoperatively with a one-week history of epiphora and photophobia in his right eye. Our examination showed that his decimal best-corrected visual acuity (BCVA) was 1.2 and his intraocular pressures was 19 mmHg bilaterally. His right eye had conjunctival hyperemia, fine keratic precipitates, and grade 1+ inflammatory cells in the anterior chamber. The vitreous and retina had no lesions bilaterally. His general health was good from birth. An initial diagnosis of iritis was made, and he underwent steroid therapy with the methods of eye drops and subconjunctival injection. The symptoms in his right eye improved only slightly. However, he had eye pain and recurrent hyperemia 3 days later. Because postoperative bacterial endophthalmitis without inflammation in the vitreous was suspected, the anterior chamber was tapped. He received repeated subconjunctival injections of vancomycin 5 mg/0.5 ml and ceftazidime 11.25 mg/0.5 ml, as well as topical cefmenoxime and 200 mg of oral minocycline. The condition in the right eye deteriorated still more, and the results of both culture and multiplex PCR examination (outside laboratory) were negative. Considering the possibility of low-grade bacterial or fungal infection, the anterior chamber was tapped a second time (Figure 1). The second PCR examination at the Tokyo Medical University targeted Actinomycetales and whole fungus. The PCR amplification and direct sequencing showed that *B. paraconglomeratum* was present in the aqueous.

Treatment was initiated with topical cefmenoxime and betamethasone, 750 mg/day of oral amoxicillin, and erythromycin ointment. The number of cells in the anterior chamber gradually decreased, and the patient had no signs of inflammation in the anterior chamber over the next 8 months. The final BCVA was 1.2 bilaterally.

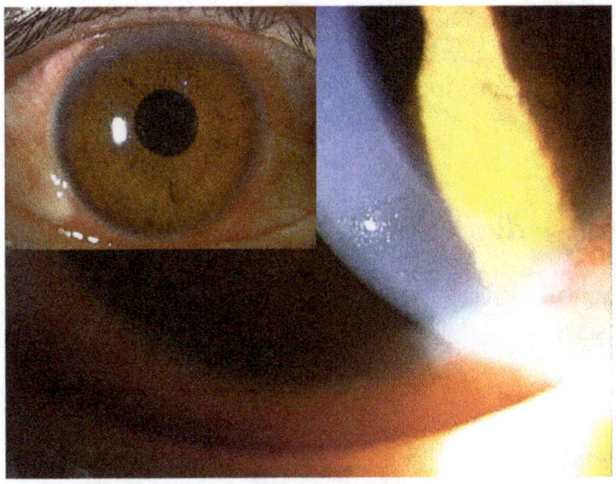

FIGURE 1: Photographs (insert: fluorescent staining) before the second anterior chamber examination. His right eye has conjunctival hyperemia, fine keratic precipitates, and inflammatory cells in the anterior chamber.

3. Discussion

Brachybacterium has been isolated from poultry deep litter by Collins et al. in 1988 [3]. The *Brachybacterium* spp. belong to the Actinomycetales and are nonsporing gram-positive rods [3]. They are considered to be nonharmful environmental bacteria [1]. The *Brachybacterium* spp. are presently confirmed to be made up of 20 strains [4].

B. paraconglomeratum was first reported by Takeuchi et al. [5]. The colonies were circular, entire, low convex, smooth, opaque, and pale brown [5]. *B. paraconglomeratum* has a slower growth rate in culture than other *Brachybacterium* spp. [5].

A human infection related to *Brachybacterium* spp. was first proposed by Tamai et al. in 2018, but there are only a few reports of *Brachybacterium* spp. isolated from human samples [1, 6–8]. It is not known why human infections by *Brachybacterium* spp. are rare.

Brain-Heart Infusion (BHI) agar is recommended as a universal medium for aerobic bacteria and for the primary recovered fungi and Actinomycetales [9, 10]. Takeuchi et al. also performed a taxonomic study including *B. paraconglomeratum* with BHI agar [5]. However, the laboratories of many hospitals and outside institutions generally use 5% sheep blood agar, chocolate agar, and Sabouraud dextrose agar as conventional agars [1].

Tamai et al. reported that the results of culture and PCR examinations of blood samples were positive for *B. paraconglomeratum*, but cultures of samples of the intervertebral disc were negative for *B. paraconglomeratum* in cultures and microscopic examinations [1]. Our sample from the anterior chamber tap was very small and was negative in culture and PCR examination.

Considering these circumstances, *Brachybacterium* spp. may need more suitable environment for growth than other microorganisms. For example, one may be enriched by nutrition agar and/or other many colleagues, although it is unclear that perhaps *Brachybacterium* spp. may have characteristics of quorum sensing. Culturing of small volume samples of presumed low-grade pathogen should have been performed with BHI agar having high nutritive value.

The advancements of the PCR method has opened the way for further development of the diagnosis level to human infections. However, the detection rate of the whole bacteria and fungi with multiplex PCR examinations is approximately 60 to 80% and not 100% [11]. A rare microorganism or small sample volume can lead to negative results even by PCR examinations. In our patient, the first multiplex PCR examination was unable to detect a pathogen. The primer used was unsuitable to the pathogen. Moreover, the sample volume might be too small after being distributed between the PCR examination and culture. Considering these factors, the sample from the second anterior chamber tap was used for PCR examination only. In addition, the second PCR examination targeted the whole fungi and Actinomycetales referring to the previous reports related to delayed-onset postoperative endophthalmitis [12]. As a result, the pathogen was identified as *B. paraconglomeratum*.

Brachybacterium spp. were reported to be susceptible to ampicillin, cefazolin, vancomycin, erythromycin, and rifampicin, and the susceptibilities to gentamicin, clindamycin, and tetracycline varied among the strains. [1, 13–16]. On the other hand, antimicrobial susceptibility of *B. paraconglomeratum* is unknown. Moreover, the antimicrobial susceptibility of our specimen could not be determined because of the negative culture. Our patient was initially treated with oral minocycline but had no sign of improvement. Therefore, after identifying *B. paraconglomeratum*, oral amoxicillin was administered as reported by Tamai et al. [1]. Then, the inflammation in the anterior chamber gradually improved with no recurrences.

Souli et al. reported that the peak level of vancomycin in the aqueous humor was $24.82 \pm 3.55\,\mu$g/ml at 5 h after a subconjunctival administration [17]. Tamai et al. reported that minimum inhibitory concentration of the isolated *Brachybacterium* spp. was $0.5\,\mu$g/ml [1]. Our patient had two subconjunctival injection with vancomycin; however, his eye condition did not improve. Although the reason of deterioration remained to be resolved, the microorganism *B. paraconglomeratum* might have been resistant to vancomycin.

In conclusion, *B. paraconglomeratum* should be considered in the differential diagnosis of organisms related to delayed postcataract endophthalmitis. Further accumulation of cases is needed to provide appropriate treatment to *Brachybacterium* sp. infections in humans.

Acknowledgments

We thank Professor Duco Hamasaki for editing this manuscript.

References

[1] K. Tamai, Y. Akashi, Y. Yoshimoto et al., "First case of a bloodstream infection caused by the genus *Brachybacterium*," *Journal of Infection and Chemotherapy*, vol. 24, no. 12, pp. 998–1003, 2018.

[2] T. Tsushima, N. Ishii, S. Matsuzaka et al., "Culture-negative group B streptococcal pericarditis: a case report and literature review of the diagnostic use of polymerase chain reaction," *Clinical Case Reports*, vol. 7, no. 3, pp. 509–514, 2019.

[3] M. D. Collins, J. Brown, and D. Jones, "*Brachybacterium faecium* gen. nov., sp. nov., a coryneform bacterium from poultry deep litter," *International Journal of Systematic Bacteriology*, vol. 38, no. 1, pp. 45–48, 1988.

[4] "The list of prokaryotic names with standing in nomenclature," https://www.bacterio.net/.

[5] M. Takeuchi, C. X. Fang, and A. Yokota, "Taxonomic study of the genus *Brachybacterium*: proposal of *Brachybacterium conglomeratum* sp. nov., nom. rev., *Brachybacterium paraconglomeratum* sp. nov., and *Brachybacterium rhamnosum* sp. nov," *International Journal of Systematic Bacteriology*, vol. 45, no. 1, pp. 160–168, 1995.

[6] I. S. Mages, R. Frodl, K. A. Bernard, and G. Funke, "Identities of *Arthrobacter* spp. and Arthrobacter-like bacteria encountered in human clinical specimens," *Journal of Clinical Microbiology*, vol. 46, no. 9, pp. 2980–2986, 2008.

[7] C. Cheng, J. Sun, F. Zheng, K. Wu, and Y. Rui, "Molecular identification of clinical "difficult-to-identify" microbes from sequencing 16S ribosomal DNA and internal transcribed spacer 2," *Annals of Clinical Microbiology and Antimicrobials*, vol. 13, no. 1, 2014.

[8] N. D. Vaziri, J. Wong, M. Pahl et al., "Chronic kidney disease alters intestinal microbial flora," *Kidney International*, vol. 83, no. 2, pp. 308–315, 2013.

[9] D. A. Sutton, "Specimen collection, transport, and processing: mycology," in *Manual of Clinical Microbiology*, P. R. Murray, E. J. Baron, J. H. Jorgensen, M. A. Pfaller, and R. H. Yolken, Eds., American Society for Microbiology, Washington, D.C., 8th edition, 2003.

[10] J. M. Brown and M. M. McNeil, "Nocardia, Rhodococcus, Gordonia, Actinomadura, Streptomyces and other aerobic actinomycetes," in *Manual of Clinical Microbiology*, P. R. Murray, E. J. Baron, J. H. Jorgensen, M. A. Pfaller, and R. H. Yolken, Eds., American Society for Microbiology, Washington, D.C., 8th edition, 2003.

[11] M. Siala, R. Gdoura, H. Fourati et al., "Broad-range PCR, cloning and sequencing of the full 16S rRNA gene for detection of bacterial DNA in synovial fluid samples of Tunisian patients with reactive and undifferentiated arthritis," *Arthritis Research & Therapy*, vol. 11, no. 4, article R102, 2009.

[12] A. R. Shirodkar, A. Pathengay, H. W. Flynn Jr. et al., "Delayed- versus acute-onset endophthalmitis after cataract surgery," *American Journal of Ophthalmology*, vol. 153, no. 3, pp. 391–398, 2012.

[13] J. H. Chou, K. Y. Lin, M. C. Lin et al., "*Brachybacterium phenoliresistens* sp. nov., isolated from oil-contaminated coastal sand," *International Journal of Systematic and Evolutionary Microbiology*, vol. 57, no. 11, pp. 2674–2679, 2007.

[14] Y. Liu, Q. Y. Xie, W. Shi et al., "*Brachybacterium huguangmaarense* sp. nov., isolated from lake sediment," *International Journal of Systematic and Evolutionary Microbiology*, vol. 64, no. 5, pp. 1673–1678, 2014.

[15] I. Gontia, K. Kavita, M. Schmid, A. Hartmann, and B. Jha, "*Brachybacterium saurashtrense* sp. nov., a halotolerant root-associated bacterium with plant growth-promoting potential," *International Journal of Systematic and Evolutionary Microbiology*, vol. 61, no. 12, pp. 2799–2804, 2011.

[16] V. A. Hoang, Y. J. Kim, N. L. Nguyen, and D. C. Yang, "*Brachybacterium ginsengisoli* sp. nov., isolated from soil of a ginseng field," *International Journal of Systematic and Evolutionary Microbiology*, vol. 64, no. 9, pp. 3063–3068, 2014.

[17] M. Souli, G. Kopsinis, E. Kavouklis, L. Gabriel, and H. Giamarellou, "Vancomycin levels in human aqueous humour after intravenous and subconjunctival administration," *International Journal of Antimicrobial Agents*, vol. 8, no. 3, pp. 239–243, 2001.

9

Prenatal Exophthalmia Revealing a Postnatal Orbital Teratoma

Ahgbatouhabeba Ahnoux-Zabsonre ,[1,2] Jérôme Sanou,[1,2] Yérénou Ferdinand Lankoandé,[2] Chantal Bouda,[3] Gertrude Méda,[1,2] and Assita Lamien-Sanou[1,4]

[1]*UFR/SDS University Joseph Ki Zerbo, 03 BP7021, Ouagadougou, Burkina Faso*
[2]*Yalgado Ouedraogo University Hospital Center, Department of Ophthalmology, 03 BP7022, Captain Sankara Avenue, Ouagadougou, Burkina Faso*
[3]*Yalgado Ouedraogo University Hospital Center, Department of Paediatrics, 03 BP7022, Captain Sankara Avenue, Ouagadougou, Burkina Faso*
[4]*Yalgado Ouedraogo University Hospital Center, Department of Pathological Anatomy, 03 BP7022, Captain Sankara Avenue, Ouagadougou, Burkina Faso*

Correspondence should be addressed to Ahgbatouhabeba Ahnoux-Zabsonre; ahgbatou@yahoo.fr

Academic Editor: Huban Atilla

Purpose. Teratomas are congenital tumors of stem cells derived from the three germ layers. They are frequently located in the sacrococcygeal region. Orbital teratoma is rare with less than 70 cases reported until 2016. We report the case of prenatal exophthalmia discovered by ultrasound exam which turned out to be a teratoma postnatally. The newborn in our case was female, just as described in the literature. Treatment consisted of total removal of the teratoma and the eyeball. Reconstructive surgery remains a big challenge since our medical technology is limited. *Conclusion.* A prenatal exophthalmia on fetal ultrasound should make us think of a teratoma, even if it is very rare. Fetal orbital teratoma may be associated with fetal survival. The infant will benefit from a reconstructive surgery of the orbit.

1. Introduction

Teratomas are congenital stem cell tumors derived from the three germ layers. Histological exam classifies these tumors as mature or well-differentiated teratoma and immature teratoma, depending on the degree of cell differentiation [1]. Immature teratoma has the tendency to turn into a malignant tumor [1]. Teratoma is twofold prevalent in women as compared to men. The most frequent localization of such tumor is the sacrococcygeal region [1, 2]. Teratoma is rarely localized in the orbits [2, 3]. It can appear in the orbit primitively or secondarily from the spread of intracranial teratomas [4, 5]. Teratoma is treated surgically by the exeresis of the tumor while sparing the ocular globe [6]. We report a case of antenatal exophthalmia that appeared to be a teratoma postnatally.

2. Case Report

We report the case of a newborn who was referred to the ophthalmologic clinic of Yalgado Ouédraogo University Hospital for appropriate care of a left side congenital exophthalmia that was discovered prenatally through a routine transabdominal ultrasound of the mother (Figure 1(a)). An MRI on the mother was prescribed prenatally but could not be realized due to shortage of money.

The newborn was seen on the first day of life and was a female baby who had a term vaginal delivery with an APGAR score of 9/9/10, a weight of 2,700 g, and a head circumference of 31 cm. No pathological family history was recorded. There was no consanguinity between the 19-year-old primipara mother and the 30-year-old father. Ophthalmic exam was normal for the right eye while showing on the left eye (Figure 1(b))

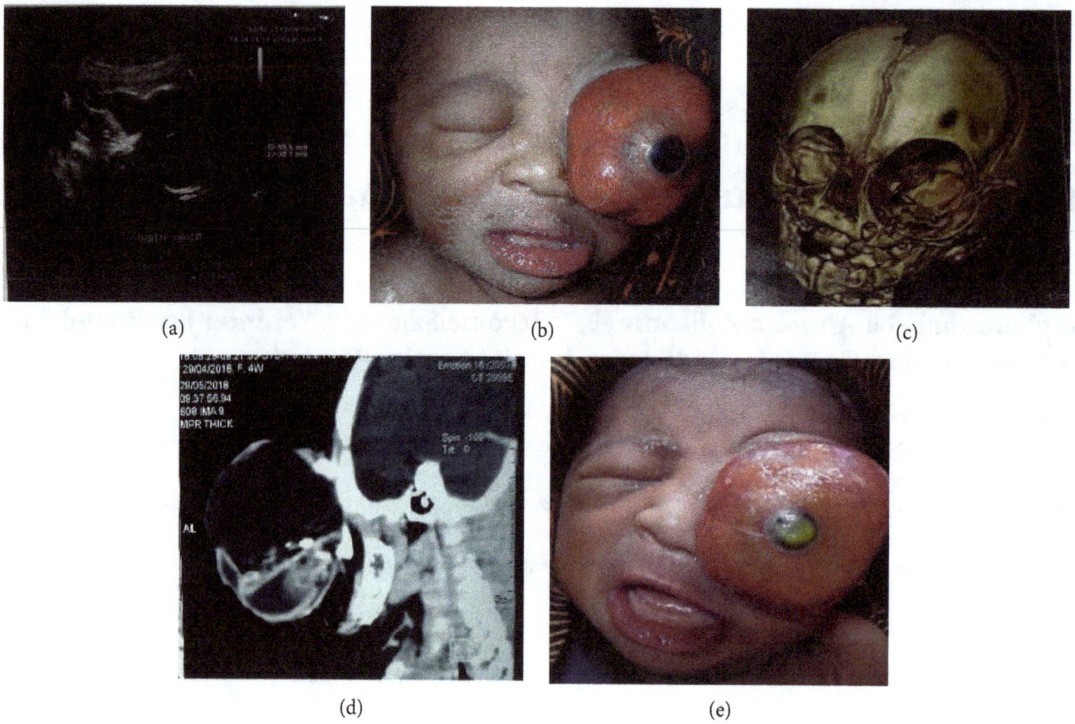

Figure 1: (a) Transabdominal ultrasound of the mother at 36 weeks of pregnancy showing a right orbital mass. (b) Congenital exophthalmia (5 cm). (c) CT scan of the head and the orbits: heterogeneous mass in the left orbit with cystic, calcified, fatty, and vascularized tissues. (d) 3D skull scan: enlarged left orbital cavity. (e) Left eye: corneal abscess with perforation.

a multilobulated hypervascularized, nonpulsatile, nonreducible massive proptosis. The cornea and the iris were normal. The anterior chamber was narrow, and the pupil was small. A thorough physical exam performed by a pediatrician did not reveal other abnormalities.

Abdominal and pelvic ultrasounds were normal. Blood cell count and biochemistry tests were normal. Computerized tomography scan of the head and orbits revealed a heterogeneous mass with cystic, calcified, fatty, and vascularized tissues (Figure 1(c)). The orbital cavity was enlarged with no bone lyses (Figure 1(d)).

Despite antibiotic treatment along with eye lubricants, the newborn developed, on his 6th day of life, corneal abscess and corneal perforation (Figure 1(e)).

Surgical treatment consisted in removing the entire mass (Figure 2(a)) while sparing the eyelids. The orbital cavity remained empty (Figure 2(b)).

Gross appearance of the mass (Figure 2(c)) revealed a multilocular cyst with clear substance and areas without endocystic vegetations. Microscopic exam showed that the cyst was boarded by a layer of mature tissues such as respiratory (Figure 3(a)) or intestinal (Figure 3(b)) type linings, keratinized malpighian epithelium (Figure 3(c)), cartilaginous nodules (Figure 3(d)), clusters of lymphoid cells, and nervous tissues (Figure 3(e)). There were no findings that were suspicious of malignancy. All findings rather pointed to a multitissular mature cystic teratoma of the left eye.

Postsurgery outcomes were without any complications (Figure 4). The remaining challenge was the reconstruction of the orbital cavity since we did not have the means of performing such a surgery.

3. Discussion

The first orbital tumor compatible with teratoma was described by Holmes in 1863 [7]. Orbital teratoma is an extremely rare tumor developed from primitive germ cells [8]. In fact, Pellerano et al. reported only 70 cases of such tumor throughout English literature until 2016 [9]. The present report is the first documented case of the disease in Burkina Faso.

Orbital teratoma can be characterized at birth by a massive unilateral exophthalmia [10–12]. Our report has the particularity of showing an exophthalmia that was noticed antenatally through ultrasound exam, so its prenatal diagnosis has been made. Such findings have prompted the prescription of an MRI on the mother but the MRI could not be run due to money shortage. Prenatal diagnosis of teratoma with voluminous exophthalmia has rarely been documented. We were able to find three documented cases. The first one had led to therapeutic abortion. Histological exam had confirmed the diagnosis of orbital teratoma [13]. The second case described a newborn who benefited from an exenteration and an orbital prosthesis [3]. The third case reported a suspicion of orbital teratoma through prenatal MRI. However, the teratoma was ruptured and led to in utero fetal death [14]. The present case report is therefore the second case in which the child was born with the tumor. However, we were not able to spare the eyeball in our treatment. The newborn of our case report was female; this corroborates with findings in other studies [2].

Massive exophthalmia may lead to exposure keratopathy and its complication such as abscess formation and eye

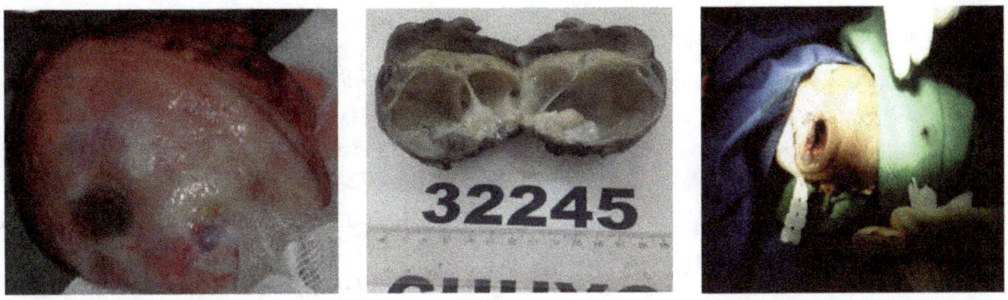

(a) (b) (c)

FIGURE 2: (a) Tumor removed. (b) Empty orbital cavity after mass exeresis. (c) Gross appearance of the mass : a multilocular cyst.

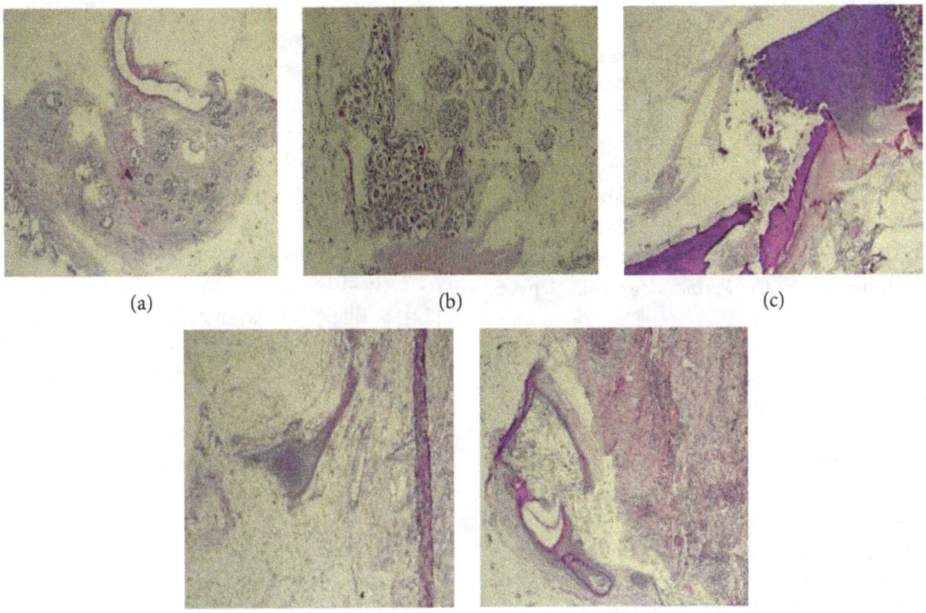

(a) (b) (c)

(d) (e)

FIGURE 3: (a) Histological examination showing respiratory tissue. (b) Histological examination showing a cluster of neuroganglion cells and nerve cells. (c) Histological examination showing cartilage tissue (top left) and bone tissue (bottom). (d) Histological examination showing a cartilaginous lobule in the middle of an adipose lobule. (e) Histological examination showing keratinized malpighian epithelium.

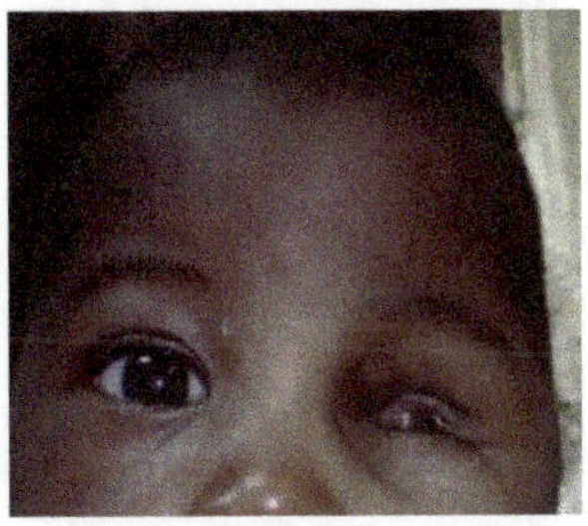

FIGURE 4: Left orbital cavity to be repaired.

perforation [9, 11, 12, 15]; this is what happened with our patient.

Postnatal CT scan of the brain, just like in our case report, usually shows an enlarged orbit with no sign of bone destruction in which can be found a heterogeneous mass containing vascularized, fatty, or calcified tissues and orbital cysts [11].

Histological exam of the removed tumor of our patient revealed various tissues (gastrointestinal, cerebral, or cartilaginous and fatty tissues) which were mature. These mature features usually rule out the risk of the tumor turning malignant [1, 16] as opposed to immature teratoma that has a high risk of malignancy [1, 16].

Common surgical treatment is the exeresis of the tumor while sparing the eyeball whenever possible [6, 17–21]. However, exenteration often appears to be the only therapeutic option [3, 11, 22]. This happened with our patient who had a prenatal massive exophthalmia with early corneal complications. Orbital reconstructive surgery is required in advance cases for esthetic purpose. This could not be recommended to the parents of our patients due to lack of adequate surgical means. Medical evacuation was therefore recommended [11, 19, 23].

Orbital teratoma is an extremely rare congenital pathology; it can be discovered prenatally using ultrasounds. Thereafter, MRI can point to this pathology when showing exophthalmia and allows early treatment of the newborn while sparing the eyeball whenever possible. Otherwise, surgery with mutilations is required with challenges of performing eyeball reconstruction on a growing child.

Consent

Consent to publish the case report was obtained.

Disclosure

All authors attest that they meet the current ICMJE criteria for authorship.

References

[1] J. R. Mann, E. S. Gray, C. Thornton et al., "Mature and immature extracranial teratomas in children: the UK children's cancer study group experience," *Journal of Clinical Oncology*, vol. 26, no. 21, pp. 3590–3597, 2008.

[2] H. M. Alkatan, I. Chaudhry, and A. Alayoubi, "Mature teratoma presenting as orbital cellulitis in a 5-month-old baby," *Annals of Saudi Medicine*, vol. 33, no. 6, pp. 623–626, 2013.

[3] T. E. Herman, A. Vachharajani, and M. J. Siegel, "Massive congenital orbital teratoma," *Journal of Perinatology*, vol. 29, no. 5, pp. 396-397, 2009.

[4] D. F. Chang, R. L. Dallow, and D. S. Walton, "Congenital orbital teratoma: report of a case with visual preservation," *Journal of Pediatric Ophthalmology and Strabismus*, vol. 17, no. 2, pp. 88–95, 1980.

[5] N. Mamalis, P. E. Garland, J. C. Argyle, and D. J. Apple, "Congenital orbital teratoma: a review and report of two cases," *Survey of Ophthalmology*, vol. 30, no. 1, pp. 41–46, 1985.

[6] J. A. Shields and C. L. Shields, "Orbital cysts of childhood–classification, clinical features, and management," *Survey of Ophthalmology*, vol. 49, no. 3, pp. 281–299, 2004.

[7] T. Holmes, "Congenital tumor removed from the orbit," *Trans. Pathol. Soc. London*, vol. 14, p. 248, 1863.

[8] R. Bernoulli, "Über ein primäres teratoides Sarkom der Orbita," *Ophthalmologica*, vol. 143, no. 5, pp. 370–377, 1962.

[9] F. Pellerano, E. Guillermo, G. Garrido, and P. Berges, "Congenital orbital teratoma," *Ocular oncology and pathology*, vol. 3, no. 1, pp. 11–16, 2017.

[10] W. F. Hoyt, "Congenital teratoid cyst of the orbit," *Archives of Ophthalmology*, vol. 68, no. 2, pp. 196–201, 1962.

[11] O. A. Ogun, G. O. Ogun, B. J. Brown, A. L. Mosuro, and A. O. Ashaye, "Congenital orbital teratoma: a case report and challenges of its management in a resource limited setting," *The Pan African Medical Journal*, vol. 12, p. 3, 2012.

[12] S. Aiyub, W. Chan, J. Szetu et al., "Congenital orbital teratoma," *Indian Journal of Ophthalmology*, vol. 61, no. 12, pp. 767–769, 2013.

[13] Y. J. Moon, H. S. Hwang, Y. R. Kim, Y. W. Park, and Y. H. Kim, "Prenatally detected congenital orbital teratoma," *Ultrasound in Obstetrics and Gynecology*, vol. 31, no. 1, pp. 107–109, 2008.

[14] A. Anami, K. Fukushima, Y. Fujita et al., "Antenatally diagnosed congenital orbital teratoma in which rupture was associated with intrauterine fetal death," *Journal of Obstetrics and Gynaecology Research*, vol. 38, no. 3, pp. 578–581, 2012.

[15] T. Kivela and A. Tarkkanen, "Orbital germ cell tumors revisited: a clinicopathological approach to classification," *Survey of Ophthalmology*, vol. 38, no. 6, pp. 541–554, 1994.

[16] L. E. Hann, S. Borden, and A. L. Weber, "Orbital teratoma in the newborn a case report," *Pediatric Radiology*, vol. 5, no. 3, pp. 172–174, 1977.

[17] M. L. Levin, C. R. Leone, and M. C. Kincaid, "Congenital orbital teratomas," *American Journal of Ophthalmology*, vol. 102, no. 4, pp. 476–481, 1986.

[18] G. A. Lee, T. J. Sullivan, G. P. Tsikleas, and N. G. Davis, "Congenital orbital teratoma," *Australian and New Zealand Journal of Ophthalmology*, vol. 25, no. 1, pp. 63–66, 1997.

[19] L. Gnanaraj, B. C. Skibell, J. Coret-Simon, W. Halliday, C. Forrest, and D. D. DeAngelis, "Massive congenital orbital teratoma," *Ophthalmic Plastic & Reconstructive Surgery*, vol. 21, no. 6, pp. 445–447, 2005.

[20] S. Khadka, G. B. Shrestha, P. Gautam, and J. B. Shrestha, "Orbital teratoma: a rare congenital tumour," *Nepalese Journal of Ophthalmology*, vol. 9, no. 1, pp. 79–82, 2017.

[21] H. M. Alkatan, O. S. AlObaidan, H. Kfoury, and Y. H. Al-Faky, "Orbital immature teratoma: a rare entity with diagnostic challenges," *Saudi Journal of Ophthalmology*, vol. 32, no. 1, pp. 75–78, 2018.

[22] S. Bilgiç, V. Dayanir, H. Kiratli, and Y. Güngen, "Congenital orbital teratoma: a clinicopathologic case report," *Ophthalmic Plastic & Reconstructive Surgery*, vol. 13, no. 2, pp. 142–146, 1997.

[23] C. González, C. A. Restrepo, G. I. Salazar, and P. Monsalve, "Congenital orbital teratoma: case report," *Colombia Medica*, vol. 43, no. 1, pp. 82–85, 2012.

10

Induced Myopia Secondary to Blunt Trauma

Mohammad Reza Sedaghat,[1] **Hamed Momeni-Moghaddam**[2,3] **Shehzad A. Naroo,**[4] **Mohammad Etezad-Razavi,**[1] **and Majid Moshirfar**[5,6,7]

[1]*Eye Research Center, Mashhad University of Medical Sciences, Mashhad, Iran*
[2]*Health Promotion Research Center, Zahedan University of Medical Sciences, Zahedan, Iran*
[3]*Department of Optometry, School of Paramedical Sciences, Mashhad University of Medical Sciences, Mashhad, Iran*
[4]*Aston University, Ophthalmic Research Group, School of Life and Health Sciences, Aston Triangle, Birmingham B4 7ET, UK*
[5]*John A. Moran Eye Center, Department of Ophthalmology and Visual Sciences, School of Medicine, University of Utah, USA*
[6]*Utah Lions Eye Bank, Murray, UT, USA*
[7]*HDR Research Center, Hoopes Vision, 11820 S. State Street Suite #200, Draper, UT 84020, USA*

Correspondence should be addressed to Hamed Momeni-Moghaddam; hmomeni_opt@yahoo.com

Academic Editor: Huban Atilla

A 28-year-old young man presented with sudden and severe visual loss in the left eye, starting three days ago following blunt head trauma from a closed fist. Vision was not improved to better than 0.4 in the left eye. Slit lamp examinations revealed asymmetric anterior chamber depth (ACD) with shallow ACD in the left eye. The key learning in this report is the use of anterior segment optical coherence tomography (AS-OCT) to better document the anterior segment changes following the blunt trauma. AS-OCT was used to visualize the forward displacement of the iris-crystalline lens diaphragm secondary to ciliary body anterior rotation and ciliochoroidal effusion. There was a temporary myopic shift about 7.00 D which resolved after 15 days.

1. Introduction

Traumatic myopia is a clinical entity that may be seen following ocular blunt trauma and is characterized with a usual range of -1.00 to -6.00 diopters (D) in the injured eye, or occasionally in both eyes [1]. It is sudden onset and usually transient, recovering within a few weeks after the trauma, although some cases may be long-standing [2]. Possible etiologic causes for this condition are as follows: spasm of the ciliary body, increased crystalline lens effective power secondary to its forward shift, ciliochoroidal effusion causing forward displacement of the crystalline lens-iris diaphragm, axial thickening of the natural lens, and other sources of choroidals which could undoubtedly produce the same refractive issues such as varicella infection [2–4]. Although the closed head trauma may produce decreased visual acuity secondary to the bilateral spasm of accommodation, one case was reported with persistent myopia which was still present three months after trauma. Interestingly, there was no significant change in the anterior chamber depth between the two eyes (0.09 mm) and nearly absolute elimination of myopia following a cycloplegic refraction [5]. This report details the initial presentation and the outcome after two weeks of a case with traumatic myopia in one eye following the blunt head trauma from a closed fist. Although there are several reports of traumatic myopia with previously mentioned etiologies in the literature [1–3, 6–9], the key learning of this report is the use of anterior segment optical coherence tomography (AS-OCT) to better detail the anterior segment changes following the blunt trauma.

2. Case Presentation

A 28-year-old man presented with sudden and severe reduced vision in the left eye, following the blunt head trauma three days ago from a closed fist. Uncorrected distance visual acuity recorded as decimal notation was 0.9 in the right eye and 0.1 in the left eye, respectively. The

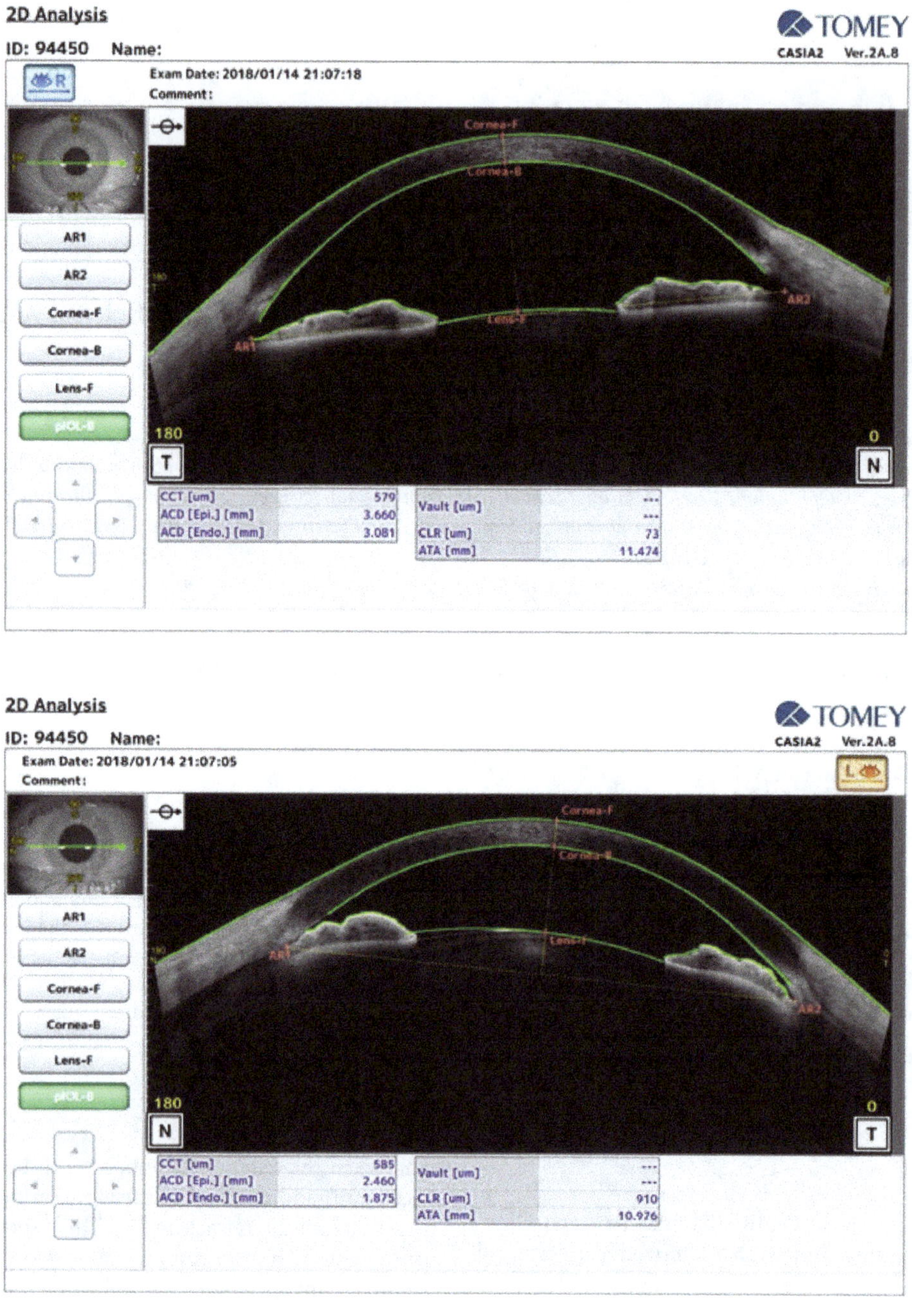

Figure 1: Anterior segment OCT three days after the trauma in the right and left eyes.

best-corrected distance visual acuity was 1.0 in the right eye with a refraction $-0.75/-0.75 \times 94°$ and 0.4 in the left eye with a refraction $-5.50/-1.00 \times 108°$.

Slit lamp examinations revealed a normal cornea and clear crystalline lens. The only abnormal finding noted was asymmetric anterior chamber depth (ACD) with shallow ACD in the left eye. This was confirmed using the CASIA2 anterior segment optical coherence tomography (Tomey Corporation, Nagoya, Japan) (Figure 1).

Assessment of pupillary reflexes showed no relative afferent pupillary defect. Intraocular pressure was 13.6 mmHg in the right eye and 7.9 mmHg in the left eye using a Topcon noncontact tonometer (Topcon Corporation, Tokyo, Japan). Dilated fundus examination showed a normal retina, macula, and optic disc in both eyes. Keratometry using Topcon Auto-KR (Tomey Corporation, Nagoya, Japan) was 44.25/44.00@55 and 44.25/44.00@168 in the right and the left eyes, respectively. Despite the difference in visual acuity between the two eyes, the unilateral and alternate cover test was performed to rule out the possibility of esodeviation secondary to the accommodative spasm. No deviation was present at the two distances.

At the initial examination after the trauma, ACD in the right and left eyes were 3.08 mm and 1.87 mm, respectively. The calculated crystalline lens rise (CLR) at this time was 73 μm in the right eye and 910 μm in the left eye (Figure 1).

Table 1: Initial wavefront analysis and two weeks later.

WF summary		Initial Ass. Entire eye OD	Initial Ass. Entire eye OS	Initial Ass. Internal optics OD	Initial Ass. Internal optics OS	Initial Ass. Cornea OD	Initial Ass. Cornea OS	2 weeks later Ass. Entire eye OD	2 weeks later Ass. Entire eye OS	2 weeks later Ass. Internal optics OD	2 weeks later Ass. Internal optics OS	2 weeks later Ass. Cornea OD	2 weeks later Ass. Cornea OS
Total		0.112	0.196	0.081	0.245	0.104	0.115	0.179	0.061	0.202	0.058	0.070	0.026
LOA	Total	0.098	0.137	0.036	0.198	0.090	0.106	0.172	0.045	0.188	0.049	0.055	0.005
	Defocus	0.0	0.0	0.0	0.0	0.0	0.0	0.0	0.0	0.0	0.0	0.0	0.0
	Astigmatism × axis°	0.098 × 179°	0.137 × 40°	0.036 × 32°	0.198 × 25°	0.090 × 168°	0.106 × 94°	0.172 × 1°	0.045 × 143°	0.188 × 9°	0.049 × 142°	0.055 × 132°	0.005 × 38°
HOA	Total	0.055	0.140	0.073	0.14[illegible]	0.052	0.045	0.050	0.042	0.074	0.030	0.043	0.026
	Coma × axis°	0.010 × 4°	0.115 × 321°	0.035 × 177°	0.110 × 306°	0.045 × 359°	0.030 × 34°	0.041 × 58°	0.039 × 234°	0.060 × 97°	0.024 × 224°	0.038 × 319°	0.016 × 249°
	Trefoil × axis°	0.049 × 39°	0.047 × 71°	0.060 × 44°	0.065 × 62°	0.016 × 118°	0.032 × 107°	0.016 × 44°	0.010 × 115°	0.031 × 40°	0.008 × 81°	0.016 × 96°	0.014 × 6°
	Spherical	0.005	-0.014	-0.013	-0.023	0.018	0.009	0.001	-0.001	-0.011	-0.014	0.012	0.013

WF: wavefront; Ass.: assessment; LOA: lower-order aberration; HOA: higher-order aberration; OD: right eye; OS: left eye.

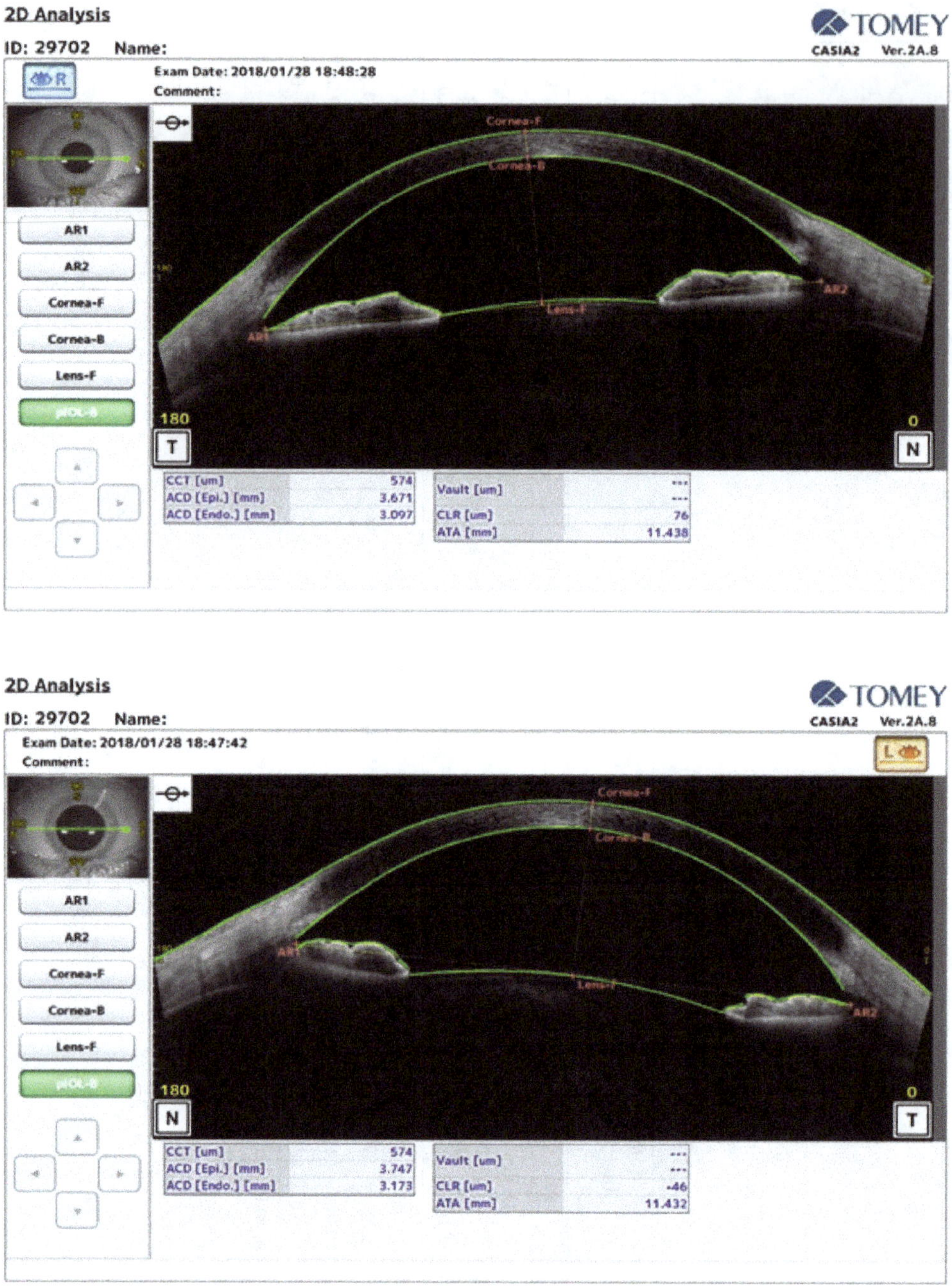

FIGURE 2: Anterior segment OCT two weeks after the trauma in the right and left eyes.

Comparison of the AS-OCTs showed the anterior rotation of the ciliary body and the anterior part of the choroid in the left eye and ciliochoroidal effusion.

The baseline wavefront analysis using iTrace aberrometer (Tracey Technologies, Houston, TX) showed a significant amount of total aberration in the internal optics in the left eye compared to the right eye (0.245 μm vs. 0.081 μm) secondary to the increased amounts of total low- and high-order aberrations (Table 1). The positional changes secondary to trauma produced considerable changes in the internal optical aberrations of the left eye mostly crystalline lens so that there is a noticeable difference in the magnitude of low-order astigmatism (0.198 μm vs. 0.036 μm) and coma (0.110 μm vs. 0.035 μm) compared to the right eye in the initial assessment.

Cycloplegic refraction was evaluated with one drop of tropicamide 1% which was instilled every five minutes for three times, and auto refraction was repeated 30 minutes after the last drop.

The patient was reevaluated two weeks later. There were no changes in the right eye while the left eye showed significant improvement in the visual acuity, refractive error, and ACD. The uncorrected distance visual acuity was 1.0 with a refraction +1.00/−0.25 × 60° in the left eye. Keratometry readings did not show changes compared to the initial assessment, and IOP increased to 13.3 mmHg in the left eye.

The left ACD increased to 1.30 mm and reached to 3.17 mm (vs. 3.09 in the right eye) while the CLR reduced by 956 μm and obtained a negative value -46 μm (Figure 2).

The next wavefront analysis at the two weeks posttrauma appointment showed a reduction of 0.187 μm in the total internal optical aberrations. The lower- and higher-orders aberrations of the internal optics reduced by 0.149 μm and 0.114 μm, respectively. Associated with these improvements, root mean square of the internal lower-order astigmatism and coma changed significantly (Table 1).

3. Discussion

In this case, the ocular nonpenetrating trauma provided a myopic shift of about 7.00 D, which resolved after 15 days. This change was associated with the narrowing of ACD and increase in the CLR in the left eye. Comparison of Figures 1 and 2 in the left eye refers to the forward displacement of the iris-crystalline lens diaphragm secondary to ciliary body anterior rotation and ciliochoroidal effusion. It has been suggested that trauma in this area can increase the permeability of the blood vessels due to the involvement of the sympathetic nerve terminating in the walls of vessels [9]. Ultrasound biomicroscopy (UBM) is the best method to display the structures behind the iris and to show the ciliary rotation and choroidal effusion [8]; however, the obtained AS-OCT images partly highlighted these changes. Figure 1 visualizes the fluid in the suprachoroidal space in the left eye. In the obtained AS-OCT cut, there was not a continuous channel between the anterior chamber and the suprachoroidal space. Despite this, there was a reduced intraocular pressure in the left eye compared to the right eye in the initial assessment (7.9 mmHg vs. 13.6 mmHg). This difference in intraocular pressures may be attributed to the posttraumatic structural alternations.

Accommodative spasm has been mentioned as an etiologic factor of pseudomyopia after trauma [1, 10]; however, lack of difference in the manifest and cycloplegic refractions in the initial assessment and no eso-shift in the cover test ruled out the ciliary spasm as the cause of the induced myopia.

In conclusion, the traumatic myopia that develops after ocular blunt trauma is mostly a transient entity and caused by a combination of different factors such as ciliochoroidal effusion and forward shift of the lens-iris diaphragm. However, the precise contribution of each of the possible causes is difficult and can have individual variations from person to person. Anterior segment optical coherence tomography (AS-OCT) provides a precise method to better illustrate the anterior segment changes following blunt trauma.

Consent

The patient has consented to the submission of the case report to the journal.

Acknowledgments

The authors would like to thank the subject and personals of Sedaghat Eye Clinic.

References

[1] N. Ikeda, T. Ikeda, and T. Kohno, "Traumatic myopia secondary to ciliary spasm after blunt eye trauma and reconsideration of its pathogenesis," *Graefe's Archive for Clinical and Experimental Ophthalmology*, vol. 254, no. 7, pp. 1411–1417, 2016.

[2] N. Ikeda, T. Ikeda, M. Nagata, and O. Mimura, "Pathogenesis of transient high myopia after blunt eye trauma," *Ophthalmology*, vol. 109, no. 3, pp. 501–507, 2002.

[3] S. I. Kim, Y. J. Cha, and S. E. Park, "A case report on the change of the refractive power after a blunt trauma," *Korean Journal of Ophthalmology*, vol. 22, no. 1, pp. 53–57, 2008.

[4] P. Rewri, G. Goyal, W. Ali, A. Sharma, and D. Sood, "Acute onset bilateral myopia in convalescence phase of varicella infection," *Oman Journal of Ophthalmology*, vol. 8, no. 1, pp. 69-70, 2015.

[5] L. M. Abraham, R. D. Keembiyage, D. Selva, and R. Casson, "Persistent unilateral myopia following blunt trauma," *Eye*, vol. 20, no. 8, p. 946, 2006.

[6] S. Doğanay, H. Er, Í. F. Hepsen, and C. Evereklioğlu, "Bilateral myopia following blunt trauma to one eye," *European Journal of Ophthalmology*, vol. 11, no. 1, pp. 83–85, 2001.

[7] M. Kuchle and G. O. Naumann, "Transient myopia after trauma," *Ophthalmology*, vol. 110, no. 7, article 1285, 2003.

[8] J. W. Lee, S. J. Kwon, S. H. Chai, and H. K. Kim, "A case of transient myopia after blunt eye trauma," *Japanese Journal of Ophthalmology*, vol. 53, no. 6, pp. 665–667, 2009.

[9] C. A. Steele, A. B. Tullo, I. B. Marsh, and J. K. Storey, "Traumatic myopia; an ultrasonographic and clinical study," *The British Journal of Ophthalmology*, vol. 71, no. 4, pp. 301–303, 1987.

[10] R. V. Chan and J. D. Trobe, "Spasm of accommodation associated with closed head trauma," *Journal of Neuro-Ophthalmology*, vol. 22, no. 1, pp. 15–17, 2002.

11

Bilateral Ampiginous Choroiditis following Presumed SARS-CoV-2 Infection

Elysse S. Tom, K. Matthew McKay, and Steven S. Saraf

Department of Ophthalmology, University of Washington, Seattle, WA, USA

Correspondence should be addressed to Steven S. Saraf; sarafs@uw.edu

Academic Editor: Stephen G. Schwartz

Purpose. To report a case of bilateral ampiginous choroiditis following presumed SARS-CoV-2 infection. *Case Description.* A 25-year-old woman presented with metamorphopsia and a paracentral scotoma in her left eye. She endorsed night sweats, headache, and new-onset anosmia beginning 1 week before her visual symptoms. She also had multiple confirmed ill COVID-19 contacts at her workplace before the onset of her symptoms. Funduscopic examination and multimodal imaging revealed placoid lesions in the macula and midperiphery of both eyes consistent with ampiginous choroiditis. COVID-19 antibody testing returned positive for IgG, and an extensive systemic evaluation was otherwise unremarkable. She was treated with oral prednisone and azathioprine with stabilization of the retinal lesions and no progression of her symptoms. *Conclusions.* Ampiginous choroiditis is an inflammatory chorioretinopathy with an unknown pathogenic mechanism that often necessitates early immunomodulatory therapy. This report suggests that SARS-CoV-2 infection may trigger chorioretinal inflammation in susceptible hosts.

1. Introduction

Severe Acute Respiratory Syndrome Coronavirus-2 (SARS-CoV-2), the novel coronavirus that causes COVID-19, is associated with a multitude of adverse systemic effects beyond acute respiratory disease. Molecular mimicry has been proposed as a contributing factor to some systemic complications, including antiphospholipid antibodies, Kawasaki disease, and Guillain-Barre syndrome. Systemic corticosteroids have shown benefit in some patients [1, 2].

Ampiginous choroiditis is an inflammatory chorioretinopathy with features of both acute posterior multifocal placoid pigment epitheliopathy (APMPPE), an often self-limited condition with good prognosis, and serpiginous choroiditis, a progressive condition with high risk of visual disability. Both can affect otherwise healthy individuals and have been hypothesized to occur due to molecular mimicry between infectious and ocular antigens. APMPPE is often preceded by a flu-like illness, and cases have been associated with vaccinations, as well as infections with group A streptococcus, adenovirus type 5, tuberculosis, Lyme disease, and mumps [3–5].

2. Case Report

A 25-year-old healthy woman presented complaining of distortion and a blind spot near the central vision of her left eye of one month duration. One week preceding visual symptom onset, she endorsed night sweats, headache, and new-onset anosmia. The night sweats and headaches lasted 3 days. The anosmia lasted 2 weeks. She had multiple confirmed ill COVID-19 contacts at her workplace before the onset of her symptoms. Best corrected visual acuity was 20/20 and 20/25 in the right and left eyes, respectively. Intraocular pressures, previously documented as normal, were 20 mmHg on the right and 24 mmHg on the left after one month of topical difluprednate therapy. The anterior chambers were both quiet with no cell or flare. Examination of the vitreous revealed rare cell and no haze in both eyes. Dilated fundus examination revealed placoid lesions in the macula and midperiphery of both eyes. Peripheral punched-out scars with Schlaegel lines were also noted. Fundus imaging (Figure 1) demonstrated hypoautofluorescent lesions in the macula and midperiphery of both eyes with irregular hyperautofluorescent borders. Hypofluorescent lesions were observed

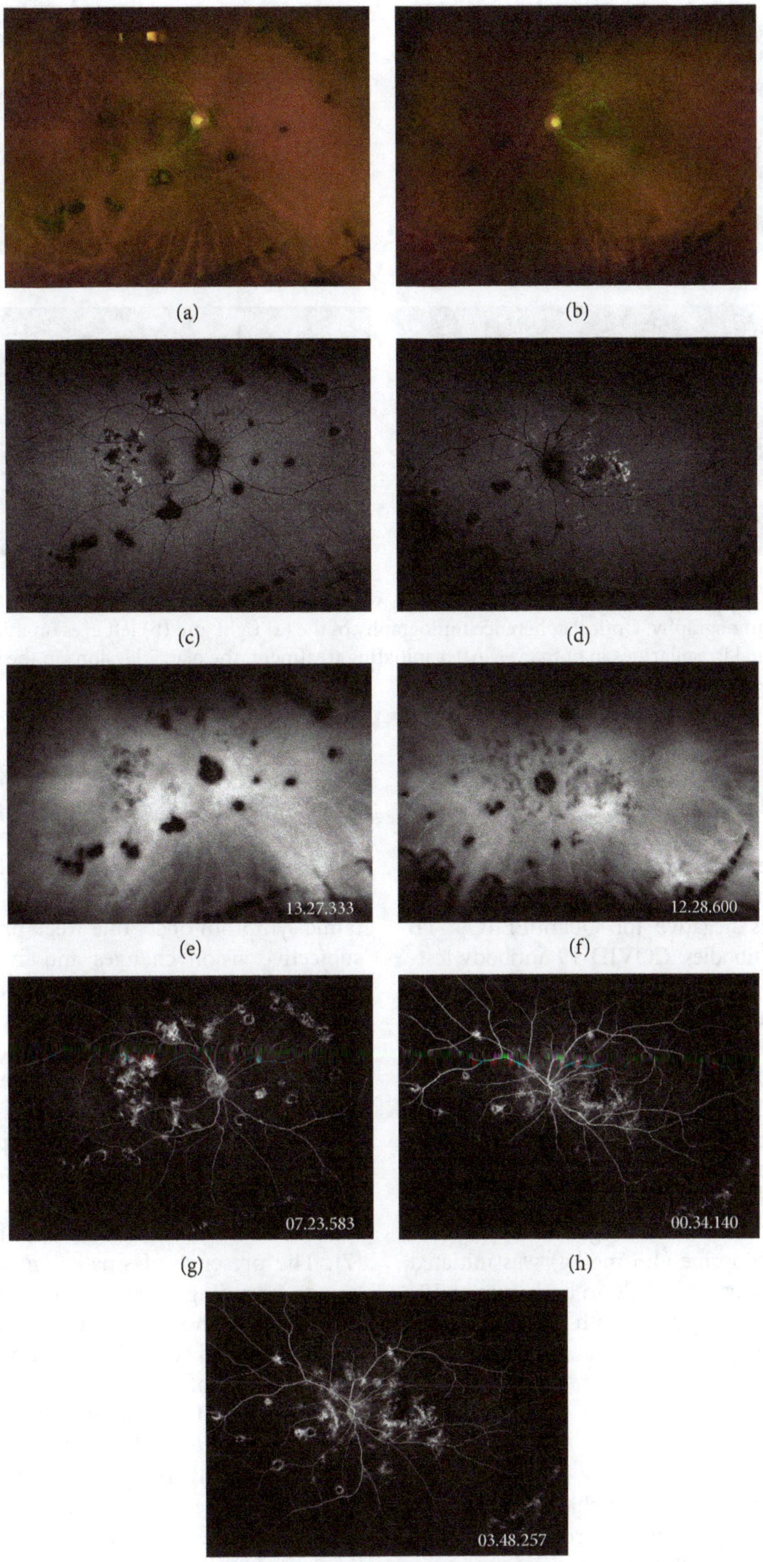

(a) (b) (c) (d) (e) (f) (g) (h) (i)

FIGURE 1: Multimodal fundus imaging. Optos fundus photos of the (a) right and (b) left eyes demonstrating placoid lesions in the macula and retinal periphery as well as peripheral punched-out scars in a Schlaegel line configuration. (c, d) Fundus autofluorescence exhibits hypoautofluorescent placoid lesions with irregular hyperautofluorescent borders in the posterior pole and midperiphery of both eyes. (e, f) Indocyanine green angiography displays hypofluorescent placoid choroidal lesions more widespread in the nasal periphery of the left eye than visible on fundus autofluorescence, signifying active inflammatory disease. Fluorescein angiography of the (g) right eye and (h) left eye early and (i) late demonstrates progressive staining and leakage from the placoid lesions.

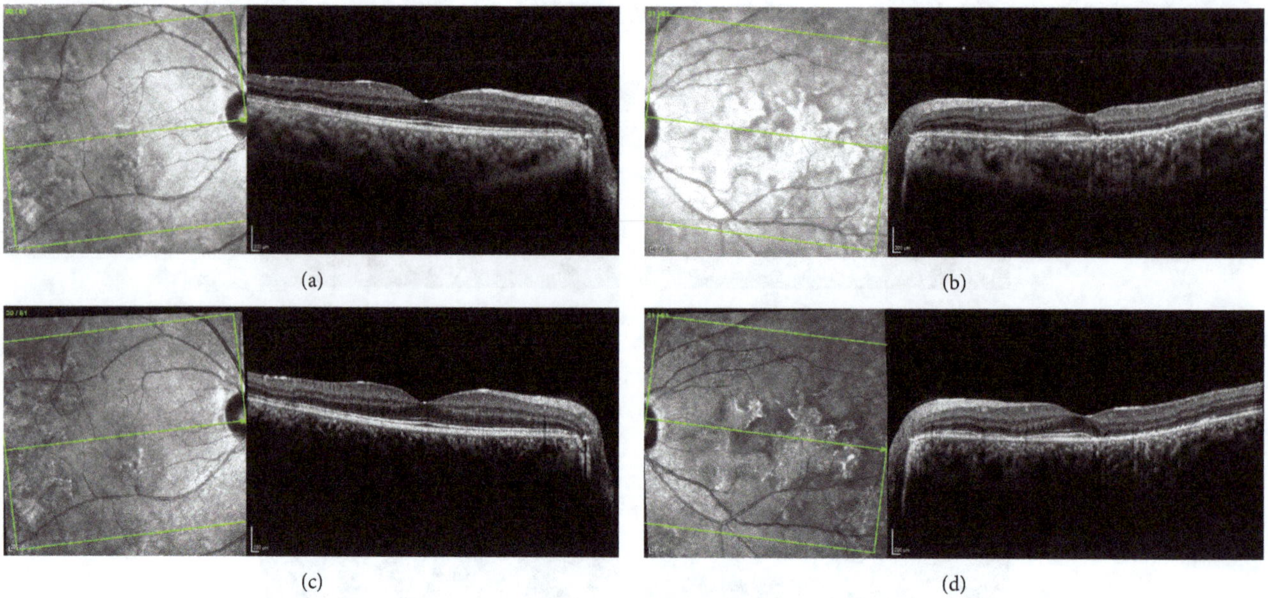

FIGURE 2: Optical coherence tomography. Optical coherence tomography of the (a) right and (b) left eyes on initial visit. The macular lesions are associated with outer retinal irregularities in both eyes. After initiating treatment, the placoid lesions in the (c) right and (d) left eyes did not progress or improve 8 weeks after the initial visit.

on indocyanine green angiography in a distribution more widespread in the left eye than appreciated on fundus examination. Fluorescein angiography (FA) demonstrated early progressive staining and leakage from the placoid lesions without significant early blockage. Optical coherence tomography demonstrated bilateral outer retinal disruption (Figure 2). Laboratory evaluation was negative for QuantiFERON-TB gold, HIV, and syphilis antibodies. COVID-19 antibody testing returned positive for IgG. COVID-19 PCR testing was not performed. The patient's systemic symptoms had occurred 4 months following the initial pandemic lockdowns in the United States when the patient's county of origin had reported a total of 450-460 cases per 100,000 inhabitants [6]. Neuroimaging was not pursued due to the resolution of headaches and absence of neurologic symptoms at the time of evaluation. She was treated with a taper of oral prednisone starting at 60 mg. The retinal lesions did not progress, and steroid-sparing therapy with azathioprine (1.5 mg/kg) was initiated at 3 weeks. Visual acuity remained 20/20 in both eyes at 10-month follow-up after completing a 3-month oral prednisone taper and continuing azathioprine.

3. Discussion

Ampiginous choroiditis is an inflammatory chorioretinopathy with high risk of visual disability that shares disease features with APMPPE and serpiginous choroiditis [7]. The disease pathogenesis is unknown, but similar processes have been observed to occur following flu-like illnesses as well as specific viral entities [3]. We present a case of ampiginous choroiditis shortly following presumed SARS-CoV-2 infection demonstrated by positive antibody testing.

To our knowledge, this is the second report of posterior uveitis potentially associated with COVID-19 . Serpiginous choroiditis was recently reported 2 weeks after onset of systemic symptoms in a case of PCR-proven COVID-19 [8]. In addition to the new serpiginous choroiditis lesions, there was documentation of preexisting peripapillary findings that could have represented an earlier manifestation of the disease. In the case of our patient, without positive PCR testing, recent SARS-CoV-2 infection was presumed based on systemic symptom onset one week prior to the development of subjective vision changes and five weeks prior to positive antibody testing. Minimally symptomatic patients may demonstrate COVID-19 antibodies for only 6 weeks after infection [9], supporting a recent primary infection in our patient, rather than a more remote, asymptomatic infection.

Differentiating APMPPE from ampiginous choroiditis is critical due to implications for prognosis and treatment. While APMPPE is often a self-limited condition with good prognosis, ampiginous choroiditis is characterized by recurrent inflammation with high risk for permanent vision loss [7]. The presence of smaller, more numerous, nonhealing lesions extending into the peripheral retina supported a diagnosis of ampiginous choroiditis in this case. Furthermore, the active lesions in the left eye did not demonstrate the classic early blocking of fluorescence on FA observed in APMPPE. The diagnosis of serpiginous-like choroiditis was also considered given the nonhealing nature of the lesions, but this possibility was less favored given negative tuberculosis testing and lack of evidence of prominent edge reactivation. Consideration of these features and the presence of fovea-threatening lesions led to the initiation of immunomodulatory therapy. Local steroids were avoided due to demonstrated steroid response and cataract risk in a young patient. Intraocular pressures normalized after topical difluprednate was discontinued, and pachymetry revealed thick corneas so further glaucoma testing was not pursued.

As reported in the serpiginous choroiditis case by Providência et al., we observed evidence of prior ocular inflammatory disease before the COVID-19-associated flare [8]. We observed inactive peripheral punched-out scars in each eye possibly associated with a history of multifocal choroiditis or ocular histoplasmosis syndrome. Multifocal choroiditis with panuveitis has been reported to overlap with other white dot syndromes [10]. Our patient had features of both active ampiginous choroiditis and chronic findings consistent with a multifocal choroiditis. It is possible that COVID-19 could serve as an immunologic trigger for the development or reactivation of ocular inflammatory disease in susceptible hosts, in this case in a patient with a propensity for overlapping white dot syndromes.

4. Conclusions

Ampiginous choroiditis is an inflammatory chorioretinopathy with unknown pathogenic mechanism that often necessitates early immunomodulatory therapy. This report suggests that SARS-CoV-2 infection may trigger chorioretinal inflammation in susceptible hosts.

Consent

Consent to publish the case report was not obtained. This report does not contain any personal information that could lead to the identification of the patient. Our institution does not require consent to be obtained for single case reports.

References

[1] F. Angileri, S. Legaro, A. Marino Gammazza, F. Conway de Macario, A. Jl Macario, and F. Cappello, "Molecular mimicry may explain multi-organ damage in COVID-19," *Autoimmunity Reviews*, vol. 19, no. 8, 2020.

[2] M. Ehrenfeld, A. Tincani, L. Andreoli et al., "Covid-19 and autoimmunity," *Autoimmunity Reviews*, vol. 19, no. 8, p. 102597, 2020.

[3] F. X. Borruat, B. Piguet, and C. P. Herbort, "Acute posterior multifocal placoid pigment epitheliopathy following mumps," *Ocular Immunology and Inflammation*, vol. 6, no. 3, pp. 189–193, 1998.

[4] T. Gonome, Y. Suzuki, T. Metoki, S. Takahashi, and M. Nakazawa, "Acute posterior multifocal placoid pigment epitheliopathy and granulomatous uveitis following influenza vaccination," *American Journal of Ophthalmology Case Reports*, vol. 4, pp. 60–63, 2016.

[5] P. Dutta Majumder, J. Biswas, and A. Gupta, "Enigma of serpiginous choroiditis," *Indian Journal of Ophthalmology*, vol. 67, no. 3, pp. 325–333, 2019.

[6] "COVID-19 Data Dashboard," 2021, https://www.doh.wa.gov/Emergencies/COVID19/DataDashboard#reports.

[7] B. E. Jones, L. M. Jampol, L. A. Yannuzzi et al., "Relentless placoid chorioretinitis: a new entity or an unusual variant of serpiginous chorioretinitis?," *Archives of Ophthalmology*, vol. 118, no. 7, pp. 931–938, 2000.

[8] J. Providência, C. Fonseca, F. Henriques, and R. Proença, "Serpiginous choroiditis presenting after SARS-CoV-2 infection: a new immunological trigger?," *European Journal of Ophthalmology*, 2020.

[9] F. J. Ibarrondo, J. A. Fulcher, D. Goodman-Meza et al., "Rapid Decay of Anti–SARS-CoV-2 Antibodies in Persons with Mild Covid-19," *New England Journal of Medicine*, vol. 383, no. 11, pp. 1085–1087, 2020.

[10] T. Kuznetcova, B. Jeannin, and C. P. Herbort, "A case of overlapping choriocapillaritis syndromes: multimodal imaging appraisal," *Journal of ophthalmic & vision research*, vol. 7, no. 1, pp. 67–75, 2012.

12

Tubulointerstitial Nephritis and Uveitis Syndrome: Case Series and Literature Review

Beatriz Oliveira Lopes,[1] **Margarida Sena Brízido**,[1] **Ana Cortesão Costa**,[2] **Mário Raimundo**,[2] **Margarida Maria Miranda**,[1] **and Susana Morais Pina**[1]

[1]*Department of Ophthalmology, Beatriz Ângelo Hospital, Loures, Portugal*
[2]*Department of Nephrology, Beatriz Ângelo Hospital, Loures, Portugal*

Correspondence should be addressed to Beatriz Oliveira Lopes; bibas.oliveiralopes@gmail.com

Academic Editor: Kamal Kishore

Tubulointerstitial nephritis and uveitis syndrome (TINU) is a rare oculorenal inflammatory entity with a probable autoimmune etiology. Interstitial nephritis may be asymptomatic and usually has a benign course with spontaneous resolution. Uveitis, instead, is classically anterior, bilateral, and nongranulomatous, but it can be unilateral and presents as posterior uveitis or panuveitis, sometimes with a chronic or recurrent evolution. The frequent time lag of ocular and renal manifestations makes this diagnosis particularly challenging. The authors describe four cases of this rare entity, two with tubulointerstitial nephritis preceding ocular manifestations and the remaining, instead, with uveitis preceding renal involvement. The therapeutic approach included systemic corticosteroids in all cases. The addition of immunosuppressive therapy was required in three patients to achieve uveitis control. TINU is probably an underrecognized entity and should always be considered in the differential diagnosis of a chronic or recurrent idiopathic uveitis, especially in young patients who may have mild and asymptomatic renal disease.

1. Introduction

Tubulointerstitial nephritis and uveitis (TINU) syndrome is a rare inflammatory autoimmune disease [1, 2], described for the first time by Dobrin et al. in 1975 [3]. It is defined by the association of uveitis and acute tubulointerstitial nephritis (TIN) and requires exclusion of infection or other potentially associated systemic diseases [4, 5]. The syndrome is an important cause of acute kidney injury, responsible for 5% of the cases of acute TIN [4, 6]. In contrast, only, 0.1-2% of uveitis had been related to TINUS [1, 7, 8]. The subclinical nature of renal manifestations [5, 7] and the possible interlude with ophthalmic presentation make this diagnosis a challenge in clinical practice.

Our purpose is to alert for the existence of this clinical entity and highlight for the importance of screening for renal disease in patients with chronic or recurrent nongranulomatous uveitis of unclear etiology reviewing a series of four clinical cases of TINU.

2. Clinical Cases

2.1. Patient 1. A 49-year-old female presented to the emergency room with lumbar pain, transitory dark urine, asthenia, anorexia, weight loss, and leg and periorbital edema (Table 1). She referred chronic use of a proton pump inhibitor and had been consuming a nonsteroidal anti-inflammatory drug (NSAID) for the previous month.

Laboratory evaluation showed elevation of the erythrocyte sedimentation rate (ESR) 140 mm/first hour and C-reactive protein (CRP) 7.75 mg/dL, normocytic and normochromic anemia (Hb 10.1 g/dL), and increased serum creatinine (3.96 mg/dL) and urea (103 mg/dL). Urinalysis showed hematuria and proteinuria (1044 mg/24 h) without cellular casts. Additional investigations were unremarkable. She underwent a kidney biopsy for declining kidney function despite intravenous hydration and discontinuation of nephrotoxins that showed, on light microscopy, normal glomeruli and diffuse mononuclear cell interstitial infiltrates, consistent with acute

TIN, which was initially deemed pharmacologic.

She started systemic corticosteroids (oral prednisolone 1 mg/kg/day) with clinical improvement and full renal function recovery in 6 months. However, at 8 months after the initial presentation, while on the final phase of steroid tapering (prednisolone 2.5 mg every other day), she presented with ciliar hyperaemia and pain in the right eye (Table 1) and unilateral anterior nongranulomatous uveitis was detected (Figure 1).

Based on the presence of uveitis and TIN, the diagnosis of TINU syndrome was confirmed. Further clinical investigation was made to rule out the main infection and inflammatory diseases considered for differential diagnosis, including hepatitis B and C, *Toxoplasma gondii*, *Mycobacterium tuberculosis*, Epstein-Barr, syphilis, cytomegalovirus, and brucellosis infections, sarcoidosis, and Behcet's disease. Examination for human leukocyte antigen (HLA) alleles showed HLADQ B1∗02∗06 HLADR B1∗02∗06 positivity. Systemic corticosteroids were optimized to 0.5 mg/kg/day, and azathioprine 2 mg/kg/day was associated, beyond topical corticosteroids, with achieved uveitis control (Table 1). Six years after being diagnosed, the patient is clinically stable under immunosuppressive therapy with prednisolone 5 mg/day and azathioprine 1 mg/kg/day.

2.2. Patient 2. A 54-year-old female presented to the emergency room with urinary frequency, asthenia, anorexia and progressive weight loss (Table 1). She had diabetes without known microvascular complications, dyslipidaemia, hypertension, and sporadic use of NSAIDs.

Analysis showed normocytic normochromic anemia (Hb 6 g/dL), metabolic acidosis, elevation of ESR (88 mm/first hour) and CRP (3.87 mg/dL), increased serum urea (171 mg/dL) and creatinine (7.7 mg/dL), nonnephrotic proteinuria (404 mg/24 h), haematuria, and leukocyturia without cellular casts. Additional investigations, namely, for autoimmune diseases and multiple myeloma, were negative, and a kidney biopsy was performed which was consistent with acute TIN (Figure 2).

She started oral steroids (1 mg/kg/day) with progressive dose tapering which resulted in clinical and kidney function improvement. One year later, treatment was discontinued motivated by apparent clinical control. However, two weeks after treatment interruption, she presented with ocular pain in the right eye (Table 1). Unilateral nongranulomatous anterior and intermediate uveitis was detected, and TINU syndrome was suspected.

Further evaluation included exclusion of infections and other autoimmune diseases. Evaluation for HLA genotypes was positive for HLADQ B1∗03∗05. Beyond topical corticosteroids and mydriatics, systemic corticosteroids (1 mg/kg/day) were reintroduced with slow progressive withdrawal, lasting two years, on account of recurrent uveitis (Table 1). Currently, the patient remains clinically stable with no new recurrences and no need for corticosteroid therapy for the last 4 years.

2.3. Patient 3. A previously healthy 32-year-old female presented to the emergency room with hyperaemia and bilateral ocular pain for a week. Ophthalmology observation revealed bilateral anterior nongranulomatous uveitis and anterior vitritis. She was prescribed topical corticosteroids, mydriatics, and NSAIDs with transitory clinical improvement. A few weeks later, uveitis recurred and she also reported asthenia, arthralgia, and myalgia (Table 1).

Investigation revealed hypergammaglobulinemia (IgG 1900 mg/dL), creatinine (1.58 mg/dL) and urea (60 mg/dL) elevation, and raised levels of ESR (61 mm/hour), CRP (2.3 mg/dL), and urine β2-microglobulin (661 mg/dL). Urinalysis showed proteinuria and hematuria. The examination for HLA genotypes was positive for HLADR B1∗01. Infections and other autoimmune diseases were ruled out.

Based on clinical criteria, TIN was considered and diagnosis of TINU syndrome was assumed. The patient started systemic corticosteroids (0.5 mg/kg/day) with a dose tapering schedule with progressive ocular resolution. Six months later, she started azathioprine (2 mg/kg/day) with subsequent need to increase the dose to 2.5 mg/kg/day on account of uveitis recurrence (Table 1). Currently, the patient is clinically stable after 2 years on immunosuppressive therapy.

2.4. Patient 4. A healthy 16-year-old male came to the emergency room with ocular pain and redness associated with bilateral diminished visual acuity for five days. He presented anterior bilateral nongranulomatous uveitis with posterior synechiae, vitritis, and diffuse scattered soft white subretinal dots compatible with multifocal choroiditis. Considering a bilateral panuveitis, an etiologic study was started and he was prescribed mydriatics and topical steroids (Table 1).

Despite slight ophthalmic improvement, 2 weeks later, he presented with fever, myalgias, anorexia and weight loss. Laboratory evaluation showed hypergammaglobulinemia (IgG 1620 mg/dL), creatinine elevation (1.5 mg/dL), nonnephrotic proteinuria (82 mg/24 h), haematuria, leukocyturia, and elevated urine β2-microglobulin (1120 mg/dL). The main infections and inflammatory diseases were ruled out. Kidney injury was attributed to TIN, and diagnosis of TINU syndrome was established. He started prednisolone (1 mg/kg/day) with progressive withdrawal and methotrexate (25 mg/week) which resulted in uveitis control and kidney function recovery within 4 months (Table 1). After two years of clinical stabilization, it was possible to discontinue immunosuppressive therapy with no new recurrences.

3. Discussion

This paper reports four cases of TINU syndrome, a rare entity with higher incidence in young females with a median age at presentation of 15 years [2, 5, 7]. Recently, cases in adults and male patients with a wider range of presentations have been described [2, 5, 9], as is evident in our case series.

The pathogenesis of the syndrome remains unclear, and it is probably multifactorial [2, 4]. An autoimmune process involving cellular and humoral immunity, possible against a common ocular and kidney antigen target, may have an important role [5, 7, 10]. A loss of T-cell tolerance may be suggested by the presence of some high-risk human leukocyte antigen genotypes (HLA-A2, HLA-A24, HLADQA1∗

Table 1: Description of the presented cases.

	Case 1	Case 2	Case 3	Case 4
Sex	Female	Female	Female	Male
Age (years)	49	54	32	16
Clinical presentation	Lumbar pain, dark urine, asthenia, anorexia, weight loss, leg and periorbital edema, unilateral anterior uveitis	Urinary frequency, asthenia, anorexia, weight loss, unilateral anterior and intermediate uveitis	Bilateral anterior and intermediate uveitis, asthenia, arthralgia, and myalgia	Bilateral panuveitis, fever, myalgias, anorexia, and weight loss
First ocular symptoms			+	+
First renal symptoms	+	+		
Clinical diagnosis			+	+
Histological diagnosis	+	+		
Ocular treatment	Topical corticosteroid, mydriatic	Topical corticosteroid, mydriatic	Topical corticosteroid, mydriatic	Topical corticosteroid, mydriatic
Systemic treatment	Oral prednisolone (1 mg/kg/day) with progressive withdrawal, azathioprine (2 mg/kg/day)	Oral prednisolone (1 mg/kg/day) with progressive withdrawal	Oral prednisolone (1 mg/kg/day) with progressive withdrawal, azathioprine (2 mg/kg/day)	Oral prednisolone (1 mg/kg/day) with progressive withdrawal, methotrexate (25 mg/week)
Follow-up	Uveitis recurrence: once	Uveitis recurrence: once	Uveitis recurrence: twice	No recurrence

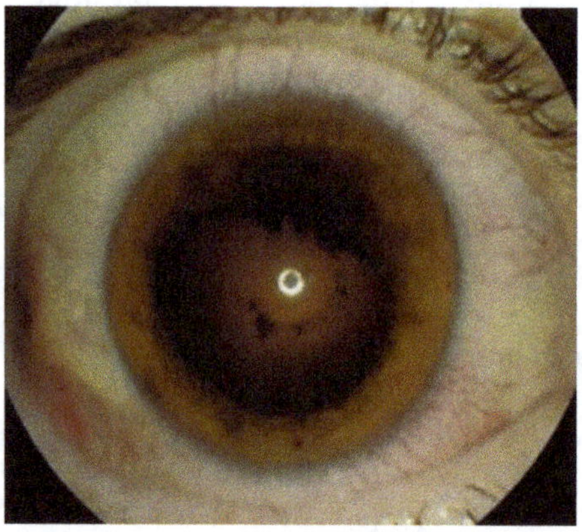

Figure 1: Photograph of the anterior segment of the right eye after pharmacological mydriases, showing posterior synechia between 12 and 2 h. Deposition of the iris pigment in the anterior capsule due to posterior synechia (patient 1).

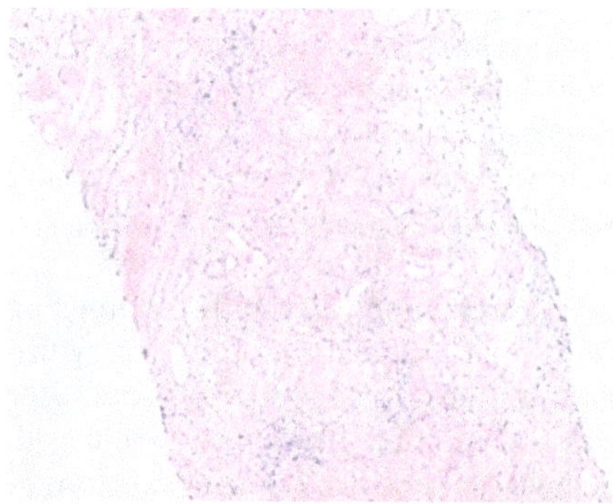

Figure 2: Pathological specimen obtained by renal biopsy (×100). Hematoxylin-eosin. Diffuse infiltration of inflammatory cells, mainly consisting of lymphocytic infiltrate, interstitial fibrosis, and tubular atrophy. The glomeruli are normal (patient 2).

01, HLADQB1*05 and HLADRB1*01, and HLADRB1 * 0102) in TINU syndrome patients, as described in the literature [1, 2, 11]. In our series, only patient 2 had one of this risk HLA alleles; however, the haplotypes identified in the other patients may contribute to the pathogenesis of the disease as well. Published papers also described the association with drugs, including some antibiotics and NSAIDs, and infections predominantly by *Toxoplasma gondii*, *Mycobacterium tuberculosis*, Epstein-Barr, and varicella-zoster viruses [2, 4, 8], risk factors involved in TINUS etiology [8]. Sporadic use of NSAIDs was documented in patients 1 and 2.

The diagnosis of this entity requires the presence of TIN and typical uveitis with no other systemic or infectious disease [8, 12]. Although kidney biopsy is considered the classic and definitive diagnostic test [1, 4, 7], TIN can be inferred by the presence of complete clinical criteria published by Mandeville et al. [2] and also found in our patients: abnormal kidney function, urinalysis alterations (elevated β2-microglobulin, low-grade proteinuria, haematuria, glycosuria, leukocyturia, urinary eosinophils, or white blood cell casts), and systemic manifestations lasting at least for two weeks, with the last one characterized by any combination of signs and symptoms such as fever, fatigue, weight loss, and laboratory abnormalities, including anemia, abnormal liver function, eosinophilia, or elevated ESR.

In the first two patients, since TIN was the first manifestation, a kidney biopsy was promptly made, and after the development of uveitis, the diagnosis was confirmed. In the last 2 patients, a kidney biopsy was not performed as kidney involvement was mild, and the procedure was not considered of clinical benefit. Early kidney function evaluation and urinalysis were imperative in these cases, as well as β2-microglobulin urinary levels. β2-Microglobulin is a low molecular weight protein which is freely filtered in the glomerulus and, in the normal condition, reabsorbed in the proximal tubule. This resorptive process is impaired in TIN, making β2-microglobulin a sensitive and specific noninvasive diagnostic test in the appropriate clinical setting [1, 4, 12].

Differential diagnosis should comprise the most common causes responsible for the coexistence of uveitis and TIN, such as sarcoidosis, tuberculosis, Sjogren's syndrome, lupus, Wegener's granulomatosis, and Behcet's disease [1, 5, 8], which always need to be ruled out.

Uveitis is typically bilateral, nongranulomatous, and anterior [1, 7, 13]. However, involvement of vitreous or choroid may also be present [4, 7, 8], as observed in patients 2, 3, and 4. In 65% of cases, uveitis takes place after the TIN [2, 12] and can occur until 12 months after its onset [12]. Less commonly (21%), it can precede nephritis, usually less than 2 months before [2]. In only 15% of patients, uveitis occurs simultaneously with TIN, which makes the diagnosis particularly challenging [2, 12].

Uveitis may be chronic or recurrent in 50% of the cases [1, 2, 7]. Prolonged treatment with immunosuppressive therapy is usually required. Kidney involvement, instead, is often subclinical and generally resolves spontaneously [2, 4, 5], although the development of chronic kidney disease may occur in 11% of patients [2, 5, 14], mostly related to treatment delay. In all presented cases, TIN was transitory with good response to systemic corticosteroids.

The best visual and renal prognosis depends on the early diagnosis and timely treatment of this medical entity. Therefore, it is essential to raise awareness of the importance of screening for renal disease in patients with chronic or recurrent uveitis of unclear cause.

Consent

Consent for publication was obtained from patients.

References

[1] K. Pakzad-Vaezi and K. L. Pepple, "Tubulointerstitial nephritis and uveitis," *Current Opinion in Ophthalmology*, vol. 28, no. 6, pp. 629–635, 2017.

[2] J. T. Mandeville, R. D. Levinson, and G. N. Holland, "The tubulointerstitial nephritis and uveitis syndrome," *Survey of Ophthalmology*, vol. 46, no. 3, pp. 195–208, 2001.

[3] R. S. Dobrin, R. L. Vernier, and A. L. Fish, "Acute eosinophilic interstitial nephritis and renal failure with bone marrow-lymph node granulomas and anterior uveitis: A new syndrome," *The American Journal of Medicine*, vol. 59, no. 3, pp. 325–333, 1975.

[4] P. Cátia, G. Joana, L. Inês, C.-R. Patrícia, S. J. E. E. Da, and S. Rosário, "Nefrite tubulointersticial e uveíte em idade pediátrica: descrição de três doentes," *Jornal Brasileiro de Nefrologia*, vol. 40, no. 3, pp. 296–300, 2018.

[5] M. A. Pinheiro, M. B. C. Rocha, B. O. Neri et al., "TINU syndrome: re-view of the literature and case report," *Jornal Brasileiro de Nefrologia*, vol. 38, 2016.

[6] M. A. Lusco, A. B. Fogo, B. Najafian, and C. E. Alpers, "*AJKD* Atlas of Renal Pathology: Tubulointerstitial Nephritis With Uveitis," *American Journal of Kidney Diseases*, vol. 69, no. 6, pp. e27–e28, 2017.

[7] M. C. Aguilar, M. Lonngi, and A. de-la-Torre, "Tubulointerstitial nephritis and uveitis syndrome: case report and review of the literature," *Ocular Immunology and Inflammation*, vol. 24, no. 4, pp. 415–421, 2016.

[8] L. O. Okafor, P. Hewins, P. I. Murray, and A. K. Denniston, "Tubulointerstitial nephritis and uveitis (TINU) syndrome: a systematic review of its epidemiology, demographics and risk factors," *Orphanet Journal of Rare Diseases*, vol. 12, no. 1, p. 128, 2017.

[9] J. M. Han, Y. J. Lee, and S. J. Woo, "A case of tubulointerstitial nephritis and uveitis syndrome in an elderly patient," *Korean Journal of Ophthalmology*, vol. 26, no. 5, pp. 398–401, 2012.

[10] S. A. Timmermans, J. J. Huitema, and J. J. Wirtz, "Keep an eye out for tubulo-interstitial nephritis," *The Netherlands Journal of Medicine*, vol. 71, no. 10, pp. 523–525, 2013.

[11] R. D. Levinson, M. S. Park, S. M. Rikkers et al., "Strong associations between specific HLA-DQ and HLA-DR alleles and the tubulointerstitial nephritis and uveitis syndrome," *Investigative Ophthalmology & Visual Science*, vol. 44, no. 2, pp. 653–657, 2003.

[12] T. Nagashima, M. Ishihara, E. Shibuya, S. Nakamura, and N. Mizuki, "Three cases of tubulointerstitial nephritis and uveitis syndrome with different clinical manifestations," *International Ophthalmology*, vol. 37, no. 3, pp. 753–759, 2017.

[13] V. H. Thomassen, T. Ring, J. Thaarup, and K. Baggesen, "Tubulointerstitial nephritis and uveitis (TINU) syndrome: a case report and review of the literature," *Acta Ophthalmologica*, vol. 87, no. 6, pp. 676–679, 2009.

[14] D. M. Hinkle and C. S. Foster, "Tubulointerstitial nephritis and uveitis syndrome," *International Ophthalmology Clinics*, vol. 48, no. 2, pp. 9–13, 2008.

13

Decentered Individualized Sphero-Cylindrical (DISC) Ablation and Corneal Crosslinking in Patient with Progressive Keratoconus

Igor Knezović and Sara Djurić

Eye Institute Knezović, Zagreb, Croatia

Correspondence should be addressed to Sara Djurić; sara.djuric@hotmail.com

Academic Editor: Stephen G. Schwartz

Aim. To report a new method with which we have treated a 29 year old patient with keratoconus and progressive bilateral visual loss during the past few years. *Methods.* The patient underwent inferotemporal decentered individualized sphero-cylindrical (DISC) ablation and crosslinking (CXL) of the left eye. After administration of topical anesthetic, the patient was subjected to phototherapeutic keratectomy (PTK) laser ablation of the central 7.0 mm optical zone with 50 μm depth of epithelial ablation. To avoid the possible outcome of corneal haze, 0.02% mitomycin C (MMC) was applied to the stromal surface for 40 seconds. Riboflavin 0.1% solution was then administered topically every 2 minutes for a 30-minute period followed by 5 cycles of corneal crosslinking, radiating with UV-A at 3 mW/cm^2, for a duration of 5 minutes. *Results.* 17 months postoperative, there was an impressive improvement in uncorrected distance visual acuity, and the cornea became more regular. Results of Fourier's analysis imply a drop of irregularity (-28.6% two months and –63% seventeen months postoperative), Zernike analysis revealed a decrease of higher order aberrations (spheric and comatic aberrations), and corneal index values in the 8 mm zone (IHD, ISV, and IVA) became lower, compared to the preoperative values. *Conclusion.* It is possible to obtain better outcome of visual function with DISC ablation through an individual approach compared to CXL solely. This approach might be a promising strategy in retrieving impaired vision in patients suffering from keratoconus.

1. Introduction

Keratoconus (KC) is a progressive corneal dystrophy commonly presenting as stromal thinning, irregular corneal steepening, and subsequent formation of conical protrusions. The process is usually bilateral and does not include cellular infiltration and vascularization. KC has a high prevalence and affects approximately 1/2000-1/50,000 in the general population [1]. KC leads to high myopia, progressive irregular astigmatism, and substantial visual distortion and significant visual function impairment due to corneal collagen weakening [2]. The etiopathogenesis remains not fully understood. However, different molecular, genomic, and gene expression analyses suggest a multifactorial origin. Certain risk factors that may be associated with disease progression are identified, such as genetic predisposition, Down syndrome, Leber congenital amaurosis, and parental consanguinity [3]. Strong associations with chronic eye rubbing, atopy syndromes, and repeated trauma occurring from contact lenses wearing are shown [4].

There are several possible approaches in KC treatment. Corneal crosslinking (CXL) is one of the promising strategies of KC progression prevention through corneal stiffening, reducing the eventual need for corneal transplantation. The CXL procedure consists of riboflavin administration followed by exposure to ultraviolet-A light (UV-A) to fortify the corneal tissue [5]. However, such an approach allows restriction of KC progression, but lacks the possibility of sight improvement, which might be a substantial necessity for the obtainment of satisfactory quality of life (QoL) in younger patients. That might be surmounted by Athens protocol (AP), another surgical procedure showing promising

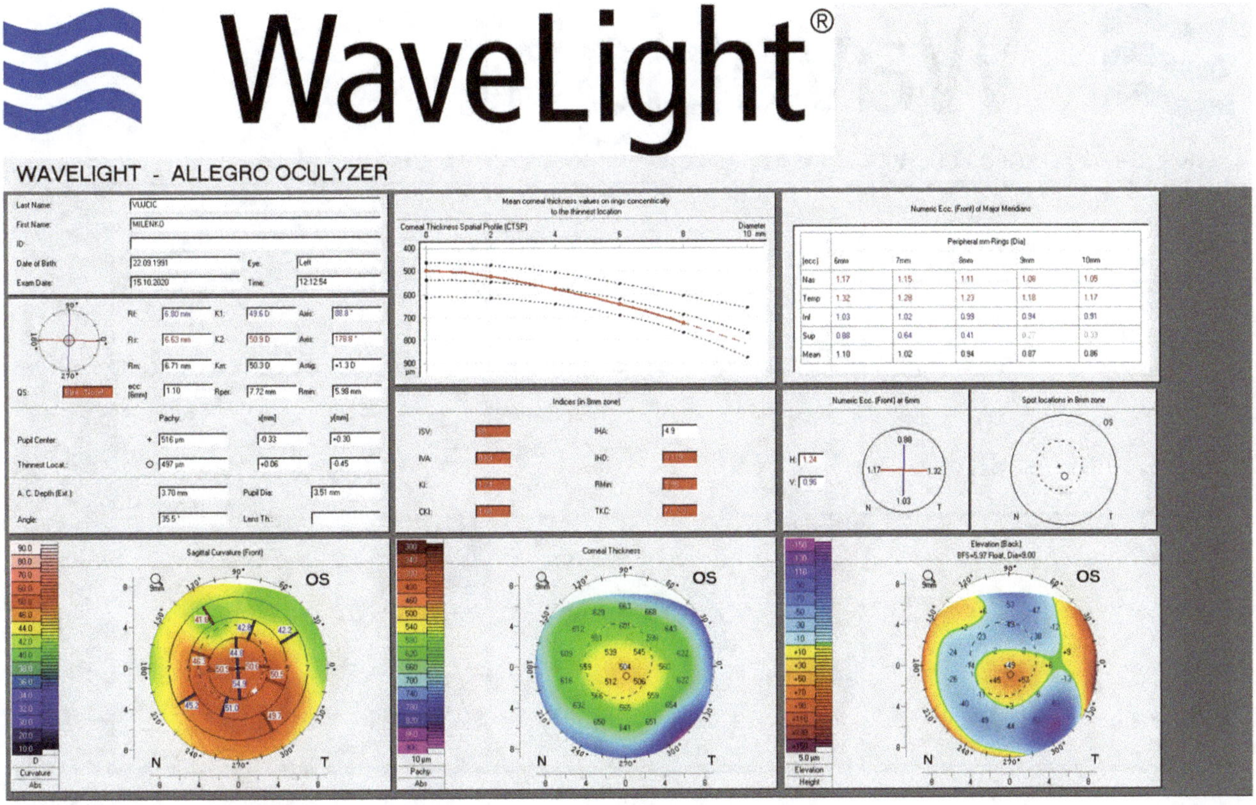

(a)

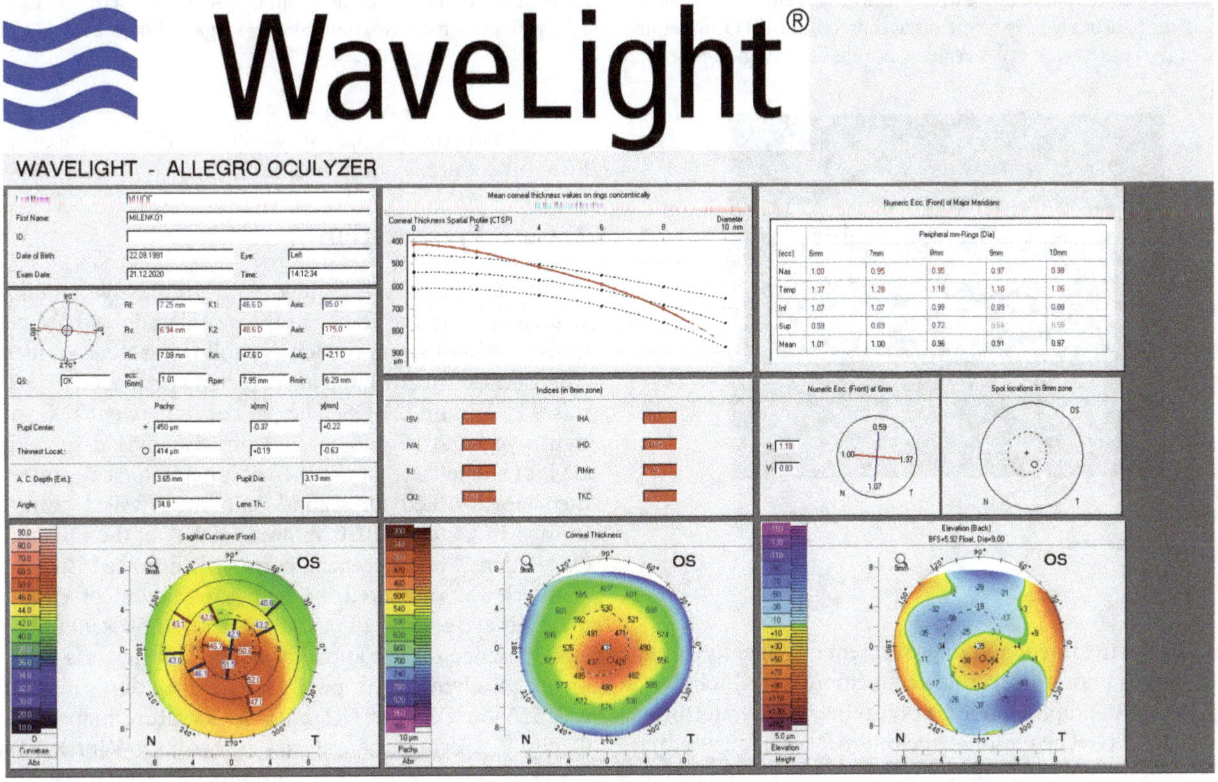

(b)

Figure 1: Continued.

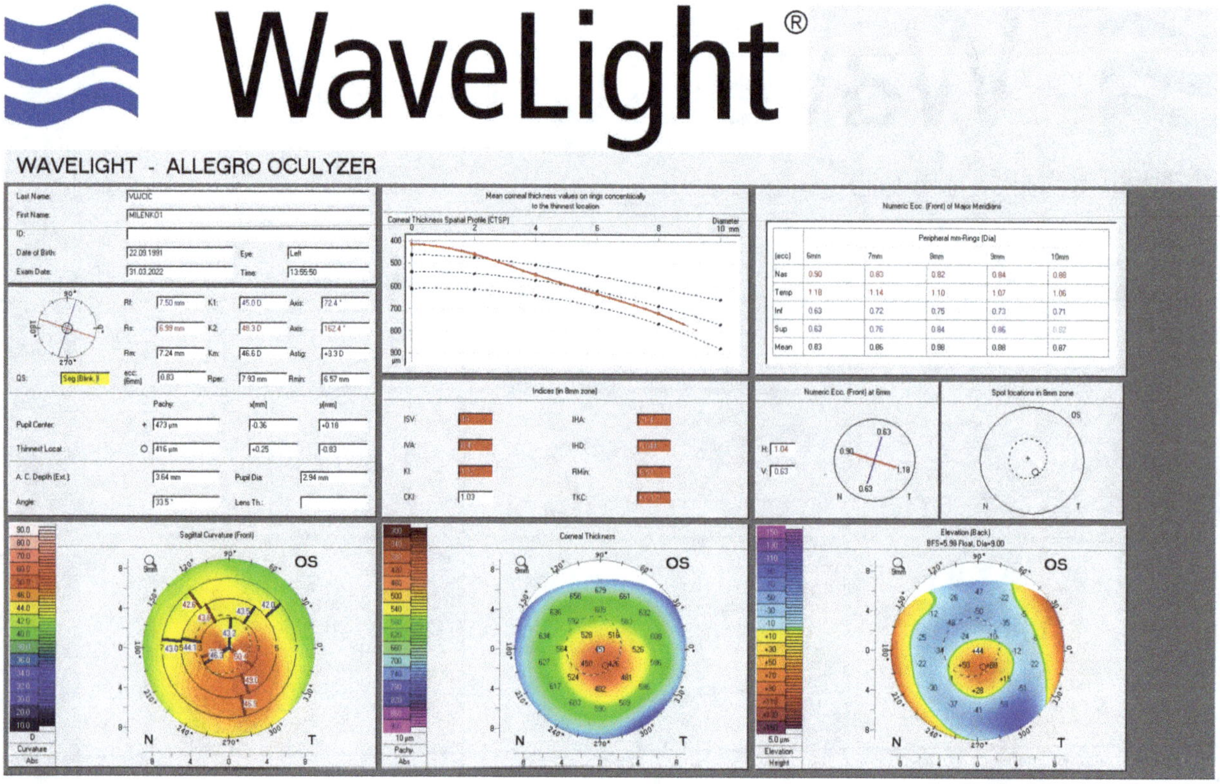

(c)

FIGURE 1: Oculyzer image of the left eye before and after DISC ablation and corneal crosslinking radiating with UV-A at 3 mW/cm^2. (a) Oculyzer image of the patient's left eye before surgical procedure. (b) Oculyzer image of the patient's left eye two months after surgical procedure. (c) Oculyzer image of the patient's left eye seventeen months after surgical procedure.

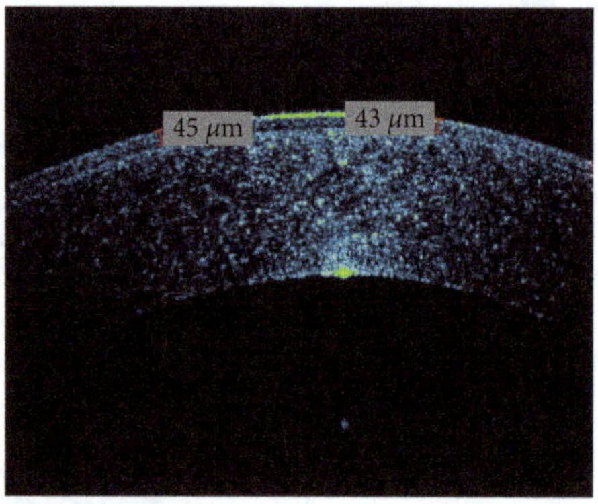

FIGURE 2: Preoperative AS-OCT of the left eye with corneal epithelium thickness.

results in KC treatment and improvement of visual function. AP combines phototherapeutic keratectomy (PTK) followed by partial topography-guided photorefractive keratectomy (PRK) and CXL. The reasoning behind AP lies in an attempt of vision function amelioration before corneal stabilization with CXL [6]. Furthermore, to avoid possible complications in eyes with low corneal thickness, another procedure protocol was introduced as the safe and effective Cretan protocol (CP). Cretan protocol manages KC performing transepithelial phototherapeutic keratectomy (PTK) followed by CXL, which has proved to be especially beneficial in cases where PRK procedure is contraindicated [7].

2. Case Presentation

A 29-year-old male presented with progressive ambilateral visual blur over the course of the past decade with exacerbation of vision loss on the left eye following a car accident in August 2020. In 2014, the uncorrected visual acuity (UDVA) was 0.2 OD and 0.4 OS. The patient underwent CXL of the right eye in 2015 and was eventually advised to perform CXL of the left eye in another ophthalmological center and thenceforth asked for second opinion. Physical exam performed in October 2020 showed UDVA of 0.2 OD and 0.1 OS. Patient's best spectacle-corrected distance visual acuity (BCVA) was measured 0.4 with a refraction of -3.00 D in the right eye and OS of 0.5 with $-3.50 - 1.50 \times 90$ in the left eye. Presence of any apparent ocular injuries was not confirmed. Pachymetry in pupil center projection preoperative was 526 μm OD and 482 μm OS. Curvature maps (Allegro Oculyzer, Alcon Laboratories Inc., Fort Worth, Texas, USA) of the left eye showed prominent inferolateral corneal protrusion (Figure 1(a)) confirming keratoconus. Central meridional 7 mm keratometric readings showed 49.6 D × 88.8 and 50.9 D × 178.8 in the left eye.

The patient underwent inferotemporal decentered customized sphero-cylindrical (DISC) ablation and crosslinking

Table 1: Fourier's analysis and Zernike analysis.

(a)

	Fourier's analysis		
	Preoperative	2 months postoperative	17 months postoperative
Irregularity	0.119	0.085	0.044

(b)

		Zernike analysis		
		Preoperative	2 months postoperative	17 months postoperative
Z_4^0	Spheric aberration	0.08	-0.062	0.05
Z_3^1	Koma 0°	-0.3	0.246	-0.082

Table 2: Preoperative and postoperative values of corneal indices in 8 mm zone of the left eye.

	Indices (in 8 mm zone)		
	Preoperative	2 months postoperative	17 months postoperative
IHD	0.119	0.085	0.044
ISV	88	71	49
IVA	0.89	0.72	0.47

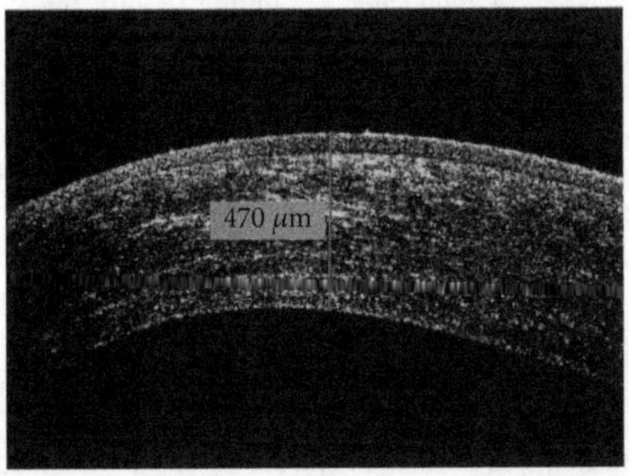

Figure 3: AS-OCT of keratoconus eye 17 months after DISC ablation and corneal crosslinking radiating with UV-A at 3 mW/cm^2.

of the left eye with riboflavin 0.1% without dextran with methylcellulose (Medio CROSS – M, Avedro). After administration of 0.4% oxybuprocaine hydrochloride eye drops as a topical anesthetic, the patient was subjected to phototherapeutic keratectomy (PTK) laser ablation of the central 7.0 mm optical zone with 50 μm depth of epithelial ablation. DISC ablation was then followed, targeting 70% of the total spherocylindrical diopter, aiming for the position 1 mm inferior and 500 μm temporal, and approximately 38% of the abnormal corneal apex distance from the pupil center which was located 3.1 mm inferior and 1.6 mm temporal from the pupil center. Excimer laser used for performing PTK and DISC ablation was Alcon/WaveLight Allegretto Eye-Q 400 Hz Excimer Laser platform (Alcon Laboratories, Ft Worth, Texas).

Decentration was performed by entering decentration laser mode which can be accessed by pressing the Set Up Key located at the Control Unit For Allegretto Eye-Q. By each joystick, movement in desired direction laser beam is decentralized for 10 micrometers. The final position of laser beam is confirmed by double pressing the OK Key which is also located at the Control Unit For Allegretto Eye-Q. Laser ablation is controlled by the Excamer Laser Eye Tracking Camera and three infrared light beams help with continuous illumination of the operating area.

Minimal remaining corneal thickness was preset to be 450 μm. To avoid the possible outcome of corneal haze, 0.02% mitomycin C (MMC) was applied to the stromal surface for 40 seconds. Riboflavin 0.1% solution was then administered topically every 2 minutes for a 30-minute period followed by a 5-cycle irradiation with a duration of 5 minutes (25 minutes in total) consisting of CXL (CSO VEGA CMB X Linker, Florence, Italy) application of UVA 370 nm at 3.0 mW/cm^2 irradiance intensity. Combined antibiotic therapy of tobramycin qid along with lubrication was included in the postoperative regimen until epithelial restoration. Dexamethasone qid was then prescribed with weekly tapering. At 2 months postoperatively, the topography showed stable results (Figure 1(b)), and UDVA was improved to 0.7 along with insignificant corneal haze on biomicroscopy. Furthermore, 17 months postoperative, there was an additional improvement in visual acuity which reached values of UDVA 0.9, with CDVA (-1.0 D) of 1.0. During the follow-up time, visual acuity of the right eye remained unchanged.

3. Discussion

The procedure that was performed in the patient's left eye was the ablation of the corneal steepening region located 1 mm inferior and 500 μm temporal from the pupil center toward the corneal apex. Such action was inspired as the patient reported for this head position adjustment to provide him better spectacle corrected vision during the examination preoperatively. The average OCT measured corneal epithelium thickness was 43.8 μm preoperatively (Figure 2), which is why a 50 μm PTK epithelium ablation was performed, removing the corneal epithelium along with some additional stromal tissue. The reasoning behind such an attempt was the previously reported PTK-related primary regularization leading to additional amelioration of visual acuity [7]. Minimal remaining corneal thickness was 450 μm after ablation. The full removal of diopters was avoided to increase safety and prevent greater result unpredictability. Another reason for refraining from such action was the expected impact of CXL on the additional corneal curvature increments over time [8].

Surprisingly, performed surgery including DISC ablation as the main part resulted in the patient's UDVA improvement from 0.1 preoperatively to 0.7 two months postoperatively and to 0.9 seventeen months after procedure. Compared to the previously treated right eye solely with CXL, which has only shown a prevention of visual deterioration and stagnant UDVA of 0.2, the results following this case report might imply promising aspects of this procedure for possible future KC treatment.

To illustrate the exact level of impact of this procedure on corneal regularization, Zernike and Fourier's analyses were conducted. Obtained pre- and postoperative data from Allegro Oculyzer revealed a significant drop of spherical aberration and amelioration of comatic aberrations in the left eye postoperatively. Results of Fourier's analysis imply a drop of irregularity (-28.6% two months and –63% seventeen months postoperative) (Table 1).

Such amelioration is accompanied by objective indicators such as corneal indices at central 8 mm corneal zone. The cornea had become more regular by the values of the corneal indices. Index of Surface Variance (ISV) is a value of curvature variation from the mean curvature, Index of Vertical Assimetry (IVA) is a value of curvature symmetry comparison of the upper and lower area, and Index of Height Decentration (IHD) is a value of the decentration of height data in vertical direction [9]. All of the 3 mentioned indexes had decreased 2 and especially 17 months postoperative compared to the preoperative values (Table 2).

Moreover, formation of demarcation line (DL), a transition zone between the crosslinked anterior and the untreated posterior corneal stroma, was present on anterior segment optical coherence tomography (AS-OCT) image 17 months after surgical procedure (Figure 3). Such formation presents an increase of the biomechanical efficacy and improvement in corneal strength after CXL performed [10].

Given all the above, especially the significant enhanced refractive effect and the evident corneal regularization after a follow-up period of 17 months after surgery, DISK ablation led to excellent results and outstanding satisfaction in the presented cases. Because CXL was performed on the right eye and DISC ablation on the left eye, this patient had the opportunity to compare the effect of two different surgical techniques on the quality of visual acuity and overall satisfaction.

4. Conclusion

This paper introduces a novel technique which might be a promising method in halting keratoconus progression as well as retrieving certain amounts of lost visual ability. Further research should be conducted for procedural optimization and better understanding of the underlying mechanisms.

References

[1] M. Romero-Jiménez, J. Santodomingo-Rubido, and J. S. Wolffsohn, "Keratoconus: a review," *Contact Lens & Anterior Eye*, vol. 33, no. 4, pp. 157–166, 2010.

[2] A. C. Ferdi, V. Nguyen, D. M. Gore, B. D. Allan, J. J. Rozema, and S. L. Watson, "Keratoconus natural progression: a systematic review and meta-analysis of 11 529 eyes," *Ophthalmology*, vol. 126, no. 7, pp. 935–945, 2019.

[3] H. Hashemi, S. Heydarian, E. Hooshmand et al., "The prevalence and risk factors for keratoconus: a systematic review and meta-analysis," *Cornea*, vol. 39, no. 2, pp. 263–270, 2020.

[4] E. Loukovitis, N. Kozeis, Z. Gatzioufas et al., "The proteins of keratoconus: a literature review exploring their contribution to the pathophysiology of the disease," *Advances in Therapy*, vol. 36, no. 9, pp. 2205–2222, 2019.

[5] K. A. Beckman, P. K. Gupta, M. Farid et al., "Corneal cross linking: current protocols and clinical approach," *Journal of Cataract & Refractive Surgery*, vol. 45, no. 11, pp. 1670–1679, 2019.

[6] A. J. Kanellopoulos, "The impact of keratoconus treatment with the Athens protocol (partial topography-guided photorefractive keratectomy combined with higher-fluence corneal collagen cross-linking) on quality of life: a long-term study," *Clinical Ophthalmology*, vol. Volume 13, pp. 795–803, 2019.

[7] G. D. Kymionis, M. A. Grentzelos, V. P. Kankariya et al., "Long-term results of combined transepithelial phototherapeutic keratectomy and corneal collagen cross linking for keratoconus: Cretan protocol," *Journal of Cataract & Refractive Surgery*, vol. 40, no. 9, pp. 1439–1445, 2014.

[8] N. Singal, S. Ong Tone, R. Stein et al., "Comparison of accelerated CXL alone, accelerated CXL-ICRS, and accelerated CXL-TG-PRK in progressive keratoconus and other corneal ectasias," *Journal of Cataract and Refractive Surgery*, vol. 46, no. 2, pp. 276–286, 2020.

[9] H. Hashemi, R. Pakzad, S. Heydarian et al., "Keratoconus indices and their determinants in healthy eyes of a rural population," *Journal of Current Ophthalmology*, vol. 32, no. 4, pp. 343–348, 2020.

[10] N. Pircher, J. Lammer, S. Holzer et al., "Correlation between central stromal demarcation line depth and changes in K values after corneal cross-linking (CXL)," *Graefe's Archive for Clinical and Experimental Ophthalmology*, vol. 256, no. 4, pp. 759–764, 2018.

Central Retinal Artery Occlusion Associated with Sildenafil Overdose

Mojtaba Abrishami,[1] Seyedeh Maryam Hosseini,[1] Hamid Mohseni,[1] Majid Razavi,[2] Amir Ghaffarian Mashhadi Nejad,[1] Mohammad Baghi Yazdi,[1] and Ghodsieh Zamani[1]

[1]*Eye Research Center, Mashhad University of Medical Sciences, Mashhad, Iran*
[2]*Department of Anesthesiology, School of Medicine, Mashhad University of Medical Sciences, Mashhad, Iran*

Correspondence should be addressed to Ghodsieh Zamani; zamanigh@mums.ac.ir

Academic Editor: Claudio Campa

Background. To report a patient with central retinal artery occlusion (CRAO) associated with sildenafil overdose. *Case Presentation.* A forty-two-year-old male presented three hours after sudden painless visual loss in the right eye. BCVA was counting finger in two meters, and relative afferent pupillary defect was positive. Fundus examination revealed retinal whiteness except in a limited area of papillomacular bundle and cherry red spot. He consumed two 100 mg film-coated sildenafil tablet (Vizarsin, Krka, d.d., Novo mesto, Slovenia) twelve hours apart, and the last one was six hours before visual loss. He was diagnosed with CRAO with cilioretinal artery sparing. Although we did not find any emboli, anterior chamber paracentesis was done. Four weeks later, BCVA improved to 20/80, with resolving of retinal edema. Cardiovascular, carotid arteries, and neurologic evaluations were negative for any predisposing factor. *Conclusion.* CRAO is a vision threatening condition that might be associated with the overdose of sildenafil.

1. Background

Sildenafil is a selective phosphodiesterase (PDE) type 5 inhibitor. It usually acts via regulation of vascular tone and relaxing vascular musculature [1]. By increasing the nitric oxide/cyclic guanosine monophosphate pathway, it is helpful in treating erectile dysfunction and pulmonary arterial hypertension [2]. The most common adverse events reported by patients using sildenafil have been mild to moderate transient headache, facial flushing, rhinitis, dyspepsia, and abnormal vision, usually bluish discoloration and impaired blue/green discrimination [3].

Central retinal artery occlusion (CRAO), as an ophthalmic emergency, is an ocular analogue of cerebral stroke. CRAO is considered as an end-organ ischemia and often associated with underlying atherosclerotic diseases [4]. Here, we present an otherwise healthy young man presented CRAO with cilioretinal artery sparing, who overdosed sildenafil with total 200 mg consumption in twelve hours.

2. Case Presentation

A forty-two-year-old man presented with a sudden painless loss of vision in the right eye since three hours ago. Visual acuity was decreased to counting finger in two meters in the right eye with relative afferent pupillary defect. Except, a limited area in papillomacular bundle in the area nourished by patent cilioretinal artery, retinal whiteness, and cherry red spot was prominent (Figures 1(a) and 1(b)). Left eye examination revealed mild retinal veins congestion and optic nerve head hyperemia. In the last night, he consumed a 100 mg film-coated sildenafil tablet (Vizarsin, Krka, d. d.,

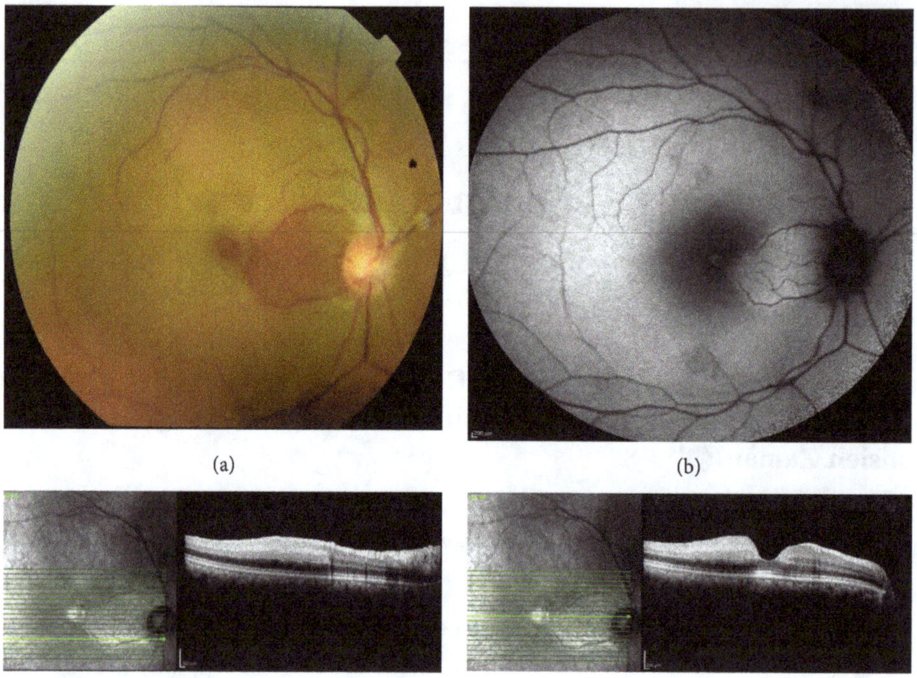

(a) (b) (c) (d)

Figure 1: At the first presentation (a). (b) Color fundus and red free photographs of the right eye: diffuse retinal edema except a limited area in papillomacular bundle (c). (d) SD OCT of the right eye: increased retinal thickness and inner retinal hyperreflectivity in the ischemic areas.

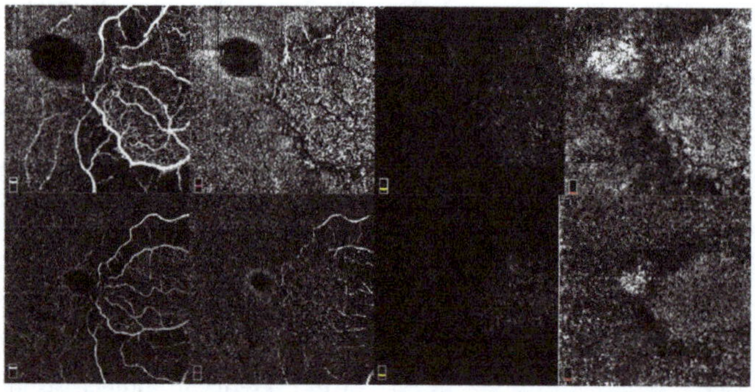

Figure 2: OCT-A of the right eye at first presentation shows no flow in superficial and deep retinal capillary plexuses microvasculature. Only the flow in cilioretinal artery is visible.

Novo mesto, Slovenia), and twelve hours later, he took another one. The last one was used six hours before visual loss. He was diagnosed with CRAO with cilioretinal artery sparing. After describing the nature of the arterial occlusion for the patient and low chance for vision recovery, although we did not find any emboli in examination, anterior chamber paracentesis was done. Unfortunately, this immediate measures taken to restore the circulation proved futile. In spectral domain optical coherence tomography (SD-OCT), inner retinal hyperreflectivity was obvious (Figures 1(c) and 1(d)) and in optical coherence tomography angiography (OCTA), both superficial and deep capillary retinal plexuses microvasculature were depleted and rendered no flow (Figure 2).

Four weeks later, resolving of retinal edema was obvious in fundus examination of the right eye, and BCVA improved to 20/60 with right head turn. In evaluation for systemic vasculitis and other rheumatologic diseases, cardiologic evaluation for cardiac or carotid vessels pathologies, and neurologic imaging, the patient was found to be healthy. He declared that he had been consuming sildenafil tablets in different doses for the past five years. In the last three years, he consumed Vizarsin 100 mg film-coated tablets, but has never taken two tablets in a short interval.

3. Discussion and Conclusion

Here, we report a patient who suffered from sudden and severe vision loss because of CRAO with a recent history of consumption of two 100 mg sildenafil tablets 12 hours apart. He was otherwise healthy and had history of sildenafil consumption for five years, but in this episode, he consumed a high dose of the medication.

Various ocular side effects have been described following the use of sildenafil. These fall into two major categories: (1) those secondary to the weak inhibitory effects of sildenafil on the isoenzyme PDE in the retina such as temporary loss of vision, green/blue tinging of vision, increased sensitivity to light, and blurred vision [5]. These symptoms are mild, dose-dependent, and completely reversible and occur in 3–11% of men taking sildenafil 25–100 mg [6]. (2) Those secondary to vascular events includes anterior ischemic optic neuropathy [7–9], cilioretinal artery occlusion [10], branch retinal artery occlusion [5], central retinal vein occlusion [11], and acute macular neuroretinopathy [12].

Murthy [13] reported a 37-year-old African American woman with a known history of sickle cell anemia and pulmonary arterial hypertension who was receiving treatment with tadalafil, a PDE5 inhibitor, developed bilateral, concurrent CRAO that persisted after exchange transfusion.

Previous studies regarding the sildenafil effect on ocular blood flow have reported inconsistent results. Most of them showed increased choroidal blood flow (CBF) with a lesser effect on the retinal vasculature. This difference may be due to discrepancy in vascular innervation. In this respect, the innervation of the choriocapillaris resembles that of the corpus cavernosum. Theoretically, because sildenafil has a strong systemic vasodilating effect that decreases systemic blood pressure, it can result in decreased CBF. Different balances of these factors among individuals can lead to variable effects on ocular blood flow [14]. In contrast to increased blood flow as a result of vasodilation by the smooth muscle relaxant effects, thrombus formation can have impaired blood flow in the vessel. Vascular insufficiency and stasis are major factors causing the initial formation and progression of thrombosis. High concentrations of cyclic guanosine monophosphate induced by the long-term use of sildenafil are known to mediate the changes in endothelial permeability and finally promote platelet adhesion and enhance thrombus formation [15].

In our case, a patient with a history of sildenafil consumption for years, he had taken two 100 mg sildenafil tablets twelve hours apart, while the standard recommended doses of sildenafil range from 25 to 100 mg three times weekly [14]. The peak plasma level after oral intake occurs at about 60 min with an elimination half-life of 3–5 h [14]. Although the occurrence of CRAO in our patient after sildenafil use may be coincidental, a possible association should not be overlooked. In this case, it seems to be a dose-response and temporal relationship between the sildenafil and the side effect, CRAO, in terms of occurrence within a reasonable amount of time after high dose drug ingestion. Although it cannot be explicitly proven that sildenafil was the cause of CRAO in this patient as other factors could also have been involved in CRAO, the close temporal relationship strongly suggests this.

Our hypotheses for mechanisms that may contribute to the CRAO in this patient include (1) a thrombotic event in artery due to enhanced platelet adhesion as a consequence of long-term sildenafil use or (2) the compressive effect of dilated vein on artery leading to decreased arterial blood flow. At the first presentation, we noted mild retinal veins congestion and optic nerve head hyperemia in the left eye. Such an event may have happened in the right eye and eventually led to CRAO.

CRAO as a sight threatening condition may be a complication associated with the use of sildenafil. Physicians should be aware of this side effect and should seek other alternatives in patients with high risk of developing CRAO. The patients using sildenafil should closely collaborate with the ophthalmologist and appeal to them when any visual symptom is experienced.

Abbreviations

PDE: Phosphodiesterase
CRAO: Central retinal artery occlusion
BCVA: Best corrected visual acuity
EDI-OCT: Enhanced depth imaging optical coherent tomography
SD-OCT: Spectral domain optical coherent tomography
CBF: Choroidal blood flow
DCP: Deep capillary plexus
SDP: Superficial capillary plexus.

Consent

Written consent for images and data publication and identifying clinical details was obtained from the patient.

Authors' Contributions

All the authors contributed significantly to this report, and all authors agree to be accountable for all aspects of the work. All authors have read and approved the manuscript.

References

[1] P. Krishnappa, E. Fernandez-Pascual, J. Carballido, and J. I. Martinez-Salamanca, "Sildenafil/Viagra in the treatment of premature ejaculation," *International Journal of Impotence Research*, vol. 31, no. 2, pp. 65–70, 2019.

[2] I. A. Abdel-Hamid, E. A. Jannini, and K. E. Andersson, "Premature ejaculation: focus on therapeutic targets," *Expert Opinion on Therapeutic Targets*, vol. 13, no. 2, pp. 175–193, 2009.

[3] A. Laties and I. Sharlip, "Ocular safety in patients using sildenafil citrate therapy for erectile dysfunction," *The Journal of Sexual Medicine*, vol. 3, no. 1, pp. 12–27, 2006.

[4] D. D. Varma, S. Cugati, A. W. Lee, and C. S. Chen, "A review of central retinal artery occlusion: clinical presentation and

management," *Eye (London, England)*, vol. 27, no. 6, pp. 688–697, 2013.

[5] A. Tripathi and N. P. O'Donnell, "Branch retinal artery occlusion; another complication of sildenafil," *The British Journal of Ophthalmology*, vol. 84, no. 8, pp. 934-935, 2000.

[6] F. Azzouni and K. Abu samra, "Are Phosphodiesterase Type 5 Inhibitors Associated with Vision-Threatening Adverse Events? A Critical Analysis and Review of the Literature," *The Journal of Sexual Medicine*, vol. 8, no. 10, pp. 2894–2903, 2011.

[7] A. J. Bella, W. O. Brant, T. F. Lue, and G. B. Brock, "Non-arteritic ischemic optic neuropathy and phosphodiesterase type 5 inhibitors," *The Canadian Journal of Urology*, vol. 13, pp. 3233–3236, 2006.

[8] M. J. Thurtell and R. L. Tomsak, "Nonarteritic anterior ischemic optic neuropathy with PDE-5 inhibitors for erectile dysfunction," *International Journal of Impotence Research*, vol. 20, no. 6, pp. 537–543, 2008.

[9] L. Gorkin, K. Hvidsten, R. E. Sobel, and R. Siegel, "Sildenafil citrate use and the incidence of nonarteritic anterior ischemic optic neuropathy," *International Journal of Clinical Practice*, vol. 60, no. 4, pp. 500–503, 2006.

[10] R. Akash, D. Hrishikesh, P. Amith, and S. Sabah, "Case Report:Association of combined Nonarteritic Anterior ischemic optic neuropathy (NAION) and obstruction of cilioretinal artery with overdose of Viagra®," *Journal of Ocular Pharmacology and Therapeutics*, vol. 21, no. 4, pp. 315–317, 2005.

[11] S. Gedik, G. Yilmaz, and Y. A. Akova, "Sildenafil-associated consecutive nonarteritic anterior ischaemic optic neuropathy, cilioretinal artery occlusion, and central retinal vein occlusion in a haemodialysis patient," *Eye*, vol. 21, no. 1, pp. 129-130, 2007.

[12] A. Kolomeyer and B. Kim, "High-Dose Sildenafil-associated Acute Macular Neuroretinopathy Variant," *Ophthalmology Retina*, vol. 2, no. 7, p. 711, 2018.

[13] R. Murthy, L. Perez, J. Priluck, S. Grover, and K. Chalam, "Acute, bilateral, concurrent central retinal artery occlusion in sickle cell disease after use of tadalafil (Cialis)," *JAMA Ophthalmology*, vol. 131, no. 11, pp. 1471–1473, 2013.

[14] N. F. Santas da Cruz, M. U. Polizelli, L. M. Cezar et al., "Effects of phosphodiesterase type 5 inhibitors on choroid and ocular vasculature: a literature review," *International Journal of Retina and Vitreous*, vol. 6, no. 1, 2020.

[15] Y. Ramot, A. Nyska, and G. Spectre, "Drug-induced thrombosis: an update," *Drug Safety*, vol. 36, no. 8, pp. 585–603, 2013.

15

Acute Anterior Uveitis with HLA-B27 Positivity after Corneal Cross-Linking with Previous Intrastromal Corneal Ring Segment

Asher Khan[1,2] **Charles D. McGuffey**[1] **Andrew T. Melson**[1] **and Kamran M. Riaz**[1]

[1]*Dean McGee Eye Institute, 608 Stanton L. Young Blvd, Oklahoma City, OK 73104, USA*
[2]*College of Medicine, University of Oklahoma, 800 Stanton L. Young Blvd, Oklahoma City, OK 73117, USA*

Correspondence should be addressed to Kamran M. Riaz; kamran-riaz@dmei.org

Academic Editor: Hsin Yi Chen

Purpose. To describe a case of acute anterior uveitis (AAU) with HLA-B27 positivity following epithelium-off corneal cross-linking (CXL) in a patient with a previous intrastromal corneal ring segment. *Observations.* A 28-year-old male with keratoconus (KCN) developed ophthalmalgia, perilimbal injection, hypopyon, and decline in corrected distance visual acuity (CDVA) 3 days after CXL. A working diagnosis of inflammatory versus infectious AAU was made, and the patient was treated with topical tobramycin, polymyxin B/trimethoprim, prednisolone, and oral valacyclovir. Clinical appearance and CDVA improved, ultimately returning to baseline by two weeks postoperatively. Diagnostic laboratory workup revealed HLA-B27 positivity. *Conclusions and Importance.* A comprehensive laboratory workup is helpful to identify potential causative and associated systemic conditions when encountering AAU after CXL. Given the overlap in patient demographics for KCN and HLA-B27 positivity, clinicians should consider this entity in the differential diagnosis and treatment of such cases.

1. Introduction

Acute anterior uveitis (AAU) is a type of intraocular inflammation of the iris and/or ciliary body, defined by the presence of cells or cellular aggregates in the anterior chamber. AAU may be primary or secondary to a variety of etiologies, including infectious, noninfectious, and masquerade diseases. AAU has a well-recognized association with HLA-B27, an antigen located on the surface of white blood cells, especially in young- to middle-aged males [1].

Several treatment options exist for the treatment of mild-moderate keratoconus (KCN). Intrastromal corneal ring segments (ICRS) are small, crescent-shaped polymethylmethacrylate rings placed in the deep, peripheral corneal stroma to flatten the cornea and decrease refractive error in ectatic corneas [2]. Corneal cross-linking (CXL) involves treatment of the cornea with riboflavin followed by photoactivation with UVA light, leading to corneal strengthening. CXL can be performed with or without removing the corneal epithelium. The former technique is well-documented in the literature as a protocol to halt the progression of KCN and is the only technique approved for on-label CXL use in the United States at this time [3]. While a number of noninfectious complications can occur after CXL, post-CXL AAU has been reported only twice before in the literature: once in association with X-linked chronic granulomatous disease (CGD) and once following a combined CXL/ICRS procedure [4, 5].

We present a case of post-CXL AAU in a KCN patient with preexisting ICRS wherein laboratory testing revealed HLA-B27 positivity without previous diagnosis or systemic pathology. Although our patient's condition resolved with treatment, we bring special attention to post-CXL AAU as a clinical finding that merits comprehensive laboratory testing for appropriate diagnosis and long-term management.

2. Case Report

A 28-year-old white male with moderate KCN had previously undergone epithelium-off CXL of the right eye approximately 8 years prior with an unremarkable postoperative course. At our institution, the patient underwent ICRS placement (Intacs-Addition Technology, Inc., Sunnyvale, CA, USA) in the left eye 8 months prior with an unremarkable postoperative course. Besides KCN, the patient had no significant ocular history, ocular surgery history, medical history, family history, social history, or medication use. The patient's last known refraction in the left eye prior to CXL was −11.50 + 0.75 × 15 with a corrected distance visual acuity (CDVA) of 20/40. A diagnosis of progressive KCN was made based on serial tomography measurements demonstrating approximately 1.8 D worsening of maximum keratometry (KMax) over the past eight months. The ultrasonic pachymetry at this time was 459 μm.

The patient subsequently underwent epithelium-off (Dresden protocol) CXL in the left eye (OS). Postoperatively, a bandage contact lens (BCL; AirOptix Night and Day, BC 8.4, diameter 13.8; Alcon Laboratories, Fort Worth, TX, USA) was placed, and the patient was instructed to use topical moxifloxacin 4 times daily with postoperative follow-up five days later. Three days later (two days before the scheduled follow-up visit), the patient presented with significant ophthalmalgia, perilimbal injection, hypopyon, and a decline in corrected distance visual acuity (CDVA).

At presentation, CDVA was 20/1000 OS. Pupils were equally reactive in both eyes with no relative afferent pupillary defect. Intraocular pressure measured 6 mmHg and ultrasound pachymetry measured 401 μm OS. Slit-lamp exam of the left eye revealed 2+ perilimbal injection and a well-placed ICRS without extrusion or epithelial defect. Notably, there was no corneal infiltrate appreciated on exam. Anterior chamber exam was notable for 2+ cells and a 1-1.5 mm inferior hypopyon (Figure 1). Anterior segment exam of the right eye and dilated fundus exam of both eyes were without evidence of intraocular inflammation.

The patient denied any previous history of intraocular inflammation, infectious keratitis, or receiving any vaccine (including recent influenza or COVID-19 vaccination) within the month leading up to symptoms but did endorse a remote history of occasional cold sores around the mouth and nose. Anterior chamber paracentesis was offered at this time, but the patient declined this invasive procedure. A working diagnosis of inflammatory versus infectious AAU was made, and the patient was started on topical tobramycin 0.3%, polymyxin B/trimethoprim, prednisolone acetate 1%, and oral valacyclovir 1 gram, all to be taken three times daily. As there were no overt signs of corneal infection such as corneal ulcer, epithelial defect, or infiltrate, corneal cultures were not obtained with consideration to avoid violation of the corneal epithelium. The patient tolerated this medication regimen without any adverse effects. Three days later, CDVA improved to 20/60, and regression of the hypopyon and perilimbal injection was noted (Figure 2). Tobramycin was discontinued, polymyxin B/trimethoprim and valacyclovir were continued, and prednisolone was increased to 6 times daily. At postoperative week 2, intraocular pressure measured 6 mmHg OS, and the ophthalmalgia, hypopyon, and perilimbal injection had completely resolved. Consequently, topical antibiotics were stopped, a prednisolone taper was initiated, and valacyclovir was reduced to once every other day dosing. All medications were stopped by three months postoperatively. No recurrences of AAU were noted over the next 6 months. Tomography imaging of the left eye revealed stability of KCN before and after CXL at the last follow-up (Figure 3).

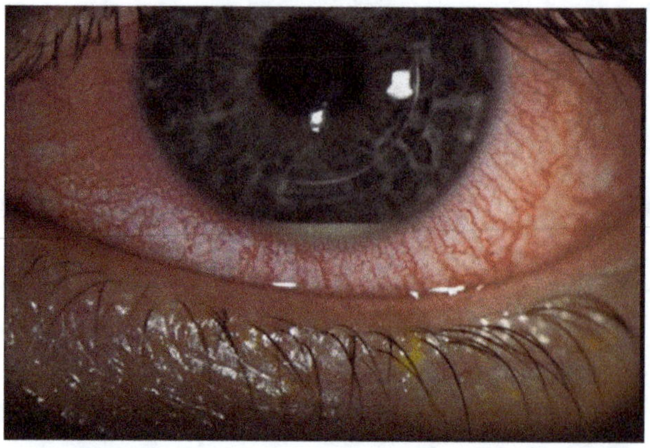

FIGURE 1: Slit beam photograph of the left eye. This photograph demonstrates 2+ perilimbal injection and 1-1.5 mm inferior hypopyon observed at the time of initial presentation. There is no overlying epithelial defect or appreciable infiltrate in the cornea. Both intrastromal corneal ring segments are in place.

Due to the unexpected AAU after CXL, the patient underwent comprehensive laboratory testing (Appendix) on the postoperative day three visit. All were normal besides HLA-B27, which was positive. Notably, the patient denied any previous history of extraocular inflammatory symptoms commonly associated with HLA-B27 positivity, including low back pain, arthritis, urethritis, and gastrointestinal changes [6]. The patient was educated on the systemic significance of the diagnosis, informed about the need for continued KCN monitoring, and subsequently referred to his primary care physician and a rheumatologist for continuity of care.

3. Discussion

While AAU can be secondary to several different etiologies, it has a well-established association with HLA-B27, especially in young white males [1]. Inclusive of all causes, AAU remains a relatively rare event after CXL. A previous study found that out of 153 eyes that underwent epithelium-off CXL, only 1.9% developed AAU during the first 3 postoperative months, though none of the patients had an ocular or systemic etiology typically associated with uveitis [7].

The use of topical steroids after CXL is a matter of debate. While many surgeons routinely employ topical steroids to control postoperative inflammation, a recent systematic review reported that a combination of steroids and bandage contact lenses postoperatively is associated with infectious keratitis after CXL [8]. The treating surgeon's (KMR) protocol is to only use topical antibiotics after CXL with BCL placement, and patients start topical steroids on the postoperative day 5-7 visit, after BCL removal and confirmation of epithelialization. It is plausible that the lack of topical steroids immediately after CXL contributed significantly to the development of AAU.

HLA-B27-associated AAU typically affects young males and may be associated with extraocular inflammatory disease [1, 9]. Our patient's AAU presentation was characteristic since there was an acute onset of blurred vision, ocular redness, pain, and hypopyon. This last finding is significant

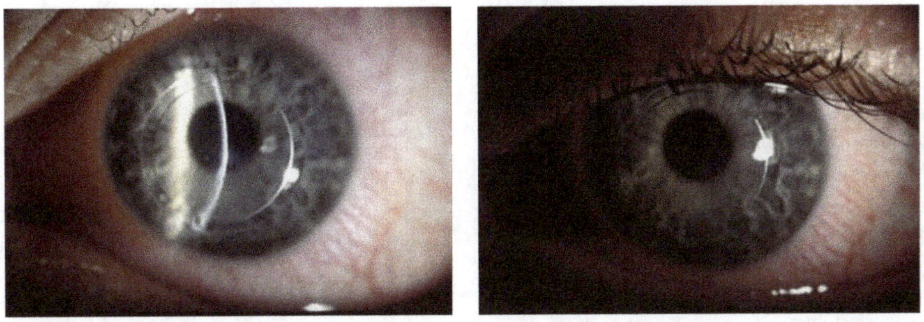

(a) (b)

FIGURE 2: Slit beam (a) and broad beam (b) photographs of the left eye. These photographs demonstrate regression of the perilimbal injection and inferior hypopyon observed in Figure 1.

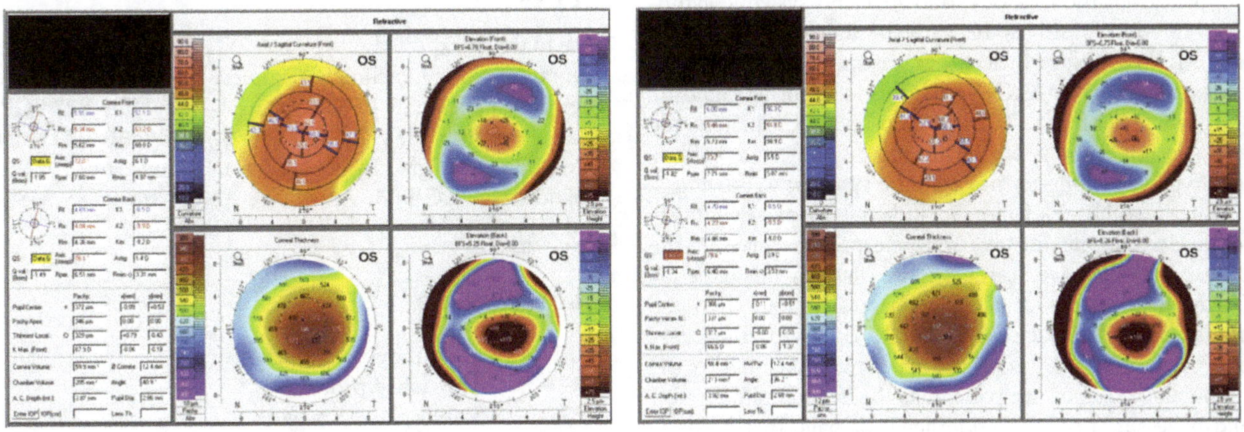

(a) (b)

FIGURE 3: Tomography images of the left eye before (a) and after (b) cross-linking at the last follow-up 6 months postoperatively demonstrate the stability of keratoconus over the time course from before and after surgery.

as hypopyon rarely develops in the context of noninfectious uveitic etiologies with a notable exception of HLA-B27, Behcet's disease, or drug use [10]. Furthermore, the patient's symptoms were unilateral and lasted for a limited duration, both additional typical characteristics of HLA-B27-associated AAU [11]. Treatment strategies for HLA-B27-associated AAU most frequently involve topical corticosteroids, with or without topical anticholinergic agents, which are slowly tapered over 8-10 weeks [1, 9, 11].

Several lessons may be of interest from our case. First, our case adds unique knowledge to the literature as it reports HLA-B27 positivity in laboratory workup for AAU after CXL in a patient without prior systemic disease and with preexisting ICRS. Our search protocol consisted of a PubMed search without any filters, using the search terms "uveitis", "crosslinking", "HLA-B27", and "keratoconus." Second, we note that for patients presenting with unexpected intraocular inflammation after CXL, a thorough laboratory workup may be of significant utility in identifying common etiologies of AAU, including HLA-B27 positivity. We emphasize that such cases should not be presumed as idiopathic. Diagnostic testing, while seemingly cumbersome and expensive, can assist clinicians to identify associated etiology and prompt appropriate systemic evaluation. A multidisciplinary approach may be needed to manage both ocular and systemic pathology in such cases, especially if the causative etiology is known to cause significant morbidity.

Previous authors have reported AAU following CXL, but in one report, the AAU was thought to be attributable to X-linked CGD [4]. In the other report, the patient developed AAU after a simultaneous CXL/ICRS procedure, thought to be due to a combination of the patient self-replacing the BCL, sterile corneal epithelial defect, and inflammation secondary to free radical formation by riboflavin [5]. The authors did not report any systemic causes or positive diagnostic testing and attributed the anterior chamber inflammation to be similar to sterile anterior chamber reaction after laser refractive surgery. In our case, since there was no known history of systemic autoimmune disease and the ICRS was preexisting, we suspect that the postsurgical inflammatory state exacerbated a relatively dormant hyperimmune state that led to the AAU episode. While CXL is not an intraocular procedure, there are numerous aspects of the procedure that may incite ocular inflammation, such as potential free radical damage by riboflavin and mechanical damage from epithelial removal upregulating ocular surface inflammation [12].

Although our patient underwent CXL of the right eye approximately 8 years prior at a different institution, there were no postoperative uveitic changes observed at that time. Since the CXL in both eyes was performed using the same protocol (Dresden protocol), it is unlikely that differences between the surgeries, such as different institutions or surgeons, account for the dissimilarity in postoperative courses. Instead, one variable that changed between the surgeries and may help explain the different outcomes is the patient's age. Other authors have reported the average age of onset for HLA-B27-positive ankylosing spondylitis (AS) in males as 25.7 years [13]. Since our patient was 20 years old at the time of the first CXL and 28 years old at the time of the second CXL, we postulate that the patient may have been more prone to developing uveitic changes associated with HLA-B27 positivity. However, we acknowledge that this is a tenuous explanation at best, and it remains unclear as to why AAU did not develop in the first eye after CXL. Furthermore, given the lack of extraocular and systemic symptoms, HLA-B27 positivity may not be the sole etiology for post-CXL AAU. Nevertheless, our case sheds light on how the appearance of post-CXL AAU led us to perform diagnostic testing which confirmed HLA-B27 positivity. Ultimately, the diagnostic implications are of the most significance as they relate to patients' long-term ocular and systemic well-being.

Other possible risk factors include the use of a BCL postoperatively. Despite the relatively steep base curve of the BCL used, it may have been too loose (flat) for this patient's KCN cornea, further causing mechanical irritation to the denuded corneal surface. Additionally, corneal trauma sustained from the CXL procedure itself may have led to the inflammation seen in our patient, as the irradiance delivered could have surpassed the endothelial damage threshold [5, 12, 14].

In both cases of AAU following CXL in the existing literature, corneal specimens were sent for gram stain, bacterial culture, and herpes simplex virus polymerase chain reaction, with all tests yielding negative results in both patients [4, 5]. Other authors have reported that herpetic keratitis reactivation can occur after CXL, and given our patient's remote history of cold sores, we chose to treat with oral valacyclovir empirically [15, 16]. As there were no corneal exam findings to suggest an infectious etiology, corneal scraping and/or an anterior chamber tap were deferred. Instead, we based our management on the clinical exam findings and laboratory workup as detailed in the Appendix. Clinicians may want to modify or expand this workup to include invasive testing in recalcitrant cases to rule out atypical or infectious causes of AAU.

Patients diagnosed with HLA-B27-associated AAU carry an almost sevenfold increased relative risk of concomitant AS [9]. Interestingly, the demographic predilection of both KCN and AS involves a similar cohort of patients, namely, young males. While previous views held that KCN is primarily a noninflammatory disease, there is increasing evidence to confirm the role of ocular and systemic inflammation in its pathogenesis and progression [17]. Prior studies emphasize additional overlap between KCN and AS by depicting how AS induces corneal biomechanical changes similar to those seen in KCN, characterized by decreases in corneal thickness, stiffness, and hysteresis [14, 18, 19]. This knowledge may allow providers to consider appropriate coinvolvement of corneal, uveitis, and systemic specialists when clinical and laboratory findings are present.

4. Conclusions

AAU is a complication that clinicians should be aware of when performing CXL. A thorough ocular and systemic history should be obtained before CXL. If clinicians observe AAU postoperatively, the intraocular findings should not be simply assumed to be idiopathic or routine postsurgical inflammation. In such cases, a thorough yet tailored laboratory workup should be considered, as it may have implications for the future management of ocular and systemic disease.

Appendix

Due to the unexpected AAU after CXL, the patient underwent laboratory testing, including complete blood count, complete metabolic panel, ESR, CRP, RPR, FTA-ABS, HLA-B27, IGRA, ACE, lysozyme, HSV IgG/IgM, HZV IgG/IgM, CMV IgG/IgM, EBV IgG/IgM, Lyme IgG/IgM, Toxoplasma IgG/IgM, Toxocariasis IgG/IgM, ANA, RF, ANCA titers, SS-A/SS-B, and HIV-1/2.

Abbreviations

ESR: Erythrocyte sedimentation rate
CRP: C-reactive protein
RPR: Rapid plasma reagin
FTA-ABS: Fluorescent treponemal antibody absorption
HLA-B27: Human leukocyte antigen B27 (subtypes B* 2701-2759)
IGRA: Interferon-gamma release assay
ACE: Angiotensin-converting enzyme
IgG/IgM: Immunoglobulin G/M
HSV: Herpes simplex virus
HZV: Herpes zoster virus
CMV: Cytomegalovirus
EBV: Epstein-Barr virus
ANA: Anti-nuclear antibody
RF: Rheumatoid factor
ANCA: Anti-neutrophil cytoplasmic antibody
SS-A: Sjögren's syndrome-related antigen A
SS-B: Sjögren's syndrome type B antigen
HIV: Human immunodeficiency virus.

Consent

The patient consented to the publication of the case in writing. This report does not contain any personal information that could be used to identify the patient.

Disclosure

The funding source had no involvement in the study design, in the collection, analysis, and interpretation of data, in the writing of the report, and in the decision to submit the article for publication.

Authors' Contributions

All authors attest that they meet the current ICMJE criteria for authorship.

Acknowledgments

This research is supported in part by an unrestricted grant from Research to Prevent Blindness.

References

[1] J. H. Chang, P. J. McCluskey, and D. Wakefield, "Acute anterior uveitis and HLA-B27," *Survey of Ophthalmology*, vol. 50, no. 4, pp. 364–388, 2005.

[2] K. Zadnik, S. Money, and K. Lindsley, "Intrastromal corneal ring segments for treating keratoconus," *Cochrane Database of Systematic Reviews*, vol. 2019, no. 5, article CD011150, 2019.

[3] S. Kolli and I. M. Aslanides, "Safety and efficacy of collagen crosslinking for the treatment of keratoconus," *Expert Opinion on Drug Safety*, vol. 9, no. 6, pp. 949–957, 2010.

[4] C. E. Wisely and M. Daluvoy, "Anterior uveitis following collagen crosslinking in a patient with X-linked chronic granulomatous disease," *Canadian Journal of Ophthalmology*, vol. 56, no. 2, pp. e60–e62, 2021.

[5] Y. Goldich, U. Elbaz, and D. S. Rootman, "Anterior uveitis after collagen cross-linking for keratoconus," *International Journal of Keratoconus and Ectatic Corneal Diseases*, vol. 4, no. 3, pp. 110–114, 2015.

[6] P. Parameswaran and M. Lucke, *HLA B27 Syndromes*, StatPearls Publishing, Treasure Island (FL), 2021.

[7] N. Cagil, O. Sarac, H. B. Cakmak, G. Can, and E. Can, "Mechanical epithelial removal followed by corneal collagen crosslinking in progressive keratoconus: short-term complications," *Journal of Cataract and Refractive Surgery*, vol. 41, no. 8, pp. 1730–1737, 2015.

[8] C. E. Murchison, W. M. Petroll, and D. M. Robertson, "Infectious keratitis after corneal crosslinking: systematic review," *Journal of Cataract and Refractive Surgery*, vol. 47, no. 8, pp. 1075–1080, 2021.

[9] E. M. D'Ambrosio, M. La Cava, P. Tortorella, M. Gharbiya, M. Campanella, and L. Iannetti, "Clinical features and complications of the HLA-B27-associated acute anterior uveitis: a metanalysis," *Seminars in Ophthalmology*, vol. 32, no. 6, pp. 689–701, 2017.

[10] A. A. Zaidi, G. S. Ying, E. Daniel et al., "Hypopyon in patients with uveitis," *Ophthalmology*, vol. 117, no. 2, pp. 366–372, 2010.

[11] D. Wakefield, D. Clarke, and P. McCluskey, "Recent developments in HLA B27 anterior uveitis," *Frontiers in Immunology*, vol. 11, article 608134, 2021.

[12] S. Çakmak, M. E. Sucu, Y. Yildirim et al., "Complications of accelerated corneal collagen cross-linking: review of 2025 eyes," *International Ophthalmology*, vol. 40, no. 12, pp. 3269–3277, 2020.

[13] E. Feldtkeller, M. A. Khan, D. van der Heijde, S. van der Linden, and J. Braun, "Age at disease onset and diagnosis delay in HLA-B27 negative vs. positive patients with ankylosing spondylitis," *Rheumatology International*, vol. 23, no. 2, pp. 61–66, 2003.

[14] D. Ozarslan Ozcan, S. C. Ozcan, and G. Kimyon, "Corneal biomechanical parameters in systemic autoimmune diseases," *Clinical & Experimental Optometry*, vol. 105, no. 1, pp. 61–64, 2022.

[15] G. D. Kymionis, D. M. Portaliou, D. I. Bouzoukis et al., "Herpetic keratitis with iritis after corneal crosslinking with riboflavin and ultraviolet A for keratoconus," *Journal of Cataract and Refractive Surgery*, vol. 33, no. 11, pp. 1982–1984, 2007.

[16] A. Al-Qarni and M. AlHarbi, "Herpetic keratitis after corneal collagen cross-linking with riboflavin and ultraviolet-A for keratoconus," *Middle East African Journal of Ophthalmology*, vol. 22, no. 3, pp. 389–392, 2015.

[17] A. Y. Nemet, S. Vinker, I. Bahar, and I. Kaiserman, "The association of keratoconus with immune disorders," *Cornea*, vol. 29, no. 11, pp. 1261–1264, 2010.

[18] M. Caglayan, O. Sarac, P. Kosekahya, S. Erten, B. Ayan, and N. Cagil, "Biomechanical evaluation of cornea in patients with ankylosing spondylitis," *International Ophthalmology*, vol. 37, no. 4, pp. 1017–1024, 2017.

[19] B. M. Fontes, R. Ambrósio Jr., G. C. Velarde, and W. Nosé, "Ocular response analyzer measurements in keratoconus with normal central corneal thickness compared with matched normal control eyes," *Journal of Refractive Surgery*, vol. 27, no. 3, pp. 209–215, 2011.

16

A New Mechanism of Silicone Oil-Induced Glaucoma and its Management

Harsh Kumar,[1] Dinesh Talwar,[2] Mithun Thulasidas,[1] and Surbi Taneja[1]

[1]*Glaucoma Services, Centre for Sight, B-5/24, Safdarjung Enclave, New Delhi, India*
[2]*Vitreoretinal Services, Centre for Sight, B-5/24, Safdarjung Enclave, New Delhi, India*

Correspondence should be addressed to Mithun Thulasidas; mithun.thulasidas@gmail.com

Academic Editor: Sandra M. Johnson

Purpose. To describe a case of secondary acute angle closure glaucoma due to silicone oil migration into the posterior chamber causing entrapment of aqueous and its successful management. *Case Presentation.* A 69-year-old female presented with decreased vision and pain in the left eye (LE) for one month. She had a history of complicated phacoemulsification with nucleus drop and retinal detachment in LE, for which vitreoretinal surgery with silicone oil endotamponade was done. She was also a known case of primary open angle glaucoma on medications. The corrected distance visual acuity was 20/20 and 20/125 in the right eye (RE) and LE, respectively. The intraocular pressure (IOP) was 18 mmHg in RE and 45 mmHg in LE. Anterior segment examination of LE revealed 270° of iridocorneal apposition in the periphery of the anterior chamber. Fundus examination of LE showed silicone oil filled vitreous cavity with attached retina. Given the recent history of silicone oil injection and elevated IOP despite maximum antiglaucoma medications, we decided to perform laser peripheral iridotomy (LPI) in the area of iridocorneal apposition. Following LPI, the IOP in LE came down to 17 mmHg and remained stable within the normal range for one month, after which the patient was taken up for silicone oil removal. *Conclusion.* This case report highlights a new mechanism of silicone oil-induced glaucoma and the technique of performing LPI in the area of iridocorneal apposition, for the first time in the literature. Silicone oil migration into the posterior chamber from the vitreous cavity in the presence of zonular dehiscence can push the iris forward and lead to iridocorneal apposition, resulting in an acute rise in IOP. Performing LPI within the area of iridocorneal apposition can help the aqueous seep into the anterior chamber and release the silicone oil globule trapped behind the iris to enter the anterior chamber, thus relieving the iridocorneal adhesions and lowering the IOP.

1. Introduction

Secondary glaucoma after vitreo-retinal (VR) surgery with silicone oil injection is a relatively common complication. Secondary glaucoma can develop at any time in the postoperative phase and can manifest with a wide range of intraocular pressure (IOP) and loss of vision. Silicone oil is a vitreous substitute used for long-term intraocular tamponade in VR surgery, usually for a period of 3-6 months, depending on the viscosity of silicone oil, retinal detachment, and surgeon's choice. Silicone oil may be left for a long-term period also in a few cases. Two main types of silicone oil available are low viscosity oil (lighter than water) and high viscosity oil (heavier than water). Low viscosity oil floats in the eye, and high viscosity oil provides long-term tamponade for inferior retinal pathologies as the oil sinks in the vitreous cavity [1–3].

Secondary glaucoma following silicone oil injection can occur due to different mechanisms, including pupillary block, migration of silicone oil into the anterior chamber, inflammation, preexisting glaucoma, trabecular meshwork infiltration by silicone oil bubbles, synechial angle closure, and rubeosis iridis [4–8].

Here, we describe a case of silicone oil-induced glaucoma due to a new mechanism and its successful management.

2. Case Presentation

A 69-year-old female presented to our outpatient services with decreased vision, pain, and discomfort in the left eye (LE) for one month. She had a history of phacoemulsification with intraoperative posterior capsule rupture and nucleus drop into the vitreous cavity in the LE, for which pars plana vitrectomy followed by nucleus removal (using a fragmatome) was performed, and a three-piece intraocular lens (IOL) was implanted in the ciliary sulcus a month ago. During the postoperative period, the patient developed retinal detachment, for which she underwent VR surgery with silicone oil endotamponade. The patient was also a known case of open angle glaucoma on four antiglaucoma medications (Latanoprost 0.005%, Timolol Maleate 0.5%, Brimonidine Tartrate 0.2%, and Ripasudil 0.4%) in both eyes prior to the cataract surgery. She was asked to stop Latanoprost 0.005% eye drops in LE one week before the surgery and continued the rest of the medications.

On examination, the corrected distance visual acuity (CDVA) was 20/20 and 20/125 in the right eye (RE) and LE, respectively. The IOP was 18 mmHg in RE and 45 mmHg in LE on Goldman applanation tonometry (GAT). Anterior segment examination of RE revealed in-the-bag IOL. LE showed circumcorneal congestion, mild corneal epithelial edema, 270° of iridocorneal apposition in the periphery of the anterior chamber 2-3 mm from the limbus, and in-the-sulcus IOL (Figure 1(a)). No silicone oil in the anterior chamber was observed. Fundus examination showed a cup-disc ratio (CDR) of 0.8 with bipolar neuroretinal rim thinning, normal macula, and attached retina in RE and a CDR of 0.6 with inferior neuroretinal rim thinning with silicone oil-filled vitreous cavity and attached retina in LE. Preoperative visual fields with a Humphrey Field Analyzer 3 24-2 Swedish Interactive Thresholding Algorithm Standard programme showed a visual field index of 51% in RE and 87% in LE. Central corneal thickness was 536 μ and 505 μ in RE and LE, respectively. Iridocorneal apposition was observed on anterior segment optical coherence tomography (AS-OCT) of LE (Figure 1(b)). A diagnosis of secondary angle closure due to silicone oil in LE was made.

The patient was given 200 cc intravenous mannitol 20% and was started on maximum antiglaucoma medications adding Pilocarpine 2% eye drops thrice daily, Latanoprost 0.05% at bedtime in LE, and oral acetazolamide 250 mg three times a day with potassium supplementation, along with the previous medications. The next day, she had an IOP of 40 mmHg in LE on GAT. Syrup Glycerol (50%, 30 ml) thrice a day was also added. She still had an IOP of 36 mmHg in LE on the following day. The choice to remove the silicone oil either partially or completely was discussed with the VR surgeon. However, as the surgery had been done only a few days back, this posed the risk of redetachment of the retina. Hence, silicone oil removal was deferred.

As the entrapment of silicone oil between the IOL and the iris was the cause for iridocorneal apposition, we considered the possibility of performing a laser peripheral iridotomy (LPI) in the area of iridocorneal apposition, which might permit egress of aqueous into the anterior chamber. LPI was performed in the area of iridocorneal apposition on the temporal aspect between 3 and 4 o'clock, which led to the seeping of aqueous through the PI into the anterior chamber, relieving the iridocorneal apposition over the entire angle. The deepening of the anterior chamber and posterior shift of the iris was followed by the entry of the silicone oil into the anterior chamber through the pupil, where it formed a globule of around 6 mm diameter in the anterior chamber (Figure 2(a)). One hour later, the IOP in LE came down to 17 mmHg, and AS-OCT showed the release of iridocorneal apposition (Figure 2(b)). The IOP remained stable within the normal range on consecutive follow-ups for one month, after which the patient was taken up for silicone oil removal.

2.1. LPI Technique for Iridocorneal Apposition. Pilocarpine 2% eye drops were used to cause miosis, stretch the iris, and facilitate perforation. After instilling Proparacaine 0.5% eye drops, Abraham iridotomy lens was applied to the eye with a coupling gel. Neodymium-doped yttrium aluminium garnet (Nd:YAG) laser was used to create LPI. The aiming beam was defocused to 125 μ posterior focus and was then focused within the iris stroma in the area of iridocorneal apposition. The part of iris tissue between its original plane and its point of apposition with the cornea was focused at the slight recess seen in the AS-OCT in the extreme periphery.

The initial shot was made in the slight recess at the extreme peripheral area with 2 mJ of energy which helped push back the iris further away from the cornea due to the force of plasma formation. Immediately, the energy was increased to 4 mJ, and partial patency of the iridotomy was achieved. After the slight deepening due to some egress of aqueous, 6 mJ energy was used to complete the iridotomy.

3. Discussion

The incidence of elevated IOP or glaucoma following silicone oil injection varies from 2.2% to 56.0% [3, 9]. Multiple mechanisms of silicone oil-induced secondary glaucoma have been described in the literature [4–8]. In the present case, we have described a new mechanism of silicone oil-induced angle closure glaucoma and how we managed it.

Usually, overfill of silicone oil in the vitreous cavity, when associated with partial zonular dehiscence, results in the anterior movement of silicone oil into the anterior chamber. If the anterior chamber is completely filled with silicone oil, direct closure of the angle and resultant glaucoma can occur, even with intact zonules. Removal of silicone oil from the anterior chamber and partial removal from the vitreous cavity is the management option in such situations.

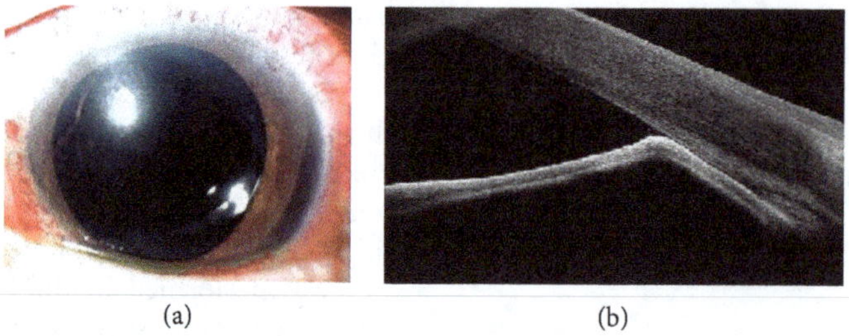

Figure 1: (a) Anterior segment photograph of the left eye showing 270° of iridocorneal apposition in the periphery of the anterior chamber. (b) Anterior segment optical coherence tomography of the left eye showing iridocorneal apposition.

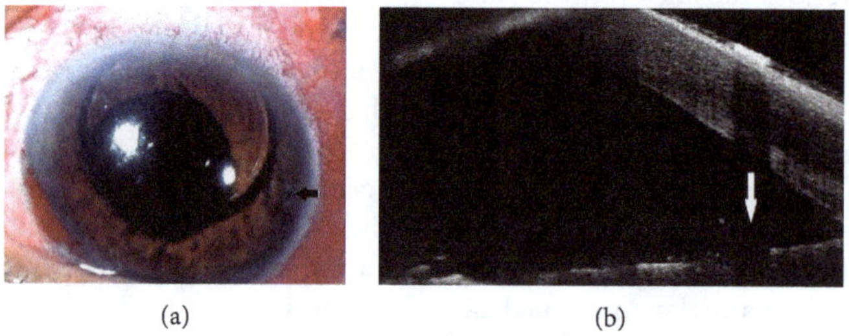

Figure 2: (a) Anterior segment photograph of the left eye showing seeping of silicone oil into the anterior chamber following laser peripheral iridotomy (black arrow). (b) Anterior segment optical coherence tomography of the left eye showing the release of iridocorneal apposition and widening of the angle following laser peripheral iridotomy (white arrow).

However, in our case, we believe that the silicone oil globule was trapped in the posterior chamber and pushing the iris forward, leading to iridocorneal touch in the periphery and a physical block of the anterior chamber angle. The silicone oil bubble trapped in the posterior chamber also possibly caused an occult pupillary block due to its surface tension preventing egress of aqueous into the anterior chamber. This possibly may have exacerbated the peripheral iridocorneal touch even further. The angle was closed 2-3 mm from the limbus temporally and caused flattening of the anterior chamber in the temporal quadrant. As the damming of the aqueous in the posterior chamber increased, the iridocorneal touch also developed in the nasal quadrant. This caused a hindrance to aqueous outflow as the conventional outflow system got blocked at the level of entry of aqueous into the trabecular meshwork. Consequently, this led to an increase in IOP. No apparent pupillary block and no iris bombe were present.

It seems likely that the silicone oil, which was injected at the end of VR surgery, partially seeped into the posterior chamber through an area of zonular dehiscence that occurred during the previous cataract surgery or VR surgery [2]. The high viscosity of silicone oil resulted in the entrapment of silicone oil behind the iris and is likely to have been aggravated by the collection of aqueous in the posterior chamber, which pushed the peripheral iris forward and flattened the anterior chamber in the periphery. This flattening further prevented the escape of silicone oil into the anterior chamber.

A prophylactic inferior surgical iridectomy is absolutely indicated in aphakic patients with silicone oil endotamponade due to the high risk of pupillary block [10]. In phakic and pseudophakic patients, there is no role of prophylactic iridectomy or iridotomy usually as the risk of silicone oil pupil block is rare [5]. However, in cases of blunt trauma or cataract surgery with subclinical zonular loss and extensive vitreous base excision, displacement of silicone oil and pupillary block could occur [11–13]. In the present case, surgical iridectomy was not done as there was no reason to believe that there was a significant loss of zonular integrity, and no air entered the anterior chamber during the fluid-air exchange, which could have suggested the likelihood of the possibility of zonular dialysis. Anterior movement of silicone oil is most likely to occur in a patient with zonular dehiscence if the patient fails to sleep in the prone position. Hence, a prophylactic surgical iridectomy or iridotomy shall be considered in cases where zonular loss is likely.

LPI is the commonly performed procedure to relieve an acute angle closure attack and to relieve the raised IOP in eyes with iris bombe due to secondary angle closure [14]. Patients with chronic unrelieved angle closure can often develop peripheral anterior synechiae, which cause closure of the trabecular meshwork and prevent aqueous outflow, thereby resulting in elevated IOP. Similarly, cases with extensive iridocorneal contact in the periphery can lead to raised IOP due to blockage of the angle. Performing LPI in an almost apposed iridocorneal situation is challenging and usually not done. The technical hitch in performing LPI in the presence of iridocorneal touch is the likelihood of localised corneal damage and the inability to complete the procedure in a nonexistent space.

However, in our case, we have decided to perform LPI in the area of iridocorneal apposition, as the patient was already on maximum antiglaucoma medications and creating a PI was the only solution to relieve the symptoms of the patient and prevent further damage to the optic nerve head. A low energy of 2 mJ was used in the initial shot, which helped push back the iris away from the cornea, resulting in our ability to increase the energy to create full penetration of the iris. After the creation of a PI in the region of iridocorneal adhesion, it was noted that the aqueous had begun to seep into the anterior chamber through it. This deepened the anterior chamber and squeezed the silicone oil trapped between the iris and the IOL, through the pupil into the anterior chamber. The high viscosity of the silicone oil, which initially prevented its movement through the pupil, now facilitated its movement when the posterior chamber of the eye between the IOL and the iris flattened. This also relieved the iridocorneal adhesions at the level of the midperiphery of the cornea. The deepening of the anterior chamber allowed further enlargement of the size of PI. The creation of an alternative passage for the flow of aqueous in the presence of an occult obstruction caused by silicone oil leads to a decrease in IOP. This outcome suggests that the passage for aqueous flow through the trabecular meshwork opened up as the iridocorneal apposition was fresh, and only the route of aqueous entry into the angle was blocked.

To the best of our knowledge, this is the first case report to describe a new mechanism of silicone oil-induced angle closure glaucoma and the unique technique of performing LPI in the area of iridocorneal apposition. Our case highlights that the clinicians should be aware of the mechanism described, and a simple procedure like LPI can give time to let the retinal reattachment become stable enough for the silicone oil to be removed from the vitreous cavity.

Consent

Written consent to publish this case has been obtained. This report does not contain any personal identifying information.

Authors' Contributions

All authors have approved the manuscript for submission.

References

[1] C. Alovisi, C. Panico, U. de Sanctis, and C. M. Eandi, "Vitreous substitutes: old and new materials in vitreoretinal surgery," *Journal of Ophthalmology*, vol. 2017, Article ID 3172138, 6 pages, 2017.

[2] R. Zivojnovic, *Silicone oil in vitreo retinal surgery*, The Netherlands, Martinus Nijhoff/ Dr W Junk, Dordrecht, 1987.

[3] M. Bhoot, A. Agarwal, S. Dubey, J. Pegu, and M. Gandhi, "Silicone oil induced glaucoma," *Silicone Oil Induced Glaucoma*, vol. 29, no. 1, pp. 9–13, 2018.

[4] P. K. Leaver, R. H. B. Grey, and A. Garner, "Silicone oil injection in the treatment of massive preretinal retraction. II. Late complications in 93 eyes," *The British Journal of Ophthalmology*, vol. 63, no. 5, pp. 361–367, 1979.

[5] K. G. Riedel, V. P. Gabel, L. Neubauer, A. Kampik, and O. E. Lund, "Intravitreal silicone oil injection: complications and treatment of 415 consecutive patients," *Graefe's Archive for Clinical and Experimental Ophthalmology*, vol. 228, no. 1, pp. 19–23, 1990.

[6] J. B. Jonas, H. L. Knorr, R. M. Rank, and W. M. Budde, "Intraocular pressure and silicone oil endotamponade," *Journal of Glaucoma*, vol. 10, no. 2, pp. 102–108, 2001.

[7] C. Ni, W. Wang, D. M. Albert, and C. L. Schepens, "Intravitreous silicone injection. Histopathologic findings in a human eye after 12 years," *Archives of Ophthalmology*, vol. 101, no. 9, pp. 1399–1401, 1983.

[8] J. H. Yeo, B. M. Glaser, and R. G. Michels, "Silicone oil in the treatment of complicated retinal detachments," *Ophthalmology*, vol. 94, no. 9, pp. 1109–1113, 1987.

[9] L. R. de Corral, S. B. Cohen, and G. A. Peyman, "Effect of intravitreal silicone oil on intraocular pressure," *Ophthalmic Surgery*, vol. 18, no. 6, pp. 446–449, 1987.

[10] W. H. Beekhuis, F. Ando, R. Zivojnovic, D. A. Mertens, and E. Peperkamp, "Basal iridectomy at 6 o'clock in the aphakic eye treated with silicone oil: prevention of keratopathy and secondary glaucoma," *The British Journal of Ophthalmology*, vol. 71, no. 3, pp. 197–200, 1987.

[11] M. B. Merriman, B. Vote, and A. McGeorge, "Silicone oil pupil-block acute angle-closure glaucoma: optimal laser position," *Retina*, vol. 23, no. 3, pp. 407–409, 2003.

[12] A. Kumar, "Silicone oil pupil-block acute angle-closure glaucoma: optimal laser position," *Retina*, vol. 24, no. 6, p. 987, 2004.

[13] I. H. Yusuf, T. H. Fung, J. F. Salmon, and C. K. Patel, "Silicone oil pupil block glaucoma in a pseudophakic eye," *Case Reports*, vol. 2014, article bcr2014205018, 2014.

[14] H. Kumar, T. Mansoori, G. B. Warjri, B. I. Somarajan, S. Bandil, and V. Gupta, "Lasers in glaucoma," *Indian Journal of Ophthalmology*, vol. 66, no. 11, pp. 1539–1553, 2018.

17

Acute Hydrops with Total Corneal Edema in a Very Young Child with Keratoconus: The Youngest Age Reported Case

Mohammad-Reza Sedaghat,[1] Hamed Momeni-Moghaddam,[2] Michael W. Belin,[3] Maryam Savardashtaki,[4] Shehzad A. Naroo,[5] and Hassan Robabi[6]

[1]*Eye Research Center, Mashhad University of Medical Sciences, Mashhad, Iran*
[2]*Health Promotion Research Center, Zahedan University of Medical Sciences, Zahedan, Iran*
[3]*University of Arizona, Department of Ophthalmology & Vision Science, Tucson, Arizona, USA*
[4]*Department of Optometry, School of Paramedical Sciences, Mashhad University of Medical Sciences, Mashhad, Iran*
[5]*College of Health and Life Sciences, Aston University, Birmingham, UK*
[6]*Department of Nursing and Midwifery, Zahedan University of Medical Sciences, Zahedan, Iran*

Correspondence should be addressed to Hamed Momeni-Moghaddam; hmomeni_opt@yahoo.com

Academic Editor: Kamal Kishore

Purpose. To present the youngest age ever reported for acute corneal hydrops with total corneal edema in a child with advanced bilateral keratoconus. *Methods.* Patient presentation in ophthalmic clinic. The patient underwent various clinical tests and examinations including anterior segment optical coherence tomography (AS-OCT) and Scheimpflug corneal tomography. *Results.* A 5-year-old girl presented with uncorrected distance visual acuity (UDVA) of 0.4 in the right eye and nonmeasurable UDVA associated with severe photophobia in her left eye of a 3-day duration. Intraocular pressure using the iCare tonometer was 14 and 5 mmHg in the right and left eyes, respectively. An old corneal hydrops scar and posterior subcapsular cataract (PSC) in the right eye and a total limbus to limbus corneal hydrops in the left eye were observed on slit-lamp examinations. Scheimpflug corneal tomography was possible in the right eye but, due to excessive irregularity and scaring, was not possible in the left eye. Corneal thinning and scarring were evident in the anterior segment optical coherence tomography in the right eye and very edematous cornea associated with stromal cleft and epithelial bullae in the left eye. A management plan consisting of topical hypertonic solution and ointment was started to reduce her symptoms. *Conclusion.* Acute corneal hydrops may be the presenting sign of keratoconus; however, extensive hydrops involving the total cornea area at a very young age is very rare and has not been previously reported in the literature.

1. Introduction

Corneal hydrops as a complication of keratoconus (KCN) is characterized by significant bullous edema of the cornea secondary to breaks in the Descemet membrane and an influx of aqueous into the stroma and epithelium of the cornea [1]. It has been postulated as a complication of eye-rubbing [2]. Various therapeutic options (medical or surgical interventions or conservative methods) were introduced to reduce patients' symptoms or shorten the healing period. These options include intracameral gas injection (air, sulfur hexafluoride (SF6) or perfluoropropane (C3F8)) to produce a gas tamponade or compression sutures such as pre-Descemet's membrane sutures [3–5]. Among the conservative approaches is the use of hypertonic saline eye drops/ointments or antiglaucoma agents, which helps to improve the condition by drawing fluid from the cornea or reducing the hydrodynamic pressure on the back surface of the cornea, respectively [6]. Corneal imaging techniques, such as anterior segment optical coherence tomography (AS-OCT), Scheimpflug tomography, and ultrasound biomicroscopy (UBM), provide both diagnostic and therapeutic guidelines. The advantages of AS-OCT are its noncontact property in delineating the location of intrastromal aqueous influx

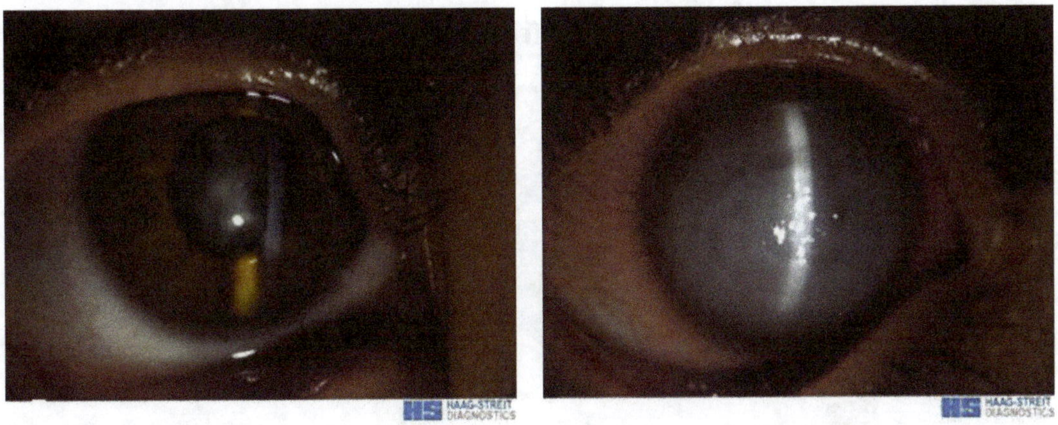

(a) (b)

Figure 1: Slit-lamp photographs in the right (a) and left (b) eyes.

through the rupture in the Descemet layer and intrastromal clefts and its ease of use in young children [7, 8]. The current study presents the youngest age ever reported for an acute corneal hydrops with total corneal edema in a case with advanced bilateral keratoconus.

2. Case Presentation

A 5-year-old girl presented to the ophthalmic clinic after her parents noticed whitish discoloration in her left eye and the child exhibiting severe light sensitivity for a three-day duration. Her clinical history was negative for any systemic, congenital/genetic disorders, atopy (recurrent rhinitis and dermatitis), and/or chronic rubbing of the eye. There was no history of topical or systemic medications, and the family history was negative for any ectatic disease. Uncorrected distance visual acuity (UDVA) recorded as decimal notation was 0.4 in the right eye and not measurable in the left eye. Intraocular pressure measured using iCare tonometer (iCare IC100, iCare Finland, Oy, Finland) was 14 and 5 mmHg in the right and left eyes, respectively.

Slit-lamp biomicroscope examination showed an old corneal scar compatible with prior hydrops and a posterior subcapsular cataract (PSC) in the right eye and limbus to limbus corneal edema with hydrops in the left eye (Figure 1).

Corneal topo/tomography was performed in the right eye, but due to excessive corneal irregularity secondary to the corneal scar, only a Scheimpflug image with an unacceptable quality specification (QS) was possible (Pentacam HR, Oculus; Wetzlar, Germany) after several attempts. A thin irregular cornea with a large posterior ectasia was noted on the corneal thickens and posterior elevation maps. The anterior elevation and anterior curvature showed milder changes with a maximum simulated keratometry of 60.7 diopters, possibly secondary to earlier scarring (Figure 2).

AS-OCT of both eyes showed a thin and scarified cornea associated with an opacity under the posterior capsular surface in the right eye. The left eye had a very edematous cornea associated with multiple stromal clefts and epithelial bullae (Casia2 AS-OCT, Tomey Corporation, Nagoya, Japan) (Figure 3).

Dilated fundus examination was not possible but the attached retina was visible in both eyes on B-scan ultrasonography.

Based on the examination of prior hydrops in the right eye, a diagnosis of acute corneal hydrops was made in the left eye. Both the slit lamp exam and AS-OCT revealed edema extending to the limbus.

Her mother was informed about the nature and course of KCN and the possible future need for penetrating keratoplasty (PKP) in her left eye. Reliable autorefraction was not possible in the presence of corneal scar and PSC in the right eye. Due to severe photophobia, the patient did not cooperate enough to achieve accurate retinoscopic refraction in the right eye, and the decision was made to postpone for subsequent sessions after corneal hydrops reduction in the left eye. A management plan consisting of topical hypertonic solution and ointment was started, and it was emphasized that hydrops in most cases of KCN is a transient condition, and the patient will be followed for changes in her visual acuity, corneal transparency, and intraocular pressure.

3. Discussion

The classic view is that KCN begins as a progressive corneal disorder during puberty and progresses to midlife. KCN is less commonly seen in the very young, and this may be related to a delay in diagnosis or the inability of the very young to verbalize or note their visual complaints [9]. It was reported that the rate of disease progression, the frequency of more advanced KCN, and ultimately the need for corneal transplantation are greater in cases with early-onset [10]. Although KCN in children may be associated with systemic or genetic disorders such as Down syndrome and myotonic dystrophy; in otherwise healthy children, eye rubbing is considered a major predisposing factor for disease progression [11, 12].

The youngest child with KCN was reported in a 4-year-old girl secondary to vernal keratoconjunctivitis and sequentially eye rubbing without evidence of hydrops [11]. A 5-year-old boy with unilateral hydrops was previously reported. The

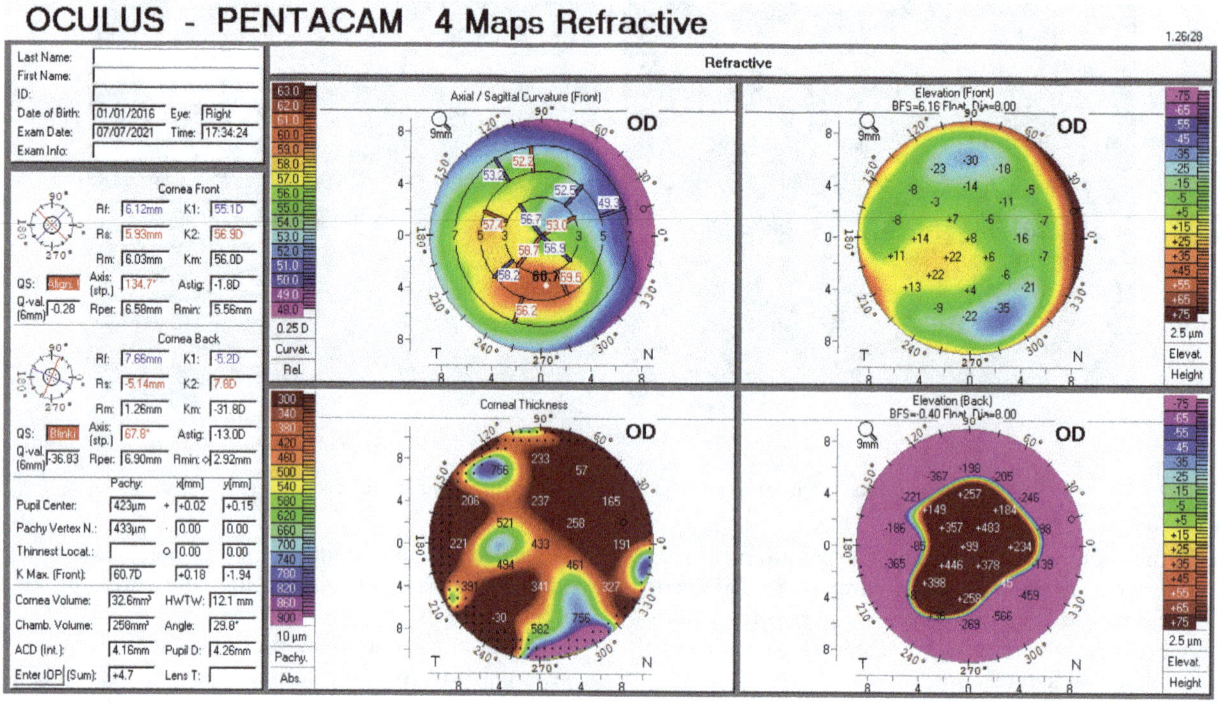

FIGURE 2: Scheimpflug image using Pentacam HR in the right eye.

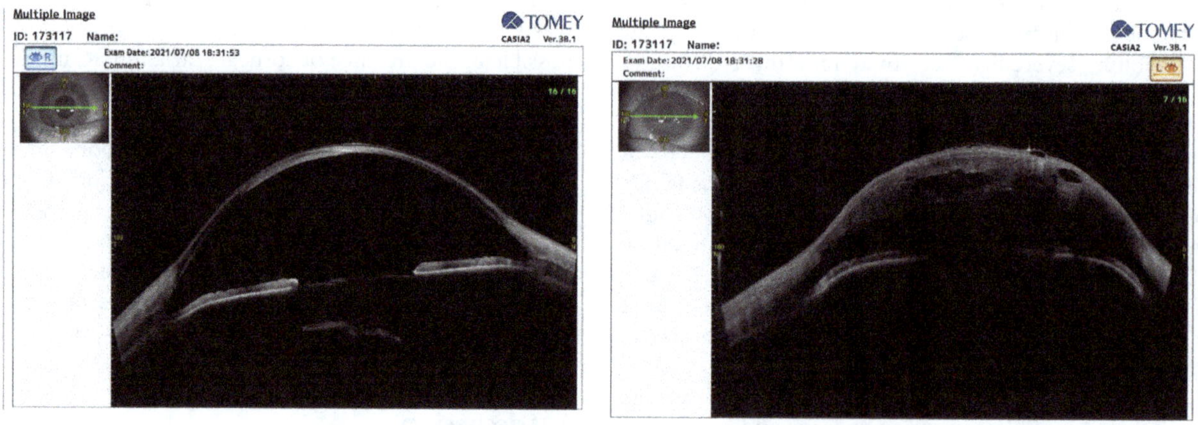

(a)

(b)

FIGURE 3: Anterior segment OCT in the right (a) and left (b) eyes.

corneal edema was limited to the temporal portion of the right cornea [13].

Although corneal hydrops can occur in various types of ectatic corneal disorders such as keratoconus, pellucid marginal degeneration (PMD), terrien marginal degeneration (TMD), and keratoglobus, it is often seen in association with keratoconus [14]. It occurs mostly in advanced stage of the disease and in younger patients, increasing the risk of visual impairment and the need for penetrating keratoplasty [15, 16].

Although with the introduction of corneal cross-linking as a treatment option for KCN by improving the mechanical strength of the cornea, the incidence of corneal hydrops appears to have decreased.

Several studies have reported corneal hydrops in children with KCN. A summary of the literature is provided in Table 1.

Gaskin and colleagues (2013) reported eye-rubbing, lower visual acuity at the first visit, and negative family history as risk factors for acute hydrops in KCN, while atopic disorders and a history of contact lens wear showed no association with hydrops. In their study, the average time to develop hydrops was 4 years following the detection of KCN [25]. In agreement with their study, our case had a negative family history of KCN. Although other studies found a higher prevalence of hydrops in severe allergic eye disease [16, 26], the mother of the present case denied chronic eye rubbing.

TABLE 1: Summary of several studies reporting corneal hydrops in children with KCN.

Study	Country	Age (years)/sex	Association
Rehany and Rumelt (1995) [13]	Israel	5/male	Bilateral advanced keratoconus, previous treatment for vernal conjunctivitis, and epithelial and stromal edema on the temporal side of the right cornea
Rahman and Anwar (2006) [17]	United Kingdom	6/female	Severe keratoconus
Rehany and Rumelt (1995) [13]	Israel	7/male	Advanced keratoconus with central stromal edema in the left eye with negative history of eye and systemic disorders and no history of habitual rubbing of the eye
Panahi-Bazaz et al. (2014) [18]	Iran	7/female	Bilateral corneal hydrops associated with eye rubbing secondary vernal keratoconjunctivitis (VKC)
Ioannidis et al. (2005) [19]	United Kingdom	7/female	Hydrops secondary to a chronic persistent eye-rubbing with no systemic involvement
Downie (2014) [20]	Australia	8/female	Bilateral acute corneal hydrops associated with severe atopy and no previous eye examination
Slim et al. (2015) [21]	Lebanon	10/male	Hydrops in an advanced KCN
Ozcan and Ersoz (2007) [22]	Turkey	11/male	Down syndrome and vigorous eye rubbing
Rehany and Rumelt (1995) [13]	Israel	11/male	Acute hydrops in the left eye in a bilateral advanced keratoconus, history of vernal conjunctivitis
Bilgin et al. (2013) [23]	Turkey	12/male	Simultaneous bilateral acute hydrops in Leber congenital amaurosis (LCA)
Khan et al. (2006) [24]	Saudi Arabia	16/male	Hydrops in a KCN patient with cornea plana
Current Study (2021)	Iran	5/female	Acute corneal hydrops associated with total limbus to limbus corneal edema, use of AS-OCT to enhance understanding of the structural corneal changes

Often, severe and chronic rubbing of the eye is considered one of the main risk factor for hydrops, sometimes very minor trauma, such as the insertion of the contact lens has been reported as causative [26].

Multimodal imaging has improved the diagnosis of acute corneal hydrops associated with the assessment of corneal integrity. The AS-OCT of the present case showed structural changes in detail such as multiple stromal clefts and epithelial bullae as evident in the left eye delineated the location and extension of the Descemet's membrane break. Another application of AS-OCT is to determine the effectiveness of interventions such as intracameral gas injection in resolving acute edema. Basu et al.'s study showed that the measurement of break dimension (size and depth) in the DM correlates with the resolution of acute hydrops after intracameral injection of C3F8 [7]. Compared to UBM, which is a contact and operator-dependent method to assess DM integrity, AS-OCT is an easy, noncontact technique and more comfortable technique in children, capable of producing high-resolution images in conditions of corneal edema [27].

In conclusion, limbus to limbus involvement in corneal hydrops is in itself an uncommon presentation. To the authors' knowledge, this is the youngest reported case of corneal hydrops (5 years of age) associated with total corneal edema reported in the literature documented with AS-OCT.

Consent

The patient's parents have consented to submit the case report along with images to the journal.

Acknowledgments

The authors would like to thank the subject and personnel of the Sedaghat Eye Clinic.

References

[1] A. Barsam, N. Brennan, H. Petrushkin et al., "Case-control study of risk factors for acute corneal hydrops in keratoconus," *The British Journal of Ophthalmology*, vol. 101, no. 4, pp. 499–502, 2017.

[2] H. Ben-Eli, N. Erdinest, and A. Solomon, "Pathogenesis and complications of chronic eye rubbing in ocular allergy," *Current Opinion in Allergy and Clinical Immunology*, vol. 19, no. 5, pp. 526–534, 2019.

[3] R. Rajaraman, S. Singh, A. Raghavan, and A. Karkhanis, "Efficacy and safety of intracameral perfluoropropane (C3F8) tamponade and compression sutures for the management of acute corneal hydrops," *Cornea*, vol. 28, no. 3, pp. 317–320, 2009.

[4] J. J. Sayadi, H. Lam, C. C. Lin, and D. Myung, "Management of acute corneal hydrops with intracameral gas injection," *American Journal of Ophthalmology Case Reports*, vol. 20, article 100994, 2020.

[5] H. Yahia Chérif, J. Gueudry, M. Afriat et al., "Efficacy and safety of pre-Descemet's membrane sutures for the management of acute corneal hydrops in keratoconus," *The British Journal of Ophthalmology*, vol. 99, no. 6, pp. 773–777, 2015.

[6] P. K. Maharana, N. Sharma, and R. B. Vajpayee, "Acute corneal hydrops in keratoconus," *Indian Journal of Ophthalmology*, vol. 61, no. 8, pp. 461–464, 2013.

[7] S. Basu, P. K. Vaddavalli, G. K. Vemuganti, M. H. Ali, and S. I. Murthy, "Anterior segment optical coherence tomography features of acute corneal hydrops," *Cornea*, vol. 31, no. 5, pp. 479–485, 2012.

[8] A. Gokul, H. R. Vellara, and D. V. Patel, "Advanced anterior segment imaging in keratoconus: a review," *Clinical & Experimental Ophthalmology*, vol. 46, no. 2, pp. 122–132, 2018.

[9] V. Anitha, M. Vanathi, A. Raghavan, R. Rajaraman, M. Ravindran, and R. Tandon, "Pediatric keratoconus - current perspectives and clinical challenges," *Indian Journal of Ophthalmology*, vol. 69, no. 2, pp. 214–225, 2021.

[10] A. Ertan and O. Muftuoglu, "Keratoconus clinical findings according to different age and gender groups," *Cornea*, vol. 27, no. 10, pp. 1109–1113, 2008.

[11] A. Gunes, L. Tok, Ö. Tok, and L. Seyrek, "The youngest patient with bilateral keratoconus secondary to chronic persistent eye rubbing," *Seminars in Ophthalmology*, vol. 30, no. 5-6, pp. 454–456, 2015.

[12] C. W. McMonnies, "Mechanisms of rubbing-related corneal trauma in keratoconus," *Cornea*, vol. 28, no. 6, pp. 607–615, 2009.

[13] U. Rehany and S. Rumelt, "Corneal hydrops associated with vernal conjunctivitis as a presenting sign of keratoconus in children," *Ophthalmology*, vol. 102, no. 12, pp. 2046–2049, 1995.

[14] A. J. Aldave, M. Mabon, D. A. Hollander, S. D. McLeod, W. H. Spencer, and R. L. Abbott, "Spontaneous corneal hydrops and perforation in keratoconus and pellucid marginal degeneration," *Cornea*, vol. 22, no. 2, pp. 169–174, 2003.

[15] J. C. Fan Gaskin, D. V. Patel, and C. N. McGhee, "Acute corneal hydrops in keratoconus–new perspectives," *American Journal of Ophthalmology*, vol. 157, no. 5, pp. 921–928.e1, 2014.

[16] S. J. Tuft, W. M. Gregory, and R. J. Buckley, "Acute corneal hydrops in keratoconus," *Ophthalmology*, vol. 101, no. 10, pp. 1738–1744, 1994.

[17] W. Rahman and S. Anwar, "An unusual case of keratoconus," *Journal of Pediatric Ophthalmology and Strabismus*, vol. 43, no. 6, pp. 373–375, 2006.

[18] M. R. Panahi-Bazaz, F. Sharifipour, and A. Moghaddasi, "Bilateral keratoconus and corneal hydrops associated with eye rubbing in a 7-year-old girl," *Journal of Ophthalmic & Vision Research*, vol. 9, pp. 101–105, 2014.

[19] A. S. Ioannidis, L. Speedwell, and K. K. Nischal, "Unilateral keratoconus in a child with chronic and persistent eye rubbing," *American Journal of Ophthalmology*, vol. 139, no. 2, pp. 356-357, 2005.

[20] L. E. Downie, "The necessity for ocular assessment in atopic children: bilateral corneal hydrops in an 8 year old," *Pediatrics*, vol. 134, no. 2, pp. e596–e601, 2014.

[21] E. A. Slim, E. F. Jarade, B. M. Charanek et al., "Acute corneal hydrops mimicking infectious keratitis as initial presentation of keratoconus in a 10-year-old child," *Case Reports in Ophthalmological Medicine*, vol. 2015, Article ID 308348, 4 pages, 2015.

[22] A. A. Ozcan and T. R. Ersoz, "Severe acute corneal hydrops in a patient with Down syndrome and persistent eye rubbing," *Annals of Ophthalmology*, vol. 39, no. 2, pp. 158–160, 2007.

[23] B. Bilgin, B. Ünal, M. Ünal et al., "Keratoconus presenting with bilateral simultaneous acute corneal hydrops," *Contact Lens & Anterior Eye*, vol. 36, no. 2, pp. 98–100, 2013.

[24] A. O. Khan, M. Aldahmesh, and B. Meyer, "Corneal ectasia and hydrops in a patient with autosomal recessive cornea plana," *Ophthalmic Genetics*, vol. 27, no. 3, pp. 99–101, 2006.

[25] J. C. Fan Gaskin, W. R. Good, C. A. Jordan, D. V. Patel, and C. McGhee, "The Auckland keratoconus study: identifying predictors of acute corneal hydrops in keratoconus," *Clinical & Experimental Optometry*, vol. 96, no. 2, pp. 208–213, 2013.

[26] S. Grewal, P. R. Laibson, E. J. Cohen, and C. J. Rapuano, "Acute hydrops in the corneal ectasias: associated factors and outcomes," *Transactions of the American Ophthalmological Society*, vol. 97, pp. 187–198, 1999.

[27] N. Sharma, R. Mannan, V. Jhanji et al., "Ultrasound biomicroscopy-guided assessment of acute corneal hydrops," *Ophthalmology*, vol. 118, no. 11, pp. 2166–2171, 2011.

18

Case Series of Recurring Spontaneous Closure of Macular Hole

Abdelrahman M. Elhusseiny,[1,2] William E. Smiddy,[1] Harry W. Flynn,[1] and Stephen G. Schwartz[1]

[1]*Department of Ophthalmology, Bascom Palmer Eye Institute, University of Miami Miller School of Medicine, 900 NW 17 Street, Miami, FL 33136, USA*
[2]*Department of Ophthalmology, Kasr Al Ainy School of Medicine, Cairo University, Egypt*

Correspondence should be addressed to William E. Smiddy; wsmiddy@med.miami.edu

Academic Editor: Maurizio Battaglia Parodi

Macular hole can undergo spontaneous reopening and reclosure. This is a retrospective review of three patients who had spontaneous reopening and reclosure of previously spontaneously closed macular hole documented by optical coherence tomography. We report the first case of nivolumab-uveitis-associated macular hole formation. The authors hypothesize that cystoid macular edema (CME) might alter the integrity of foveal tissues or conversely the orientation of the macular hole edges and play a role in formation and resolution of a macular hole.

1. Introduction

Macular holes (MH) are a common cause of decreased central vision. Most MHs are idiopathic, but secondary causes include trauma and uveitis. Surgery is usually recommended, but spontaneous closure of full thickness macular hole (FTMH) has been reported in 0-6% with one series as high as 11.5% [1].

In as much as the original pathogenesis is incompletely understood, the mechanisms of spontaneous closure and reopening are even less well understood. Certain subsets, as uveitis-induced MH, are more likely to close spontaneously and perhaps physical effects from cystoid macular edema play a role [2]. Conversely, macular edema per se, rather than inflammation, has been implicated as a causative element [3].

We present three patients who each had spontaneous MH closure, followed by reopening and reclosure; the MH closed spontaneously twice. One of these involved uveitis-associated macular edema caused by nivolumab therapy and represents the first reported case associated with MH formation.

2. Case Description

Case 1. An 80-year-old male presented with bilateral posterior uveitis and CME with onset 5 months after initiating nivolumab (Opdivo) for treatment of metastatic cancer due to an unknown primary tumor. Best corrected visual acuity (BCVA) was 20/70 OD and 20/40 OS. Oral prednisone, topical difluprednate (Durezol), and nepafenac (Nevanac) were started. CME had resolved with improved BCVA (20/30 OU) after 6 months of therapy. 9 months later, foveal thinning developed which progressed to a FTMH one month later (Figure 1(a)), reducing BCVA to 20/60 OS. Scheduled macular hole surgery (MHS) was cancelled when the vision improved to 20/40. OCT showed a closed MH, with residual subretinal fluid (SRF) (Figure 1(b)). The condition remained stable until three months later when the patient presented with decreased VA (20/150). OCT showed reopening of the MH (Figure 1(c)). The patient scheduled MHS but wanted to wait for 3 months, hoping for spontaneous resolution. 3 months later, MH spontaneously closed (Figure 1(d)) with improved VA to 20/80 OS. The condition has remained stable with 20/70 BCVA.

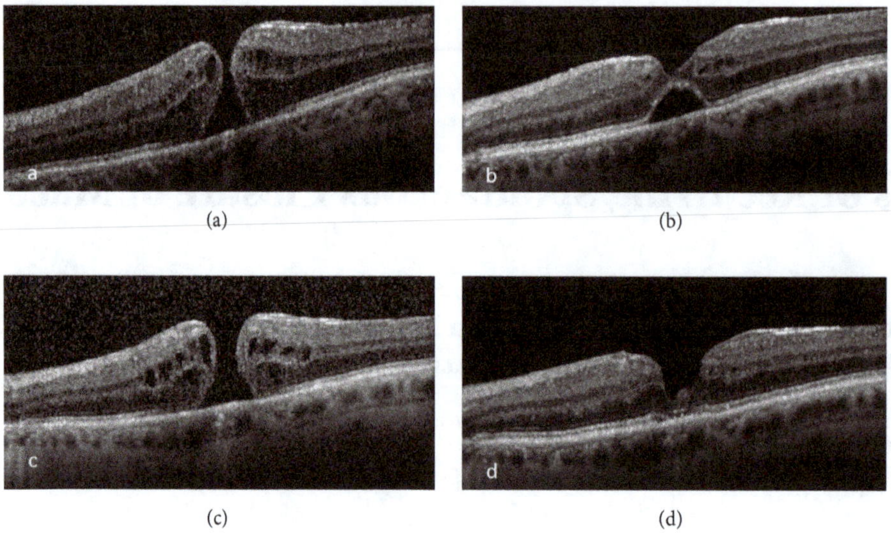

FIGURE 1: Optical coherence tomography showing (a) full thickness macular hole, (b) first closure of macular hole with residual subretinal fluid, (c) reopening of macular hole, and (d) second closure of the macular hole.

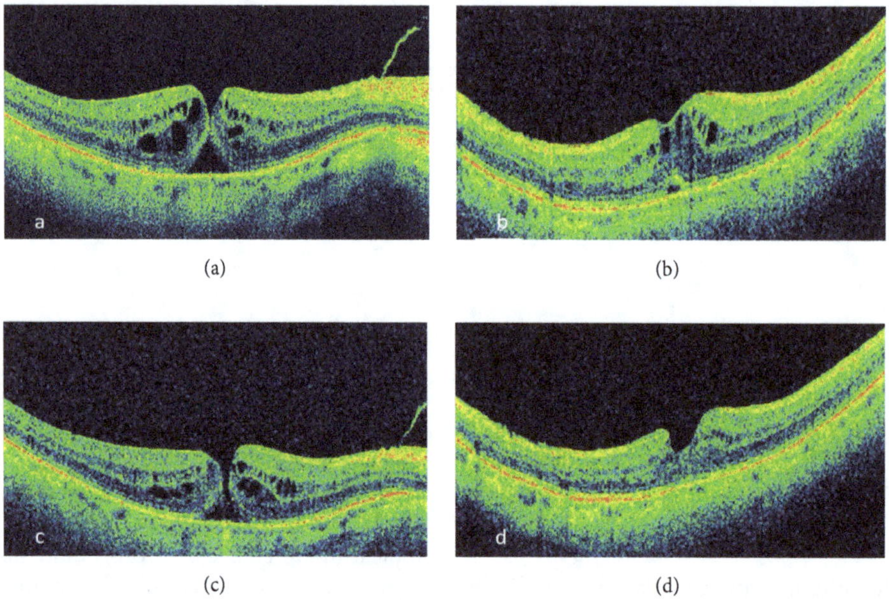

FIGURE 2: Optical coherence tomography showing (a) tiny full thickness macular hole, (b) first closure of macular hole, (c) reopening of macular hole, and (d) reclosure of macular hole.

Case 2. A 73-year-old male patient presented with a 2-month history of decreased vision OD (20/60). OCT showed a thinned fovea, progressing over 2 weeks into a tiny MH (Figure 2(a)). The patient was counseled about the treatment options and MHS was scheduled. 6 weeks later, vision improved (20/50), and OCT showed a closed MH although with residual CME (Figure 2(b)). 3 months later, MH had reopened (Figure 2(c)) with decreased vision (20/70), but the patient deferred MHS. Over 3 months, MH gradually reapproximated and closed with residual intraretinal CME and SRF which resolved slowly over 6 months (Figure 2(d)) with improved BCVA to 20/50 and remained stable during the next 7 months.

Case 3. An 85-year-old female patient with a history of pseudoexfoliative glaucoma presented with a 4-month history of decreased vision OD (20/60). OCT showed MH (Figure 3(a)). 1 month later, spontaneous closure of the MH was observed (Figure 2(b)) with BCVA of 20/50. After 3 years, patient complained of a central scotoma OD. BCVA was 20/70. OCT showed a MH with intraretinal cystic spaces (Figure 3(c)). MHS was recommended but the patient declined. 1 month

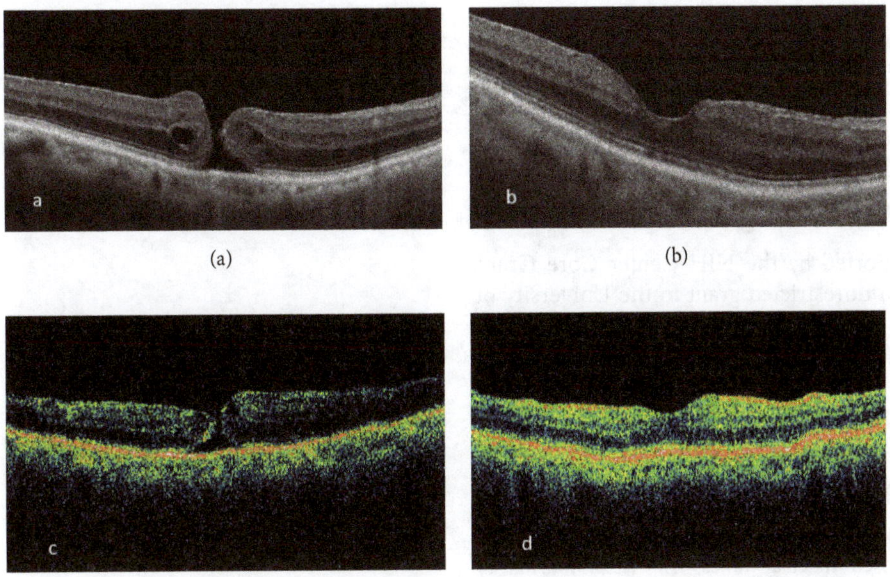

(a) (b) (c) (d)

FIGURE 3: Optical coherence tomography showing (a) full thickness macular hole, (b) first closure of the macular hole, (c) reopening of the macular hole, and (d) second closure of macular hole.

later, the MH had again spontaneously closed with a few cystic spaces and minimal SRF which resolved gradually (Figure 3(d)) although the BCVA was 20/125.

3. Conclusions

These three cases represent an unusual occurrence in which a macular hole spontaneously closed, opened, and then closed again. Spontaneous closure of a MH has been widely reported [4]. Also reopening of a previously surgically or spontaneously closed MH has been described [5]. A case with multiple spontaneous opening and closure of a myopic MH was reported [6]. Nivolumab-associated uveitis (present in Case 1) has only rarely been reported to cause CME but has never been reported in association with a MH.

The mechanism of spontaneous MH closure is unknown, but several hypotheses have been reported. OCT findings suggest that relief of anteroposterior traction after posterior hyaloid separation results in flattening of the MH edges [7]. This may then allow cells to bridge the hole and result in spontaneous MH closure. A postmortem histopathologic study suggested exposed retinal pigment epithelial (RPE) cells play a role by migrating onto the inner retinal surface, proliferate and contract circumferentially, pulling MH edges centripetally to facilitate spontaneous closure [8]. This seemed to be consistent with a clinical case report [5]. The normal accumulation of intraretinal fluid is a characteristic, but variably severe, feature of early MH formation; we hypothesize that frank CME might facilitate spontaneous closure by reapproximating the edges through physical expansion, a sort of healing by primary intention. Intercurrent CME, as in uveitis or otherwise, might exercise this effect. CME seemed to have been present in this way in case 2 when the spontaneous closure occurred.

Also, the mechanism of MH reopening is not understood. Chronic or recurrent CME might play a (different) role in some cases by weakening retinal tissue (particularly Muller cells). This may cause progressive retinal attenuation or render degenerated retina more vulnerable to incidental retinal surface or vitreous traction [3]. Gass proposed that rupture of the cystic spaces inner wall resulted in collapse of the cyst with subsequent retraction of the adjacent retinal tissue forming lamellar macular hole [9], so potentially a full thickness defect could similarly result. Uveitis has been reported to be associated with MH formation through either CME or chorioretinitis-induced structural weakening, vitreous liquefaction causing anomalous vitreomacular adhesions, or ERM formation [2].

Nivolumab is a recently approved checkpoint inhibitor, a monoclonal antibody for treatment of metastatic melanoma, renal carcinoma, and treatment-resistant cancer. It binds to programmed cell death protein 1 receptors on T-lymphocytes to enhance the host immunity against neoplastic cells [10]. Activation of the immune system may lead to adverse events such as autoimmune uveitis, hepatitis, pneumonitis, and renal failure [10]. Rarely reported ocular adverse effects of nivolumab-induced inflammatory cytokines include uveitis, Vogt-Koyanagi-Harada like syndrome, dry eye, keratitis, and CME [10]. Nivolumab-induced uveitis with CME has been sparsely reported previously, but not in association with MH formation as in Case 1. Nivolumab and ipilimumab (Yervoy) in combination have been associated with improved survival in cancer patients; ipilimumab has also been reported to cause ocular and orbital inflammation but was not used in our patient.

Disclosure

All authors attest that they meet the current ICMJE criteria for authorship.

Acknowledgments

This study was supported by the NIH Center Core Grant P30EY014801 and an unrestricted grant to the University of Miami from the Research to Prevent Blindness.

References

[1] E. Privat, R. Tadayoni, D. Gaucher, B. Haouchine, P. Massin, and A. Gaudric, "Residual defect in the foveal photoreceptor layer detected by optical coherence tomography in eyes with spontaneously closed macular holes," *American Journal of Ophthalmology*, vol. 143, no. 5, pp. 814–819.e1, 2007.

[2] N. Bonnin, P. Cornut, F. Chaise et al., "Spontaneous closure of macular holes secondary to posterior uveitis: case series and a literature review," *Journal of Ophthalmic Inflammation and Infection*, vol. 3, no. 1, p. 34, 2013.

[3] A. Lecleire-Collet, O. Offret, D. Gaucher, F. Audren, B. Haouchine, and P. Massin, "Full-thickness macular hole in a patient with diabetic cystoid macular oedema treated by intravitreal triamcinolone injections," *Acta Ophthalmologica Scandinavica*, vol. 85, no. 7, pp. 795–798, 2007.

[4] O. S. Punjabi, H. W. Flynn Jr., J. E. Legarreta, G. Gregori, R. W. Knighton, and C. A. Puliafito, "Documentation by spectral domain OCT of spontaneous closure of idiopathic macular holes," *Ophthalmic Surgery, Lasers & Imaging Retina*, vol. 38, no. 4, pp. 330–332, 2007.

[5] J. G. Gross, "Late reopening and spontaneous closure of previously repaired macular holes," *American Journal of Ophthalmology*, vol. 140, no. 3, pp. 556–558, 2005.

[6] S. Golan and A. Barak, "Third time spontaneous closure of myopic macular hole," *Retinal Cases & Brief Reports*, vol. 9, no. 1, pp. 13-14, 2015.

[7] M. Ishida, S. TakeuchI, and S. Okisaka, "Optical coherence tomography images of idiopathic macular holes with spontaneous closure," *Retina*, vol. 24, no. 4, pp. 625–628, 2004.

[8] D. R. Guyer, W. R. Green, S. de Bustros, and S. L. Fine, "Histopathologic features of idiopathic macular holes and cysts," *Retina*, vol. 11, no. 4, p. 446, 1991.

[9] J. D. Gass, "Lamellar macular hole," *JAMA Ophtalmology*, vol. 94, no. 5, p. 793, 1976.

[10] D. Richardson, B. Ellis, I. Mehmi, and M. Leys, "Bilateral uveitis associated with nivolumab therapy for metastatic melanoma: a case report," *International Journal of Ophthalmology*, vol. 10, no. 7, pp. 1183–1186, 2017.

Vision Improvement after Osimertinib Treatment in Paraneoplastic Optic Neuropathy Associated with Lung Adenocarcinoma

Masaomi Kubota,[1] **Nobumasa Tamura**,[2] **Takaaki Hayashi**,[1] **Euido Nishijima**,[3] **Haruhiko Yanagisawa**,[2] **Akira Kojima**,[2] **and Tadashi Nakano**[3]

[1]*Department of Ophthalmology, Katsushika Medical Center, The Jikei University School of Medicine, 6-41-2, Aoto, Katsushika-ku, Tokyo 125-8506, Japan*
[2]*Department of Respiratory Medicine, Katsushika Medical Center, The Jikei University School of Medicine, 6-41-2, Aoto, Katsushika-ku, Tokyo 125-8506, Japan*
[3]*Department of Ophthalmology, The Jikei University School of Medicine, 3-25-8, Nishi-shimbashi, Minato-ku, Tokyo 105-8461, Japan*

Correspondence should be addressed to Takaaki Hayashi; taka@jikei.ac.jp

Academic Editor: Alexander A. Bialasiewicz

Treatments for paraneoplastic optic neuropathy (PON), a tumor-related autoimmune disease, include immunosuppression, plasma exchange, and immunoglobulin therapies, as well as treatment of the underlying disease. Herein, we describe the clinical course of an older adult patient with PON whose loss of vision improved after switching between epidermal growth factor receptor-tyrosine kinase inhibitor (EGFR-TKI) treatments for cancer. A 76-year-old woman, who had been treated with gefitinib for lung adenocarcinoma for two years, presented with acute bilateral visual disturbances. Her decimal best-corrected visual acuity (BCVA) was 0.3 in the right eye (RE) and 0.7 in the left eye (LE). Slit-lamp examination and funduscopy showed no abnormal findings. Two weeks later, her BCVA decreased to 0.2 in the RE and 0.01 in the LE. Goldman's perimetry showed a defect in the lower nasal RE and extensive visual-field loss in the LE. Single-flash electroretinograms showed normal amplitudes. Magnetic resonance imaging revealed left optic neuritis and showed neither metastatic cancer nor multiple sclerosis. Pattern-reversal visual evoked potentials showed decreased P100 amplitudes in both eyes (BE). Based on a diagnosis of PON from clinical findings, methylprednisolone pulse treatment was administered. However, her BCVA became no light perception in BE two months after the first visit. Because the tumor tissue was found to be positive for the EGFR T790M resistance mutation by bronchoscopy, the EGFR-TKI treatment was changed to osimertinib, decreasing the size of the lung cancer lesions. Her BCVA improved to hand motion in BE. Her final BCVA was 0.01 in the RE, counting fingers 10 cm in the LE. She died at the age of 79 years. To our knowledge, no reports have shown improvement in BCVA in patients with PON after changing EGFR-TKI treatments. This report indicates that some patients may develop severe visual dysfunction without early treatment for the primary tumor.

1. Introduction

Paraneoplastic optic neuropathy (PON) is one of several tumor-related autoimmune diseases, such as cancer-associated retinopathy (CAR) and melanoma-associated retinopathy (MAR) [1, 2]. Malignant tumors, such as small-cell lung cancer and malignant lymphoma, are known to cause PON [1, 2], but it can also be caused by benign tumors, such as choroid meningioma [3]. Patients with PON usually exhibit bilateral subacute vision loss and cerebellar ataxia, and other neurologic deficits are seen in some patients [2]. It has been reported that anti-CV2/collapsin response-

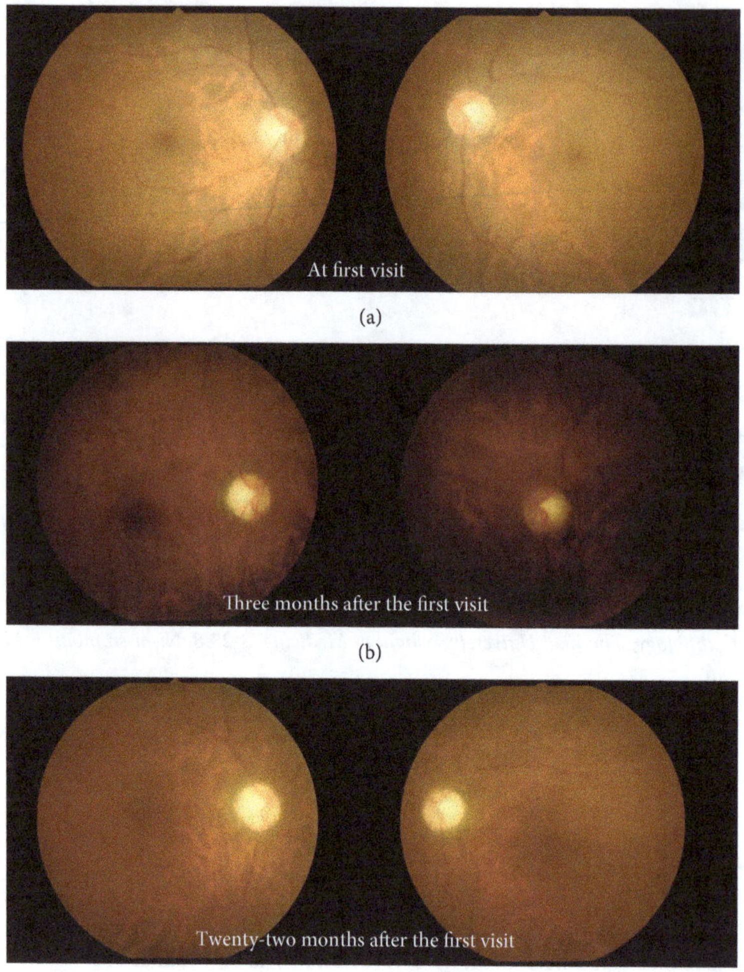

(c)

FIGURE 1: Fundus photographs. (a) At the first visit, funduscopy showed an almost normal appearance in both eyes. (b) Three months after the first visit, funduscopy showed optic disc pallor in both eyes. (c) Twenty-two months after the first visit, the optic disc pallor remained unchanged.

mediator protein-5 (CRMP-5) antibody is detected in PON associated with small-cell lung cancer [2]. In some patients with autoimmune optic neuropathies, visual function can be improved with corticosteroid treatment, and overall visual prognosis is better compared to those of CAR and MAR [1]. However, visual prognosis of PON depends upon responsiveness to treatment for the underlying malignancies [4, 5]. Herein, we describe the clinical course of an older adult patient diagnosed with and treated for PON associated with lung adenocarcinoma.

2. Case Presentation

A 76-year-old woman presented with acute bilateral visual disturbances starting one week prior to the first visit. She had been diagnosed with advanced stage 4 lung adenocarcinoma two years prior and treated with the first-generation epidermal growth factor receptor-tyrosine kinase inhibitor (EGFR-TKI), gefitinib, due to a somatic EGFR exon-19 deletion mutation.

Her decimal best-corrected visual acuity (BCVA) was 0.3 in the right eye (RE) and 0.7 in the left eye (LE). Slit-lamp examination showed mild cataracts and no inflammatory cells in the anterior chamber and media. Funduscopy revealed no abnormal findings in the optic disc, retina, or vitreous humor in both eyes (BE) (Figure 1(a)). One week after presentation, her BCVA was decreased to 0.15 in the LE with a relative afferent pupillary defect.

One week later, her BCVA was severely decreased to 0.2 in the RE and 0.01 in the LE. Goldman's perimetry (GP; Haag-Streit, Bern, Switzerland) showed a visual-field defect in the lower nasal RE and extensive visual-field loss in the LE (Figure 2(a)). However, spectral-domain optical coherence tomography (OCT; Carl Zeiss Meditec AG, Dublin, CA, USA) revealed no remarkable findings in all retinal layers nor swelling around the optic discs in BE (Figures 3(a) and 3(b)). Dark-adapted single-flash electroretinograms (ERG; LE-4000, Tomey, Nagoya, Japan) using a strong flash (200 cd s m^{-2}) showed normal amplitudes in BE (Figure 4(a)). We consulted neurologists for the possibility of retrobulbar optic neuritis, multiple sclerosis, or neuromyelitis optica. Brain and orbital

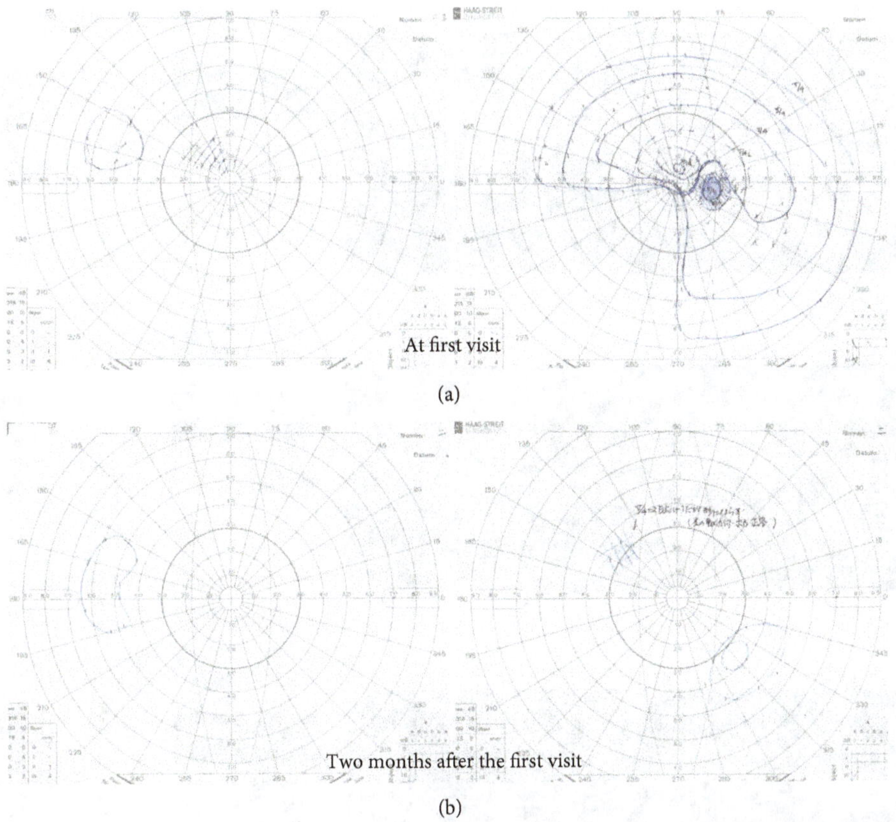

Figure 2: Visual fields. (a) At the first visit, Goldman's perimetry (GP) showed a visual-field defect of the lower nasal right eye and extensive visual-field loss in the left eye. (b) Two months after the first visit, GP showed severe visual-field defects with peripheral visual islands in both eyes.

magnetic resonance imaging (MRI) revealed left optic neuritis but showed neither metastatic cancer nor the white matter lesions seen in multiple sclerosis (Figure 5(a)). Cerebrospinal fluid examination revealed no remarkable findings. Full-field pattern-reversal visual evoked potentials (VEPs) showed decreased P100 amplitudes in BE, indicating bilateral optic neuropathy (Figure 4(e)).

Three weeks after the first visit, her BCVA had further decreased to 0.02 in the RE and no light perception (NLP) in the LE, and ERG showed slightly decreased oscillatory potentials (OPs) in BE (Figure 4(b)). Treatment with oral prednisolone was started at 30 mg per day and gradually tapered, but there was no improvement in visual function. Her BCVA decreased to light perception (LP) in the RE and NLP in the LE after the first treatment, and to NLP bilaterally one week later with dilated pupil and absence of the pupillary light reflex. Subsequently, three courses of methylprednisolone (1,000 mg per day) pulse treatment was administered for 3 days but her visual acuity did not improve; her BCVA remained NLP bilaterally at two months after the first visit.

Serum autoantibody tests were negative for anti-aquaporin-4 and anti-myelin-oligodendrocyte glycoprotein (MOG) by enzyme-linked immunosorbent assay. Autoantibodies, such as anti-Tr/DNER, anti-GAD65, anti-ZIC4, anti-TITIN, anti-SX1, anti-recoverin, anti-Hu, anti-Yo, anti-Ri, anti-PNMA (Ma2/Ta), anti-CV2/CRMP-5, and amphiphysin antibodies, were negative by immunochromatography analysis. Clinically, PON was diagnosed by exclusion diagnosis.

As transbronchial lung biopsy of the primary lesion revealed the acquired EGFR T790M resistance mutation, her EGFR-TKI treatment was changed from gefitinib to osimertinib, a third-generation EGFR-TKI. Subsequently, her primary and metastatic lung cancer lesions decreased in size.

One week after the change in EGFR-TKI treatment, her BCVA had improved to hand motion in BE. Two months after the first visit, GP showed severe visual-field defects but recovered peripheral visual islands in BE (Figure 2(b)). Orbital MRI showed improvement in the enhanced left optic nerve (Figure 5(b)); however, the ERG response had not changed in BE (Figure 4(c)).

Three months after the first visit, her BCVA further improved to counting fingers (CF) 20 cm in BE. However, pattern-reversal VEPs were nonrecordable in BE. The ERG showed markedly decreased OPs in BE (Figure 4(f)). Funduscopy revealed optic disc pallor (Figure 1(b)), and OCT showed thinning of all layers of the macula and the neuroretinal rim of the optic nerve head in BE (Figures 3(c) and 3(d)), although there was improvement of visual acuity (from NLP to CF). Additional MRI scans (Figure 5(b)) performed during the course of the disease showed no evidence of optic neuropathy or optic nerve abnormalities.

At her final visit, approximately two years after the first visit, her BCVA remained 0.01 in the RE and CF 10 cm in

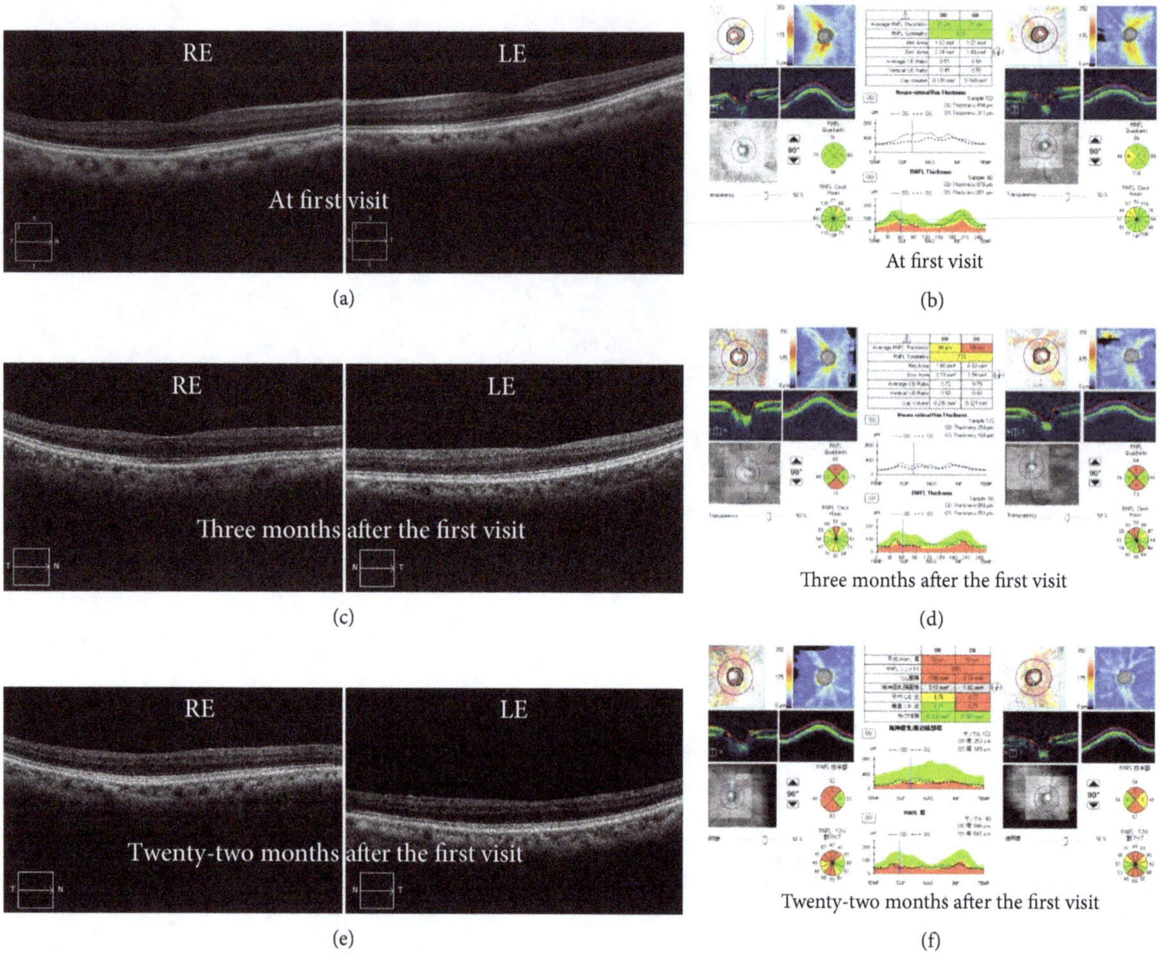

FIGURE 3: Optical coherence tomography (OCT) imaging. At the first visit, OCT revealed no remarkable findings on the macula and optic discs in both eyes (a, b). However, the macula (c, e) and optic disc head (d, f) had thinned in both eyes during the clinical course.

the LE, and funduscopy showed optic disc pallor in BE (Figure 1(c)). OCT revealed the thinned macula and optic nerve head (Figures 3(e) and 3(f)). Visual acuity and treatment timeline were described in Figure 6. She died at the age of 79 years.

3. Discussion

In this report, we describe a rare case of clinically diagnosed PON associated with lung adenocarcinoma in which visual acuity was initially improved after switching between EGFR-TKI treatments, but ultimately resulted in severe loss of visual acuity. To our knowledge, no reports have demonstrated improvement in visual acuity by changing EGFR-TKI treatments during the treatment of PON.

The differential diagnosis of a disease that causes rapid vision loss with no findings in the optic disc or retina at the first visit includes posterior ischemic optic neuropathy (PION), CAR, and PON. PION was excluded because our patient had none of the risk factors (e.g., coagulopathies; ischemic heart disease, such as angina or myocardial infarction; and stenosis of the internal carotid artery) and no inflammation; moreover, the onset was subacute and binocular, and the course was progressive.

CAR and MAR are well known for progressive retinal degeneration, which is a frequent complication in patients with cancer, and an absence of obvious abnormalities by funduscopy at the first consultation. Anti-recoverin antibodies are often detected in CAR and anti-bipolar cell antibodies (e.g., anti-TRPM1) in MAR as specific serum autoantibodies. Further, ERG shows extremely reduced a- and b-wave responses in CAR and a negative-ERG pattern in MAR. However, in our patient, CAR and MAR were excluded based on the normal ERG findings, lack of night blindness, and absence of anti-recoverin antibodies at the first visit. Furthermore, immune-mediated optic neuritis, such as MS and NMO, were ruled out as tests were negative for anti-aquaporin antibody and anti-MOG antibody. We established PON as exclusion diagnosis based on clinical findings in total. On the other hand, the T2 signal of MRI in LE at the first visit of this patient was increased. This may have been an inflammatory process, but there is also a case report of increased signal on MRI in cases of PON [6]. In this case, an increase in the signal of the left eye on the MRI T2 image was considered to be consistent with the diagnosis of PON. The enhancement of the RE is unknown because no contrast-enhanced MRI was performed, but the reason that the increase in signal was unilateral was that the onset was

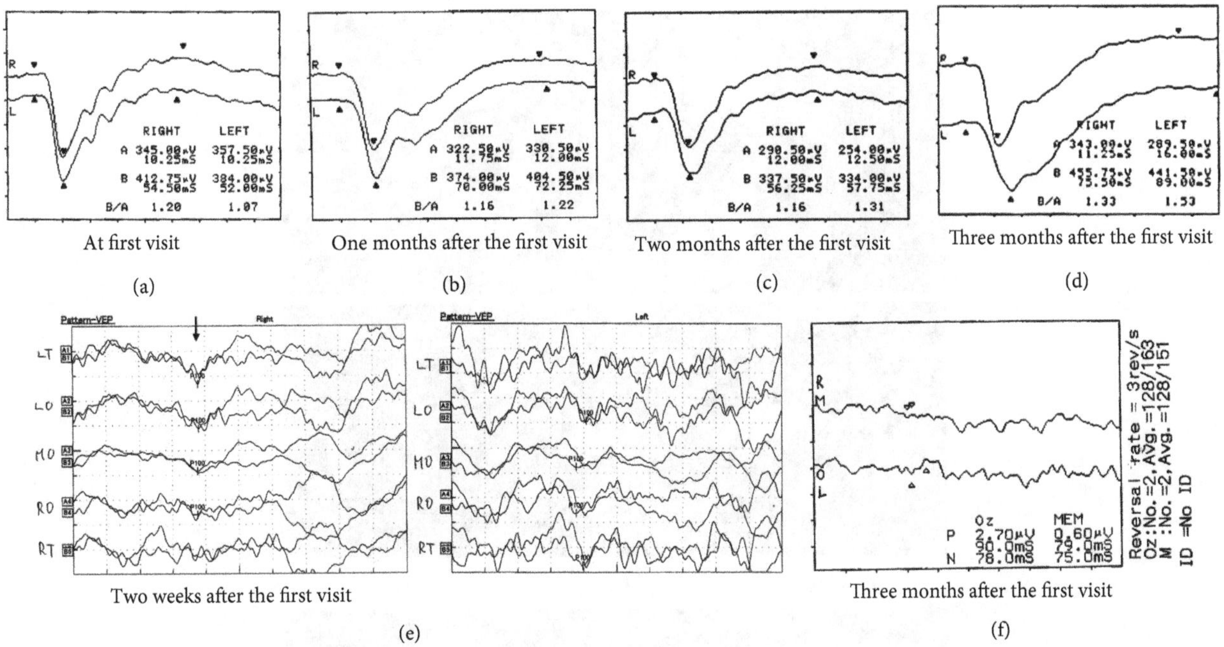

Figure 4: Dark-adapted single-flash electroretinograms (ERG) and pattern visual evoked potential (VEP) findings. (a) At the first visit, ERG showed normal amplitudes in both eyes (BE). (b) One month after the first visit, ERG showed slightly decreased oscillatory potentials (OPs) in BE. (c) After changing the EGFR-TKI treatment, the ERG response did not change in BE two months after the first visit. (d) Three months after the first visit, ERG showed markedly decreased OPs in BE. (e) VEP two weeks after the first visit had decreased P100 amplitudes in the midline occipital region of BE. (f) VEPs are non-recordable in BE.

predominantly in the LE, with marked loss of visual acuity. It is possible that the signal increase in the RE was minimal on T2-weighted MRI.

PON is an autoimmune optic neuropathy, and CRMP-5 has been most frequently reported as an autoantigen associated with PON [2, 7–9]. Anti-CRMP-5-positive PON develops as optic neuritis with anterior vitreous cells, optic disc swelling, and leakage of the optic disc on fluorescein angiography [4, 5]. On the other hand, some patients with PON do not have swelling of the optic disc [8]. Although the detection of anti-CRMP-5 gives a definitive diagnosis of PON, most patients with PON and anti-CRMP-5 antibodies have small-cell lung cancer. There are few reports of specific autoantibodies in PON due to lung adenocarcinoma [10]. In this case, serum autoantibody testing, including anti-CRMP-5, was negative and no retinal/vitreous inflammation nor optic disc swelling was observed during the clinical course. However, PON was diagnosed based on the history of lung adenocarcinoma and on clinical examination.

Because PON is an autoimmune disease, corticosteroid therapy is the first-line treatment, and plasma exchange/plasmapheresis or immunoglobulin therapies are considered second-line therapies. In a review by Chan, oral prednisolone therapy was frequently reported, the response to corticosteroids was relatively good, and the visual prognosis was better than those of CAR or MAR [1], demonstrating that 8/11 patients with PON exhibited improvement of their visual field to normal or nearly normal after treatments. Therefore, the prognosis of visual function is also thought to be dependent on responsiveness to the treatment of the underlying malignant tumors [4, 5]. There has been a report that plasmapheresis therapy in addition to immunosuppression therapies were effective to preserve visual acuity [11]. In our patient, the first treatment with prednisolone did not influence visual acuity outcomes, and three courses of methylprednisolone pulse treatment were ineffective. However, after switching from gefitinib to osimertinib for systemic treatment with anticancer drugs, the primary lung cancer lesions and systemic metastasis were reduced, and visual acuity was notably improved.

When EGFR-TKI is administered for first-line treatment of EGFR mutation-positive non-small-cell lung cancer, many patients acquire resistance, and it has been reported that the EGFR T790M mutation accounts for approximately 60% of the resistance mechanism [12, 13]. Osimertinib, an EGFR-TKI that is effective despite resistance associated with the T790M mutation, is selected as the second-line treatment. In our patient, bronchoscopy performed during steroid pulse therapy revealed acquisition of the EGFR T790M mutation.

In some cases, loss of visual acuity and visual-field defects can be improved transiently in response to corticosteroid monotherapy; however, it has been suggested that ultimate visual function cannot be preserved unless the tumor is reduced in size early after the onset of optic neuropathy. PON associated with lung adenocarcinoma may have a different mechanism from that of small-cell lung carcinoma, with which anti-CRMP-5 antibodies are associated. However, there are few reports of PON associated with lung adenocarcinoma [10, 14], and a number of autoantibodies related to autoimmune optic neuropathies are yet to be

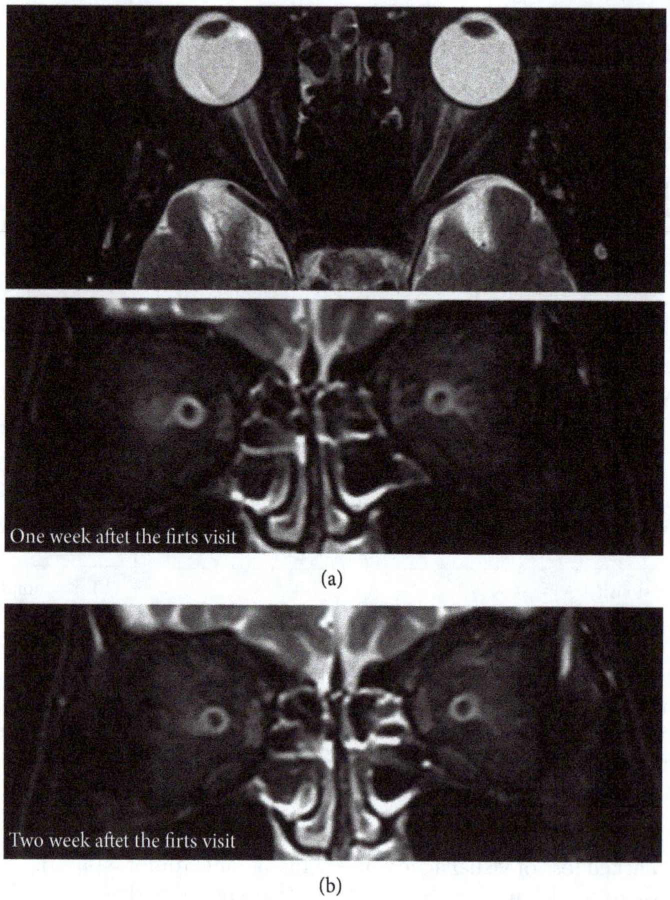

FIGURE 5: Magnetic resonance imaging (MRI). (a) One week after the first visit, T2-weighted MRI demonstrates well-marked enhancement of the left optic nerve compared to the right optic nerve. (b) Two months after the first visit, MRI showed improvement in the enhancement of the left optic nerve.

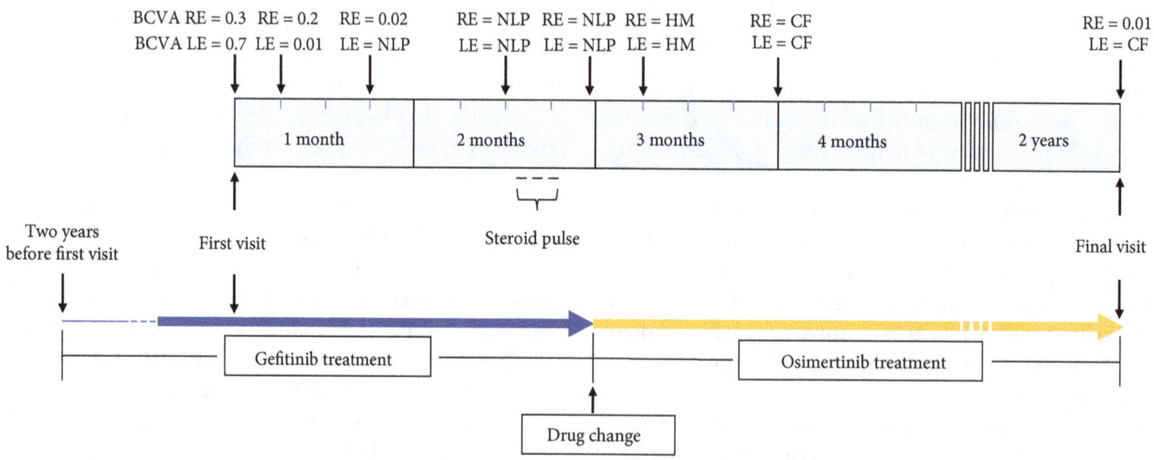

FIGURE 6: Visual acuity and treatment timeline. Decimal best-corrected visual acuity (BCVA) is described from the first visit to the final visit. RE: right eye; LE: left eye; CF: counting fingers; HM: hand motion; NLP: no light perception. Gefitinib is changed to osimertinib two months after the first visit. Three courses of steroid pulse treatment are administered before changing to osimertinib.

identified. In our patient, the reduced tumor size by osimertinib treatment might lead to a reduction of unknown autoantibody production. Further studies on autoantibodies associated with PON are needed.

4. Conclusion

Generally, although loss of vision is improved by immunosuppressive treatment, such as corticosteroids, at an early stage in some cases of PON, improved visual function cannot be preserved without treatment of the underlying tumor. In our patient, changing treatment to osimertinib for primary lung adenocarcinoma resulted in visual acuity improvement. This indicates the importance of thoroughly treating the primary cancer for the treatment of PON.

References

[1] J. W. Chan, "Paraneoplastic retinopathies and optic neuropathies," *Survey of Ophthalmology*, vol. 48, no. 1, pp. 12–38, 2003.

[2] M. W. Ko, J. Dalmau, and S. L. Galetta, "Neuro-ophthalmologic manifestations of paraneoplastic syndromes," *Journal of Neuro-Ophthalmology*, vol. 28, no. 1, pp. 58–68, 2008.

[3] S. Nakano, A. Kanamori, M. Nakamura, K. Mizukawa, and A. Negi, "Paraneoplastic optic neuropathy associated with cerebellar choroid meningioma," *Eye (London, England)*, vol. 27, no. 10, pp. 1220-1221, 2013.

[4] J. E. Luiz, A. G. Lee, J. L. Keltner, C. E. Thirkill, and E. C. Lai, "Paraneoplastic optic neuropathy and autoantibody production in small-cell carcinoma of the lung," *Journal of Neuro-Ophthalmology*, vol. 18, no. 3, pp. 178–181, 1998.

[5] V. de la Sayette, F. Bertran, J. Honnorat, S. Schaeffer, S. Iglesias, and G. Defer, "Paraneoplastic cerebellar syndrome and optic neuritis with anti-CV2 antibodies: clinical response to excision of the primary tumor," *Archives of Neurology*, vol. 55, no. 3, pp. 405–408, 1998.

[6] R. Sheorajpanday, H. Slabbynck, W. Van De Sompel, D. Galdermans, I. Neetens, and P. P. De Deyn, "Small cell lung carcinoma presenting as collapsin response-mediating protein (CRMP) -5 paraneoplastic optic neuropathy," *Journal of Neuro-Ophthalmology*, vol. 26, no. 3, pp. 168–172, 2006.

[7] Z. Yu, T. J. Kryzer, G. E. Griesmann, K. Kim, E. E. Benarroch, and V. A. Lennon, "CRMP-5 neuronal autoantibody: marker of lung cancer and thymoma-related autoimmunity," *Annals of Neurology*, vol. 49, no. 2, pp. 146–154, 2001.

[8] S. A. Cross, D. R. Salomao, J. E. Parisi et al., "Paraneoplastic autoimmune optic neuritis with retinitis defined by CRMP-5-IgG," *Annals of Neurology*, vol. 54, no. 1, pp. 38–50, 2003.

[9] G. Adamus, L. Brown, J. Schiffman, and A. Iannaccone, "Diversity in autoimmunity against retinal, neuronal, and axonal antigens in acquired neuro-retinopathy," *Journal of ophthalmic inflammation and infection*, vol. 1, no. 3, pp. 111–121, 2011.

[10] Y. Murakami, S. Yoshida, H. Yoshikawa et al., "CRMP-5-IgG in patient with paraneoplastic optic neuritis with lung adenocarcinoma," *Eye (London, England)*, vol. 21, no. 6, pp. 860-862, 2007.

[11] A. Durrani, R. J. Shah, and S. J. Kim, "Successful long-term treatment of paraneoplastic optic neuropathy with mycophenolate mofetil, prednisone, and plasmapheresis," *American journal of ophthalmology case reports*, vol. 8, pp. 31–34, 2017.

[12] S. Kobayashi, T. J. Boggon, T. Dayaram et al., "EGFR mutation and resistance of non-small-cell lung cancer to gefitinib," *The New England Journal of Medicine*, vol. 352, no. 8, pp. 786-792, 2005.

[13] W. Pao, V. A. Miller, K. A. Politi et al., "Acquired resistance of lung adenocarcinomas to gefitinib or erlotinib is associated with a second mutation in the EGFR kinase domain," *PLoS medicine*, vol. 2, no. 3, p. e73, 2005.

[14] A. Oohira, T. Inoue, N. Fukuda, and K. Uchida, "A case with paraneoplastic optic neuropathy presenting bitemporal hemianopsia," *Neuroophthalmology*, vol. 11, no. 6, pp. 61–64, 1991.

20

A Case of Cat Scratch Disease with Neuroretinitis in a 16-Month-Old Boy

Daisuke Nakata ,[1,2] Sayaka Kakehi,[1] Hiroshi Okada,[1] Atsuhiro Tanikawa ,[2] Yoshiaki Shimada,[2] Masayuki Horiguchi,[2] and Yasuki Ito[2]

[1]*Department of Ophthalmology, Toyokawa City Hospital, Toyokawa, Aichi, Japan*
[2]*Department of Ophthalmology, Fujita Health University, School of Medicine, Toyoake, Aichi, Japan*

Correspondence should be addressed to Daisuke Nakata; dnakata@fujita-hu.ac.jp

Academic Editor: J. Fernando Arevalo

Purpose. We report a case of neuroretinitis associated with cat scratch disease (CSD) in young children. *Method.* Case report. *Results.* A 16-month-old boy was admitted for a detailed examination and treatment of a fever of unknown origin. Blood tests revealed no significant findings other than a white blood cell count of $16,100/mm^3$ and C-reactive protein level of 9.89 mg/dL. Computed tomography revealed no relevant findings to determine the causative disease. Antibiotic therapy with cefotaxime was initiated; however, the fever did not resolve. The patient was referred to our department for further examination to detect the cause of the fever. Fundoscopy revealed neuroretinitis in the right eye. His mother reported a history of breeding cats. Cat scratch disease (CSD) was suspected based on the clinical course and fundus findings. Cefotaxime was discontinued, and azithromycin, rifampicin, and prednisolone were administered, following which the fever disappeared and fundus findings improved. Immunoglobulin G (IgG) and IgM antibodies against *Bartonella henselae* was positive, leading to a definitive diagnosis of CSD. *Conclusion.* Infants cannot complain of decreased visual acuity; therefore, these findings may be overlooked unless a fundus examination is performed. As in this case, the early detection of neuroretinitis by an ophthalmologist may help in the diagnosis of CSD. It is extremely difficult to capture a photograph of the fundus of an infant, and recording with a smartphone is relatively simple and useful for monitoring continuous changes. *Summary.* We describe a case of neuroretinitis associated with cat scratch disease (CSD) that was diagnosed on the basis of fundus findings. The findings suggest the importance of an aggressive ophthalmologic examination when CSD is suspected in young children who are unable to describe their symptoms.

1. Introduction

Cat scratch disease (CSD) is a zoonotic disease caused by *Bartonella henselae*, which is transmitted through cat scratches and cat fleas. It is characterized by symptoms such as fever, local lymphadenitis, and redness of the injured area. In recent years, atypical cases with central nervous system and ocular symptoms have been reported [1–10]; the frequency of the complications of neuroretinitis is approximately 1%–2% [1, 2].

It is relatively difficult to photograph the fundus in infants during examination, and it requires expensive equipment. In recent years, the usefulness of anterior segment and fundus photography using smartphones has been reported, which facilitates convenient recording of the ophthalmologic findings [11, 12].

We present a case of neuroretinitis associated with CSD that was diagnosed through the examination of the fundus. Moreover, we observed the progress of neuroretinitis by photographing the fundus using a smartphone.

2. Case Presentation

A 16-month-old boy was admitted to our department for the assessment of a fever of unknown origin. The patient's medical history was insignificant. In early October 2021, the patient visited a local doctor with a complaint of a fever of 39°C and was prescribed acetaminophen (100 mg/day). Since the fever persisted, he was admitted to the Department of Pediatrics at Toyokawa City Hospital on October 11, 2021 for a detailed examination and treatment of the fever.

Physical examination on admission revealed a body temperature of 38.2°C and no obvious lymphadenopathy or rash. Blood tests revealed no significant findings other than a white blood cell count of $16{,}100/mm^3$ and C-reactive protein level of 9.89 mg/dL, indicating an increased inflammatory response. In addition, computed tomography (CT) from the head to the pelvis revealed no lymphadenopathy, liver or intra-abdominal abscess, or any findings that could identify the cause of the fever.

Antibiotic therapy with cefotaxime (100 mg/kg/day) was initiated, but the fever persisted. Echocardiography revealed no evidence of infective endocarditis or Kawasaki disease, and an otolaryngology examination ruled out otitis media and sinusitis. The patient was referred to our department on October 13, 2021 for the assessment of the fever.

No distinct findings were noted in the anterior segment of the eye. Redness and swelling of the optic disc, serous retinal detachment from the same site to the macula, and macular star exudates were observed in the fundus of the right eye (shown in Figure 1). No abnormalities were observed in the left eye.

The next day, no intracranial lesions were observed under magnetic resonance imaging of the head; the fundus was photographed using a smartphone (iPhone8™, Apple Inc., CA, USA) and a 20-D lens, and the fundus findings were recorded. The shooting method employed was as previously reported [11, 12], and the fundus photograph was captured in the video mode of the smartphone camera application and saved as a still image. The fundus examination revealed neuroretinitis. Upon subsequent enquiry, his mother reported a history of breeding cats and his sister had a history of hospitalization for lymphadenitis. Based on the clinical course and fundus findings, neuroretinitis associated with CSD was suspected, and a *Bartonella* antibody test was performed. Treatment with cefotaxime was discontinued, and azithromycin (10 mg/kg/day), rifampicin (20 mg/kg/day), and prednisolone (1 mg/kg/day) were initiated.

The fever promptly subsided, the fundus findings improved, and the patient was discharged on October 19, 2021. Later, upon testing, the immunoglobulin G (IgG) and IgM antibodies against *Bartonella henselae* were 512 (less than the standard 64 times positive) and 80 (less than the standard 20 times positive), respectively, resulting in a definitive diagnosis of CSD. Antibiotics were administered along with steroids at a tapering dose, and the papilledema of the optic disc and retinal detachment disappeared. No recurrence of optic disc swelling or retinal detachment and no formation of hard exudates in the macula (shown in Figure 2) were observed in the 2-month follow-up. Since then, the patient has been followed-up at an outpatient clinic.

3. Discussion

We encountered a case of neuroretinitis associated with CSD, which was not accompanied by local lymphadenopathy and whose fundus findings triggered the identification of the etiology of the patient's fever of unknown origin. Although ocular symptoms are relatively rare in CSD, 5% of the ocular lesions are predominantly conjunctivitis-based anterior ocular inflammation (Parinaud's syndrome), and 1% occur following neuroretinitis or chorioretinitis, which reportedly result in eye inflammation [1–4]. In an epidemiological study of fever of unknown origin in children by Kasai et al. [5], infectious diseases accounted for 23% of all cases, with CSD being the most common. It is important to consider CSD when fever of unknown origin occurs.

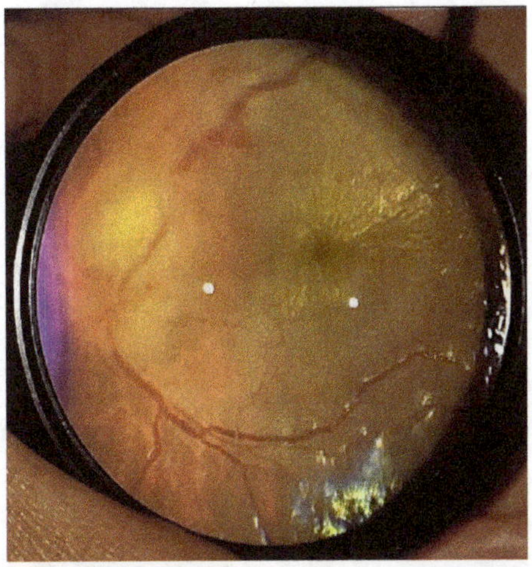

FIGURE 1: Right eye at the first visit of the examination: papilledema and macular star exudates imaged using a smartphone.

Neuroretinitis develops with papilledema and macular edema, and macular star exudates are observed over time. It is caused by various infectious diseases, including ocular toxoplasmosis, tuberculosis, syphilis, and various viral infections (herpes simplex virus, cytomegalovirus, and Epstein-Barr virus), in addition to CSD. Noninfectious diseases include hypertensive retinopathy, sarcoidosis, and Behçet's disease.

In this case, tuberculosis and various viral infections were ruled out by the appropriate blood tests. Sarcoidosis was excluded because chest CT revealed no hilar lymphadenopathy, and Behçet's disease had no extraocular symptoms. At the time of admission to the pediatric department, we did not ask for a history of cat ownership, and a fundus examination revealed optic neuroretinitis, which was additionally considered a differential for CSD. The patient's mother had a history of breeding cats, which was mentioned in another day interview, and the antibody against *Bartonella henselae* was positive at a later date, resulting in the definitive diagnosis of optic retinitis associated with CSD. The frequency of optic neuroretinitis in CSD is 1–2%, but according to Yap et al. [6], CSD is one of the most common infectious causes of infectious optic neuroretinitis.

CSD has a good prognosis with spontaneous recovery; therefore, it often requires no treatment. However, although the prognosis of visual acuity in neuroretinitis associated with CSD is generally considered good [1–3], cases with a long recovery time and fulminant visual impairment exist

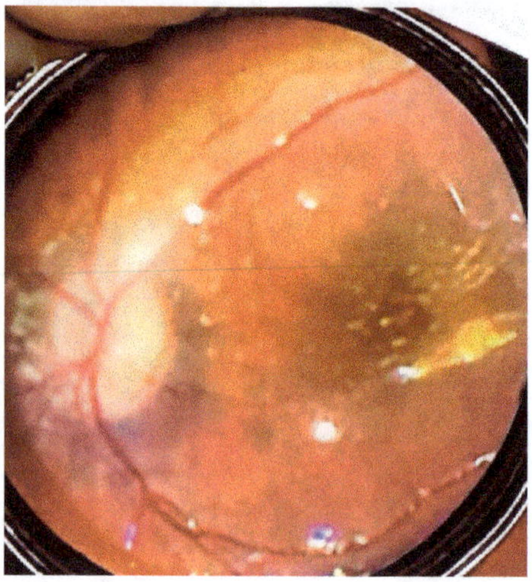

Figure 2: Right eye at the 2-month follow-up after discharge, imaged using a smartphone.

[4]. Thus, if the visual function is expected to be affected, aggressive treatment may be necessary. Some reports suggest that antimicrobial agents may alleviate symptoms and shorten the duration of the disease, and Reed et al. [2] suggest that such agents should be used as soon as the diagnosis is made. Although no established treatment exists, antibacterial agents, such as new quinolones, macrolides, and tetracyclines are often considered [1, 2, 4].

Furthermore, a certain type of immune response may be involved in the onset of the ocular lesions rather than direct infection with *Bartonella*; many studies have reported the concomitant use of corticosteroids in cases with ocular findings and strong visual dysfunction [3, 4]. However, there are no clear standards for dosage.

Although reports of pediatric cases exist [7–10], most infant cases were seen by ophthalmologists who noted subjective symptoms such as decreased visual acuity and visual field constriction. However, only a few cases of CSD have been reported in infants. Infants cannot complain of subjective symptoms (such as vision loss); therefore, these findings may be overlooked unless a fundus examination under mydriasis is performed. This may be because pediatricians do not usually consult an ophthalmologist, even in the presence of a systemic infection. In this case, the early detection of neuroretinitis by an ophthalmologist aided in the diagnosis of CSD. The change from cephem antibiotics to macrolide antibiotics, the addition of antituberculosis drugs, and the administration of steroids were effective in curbing the symptoms and restoring visual function.

Although the retinal and macular edema significantly improved, the macula may have atrophied or thinned due to the presence of hard exudates; thus, careful follow-up is required in the future. Further, photographing an infant's fundus is relatively challenging in daily medical care, and the record of the fundus findings greatly relies on the medical record description, which in turn, depends on the memory of the doctor who examined the patient. Fundus photography with a smartphone can be performed immediately without the need for expensive devices such as RetCam™ (Natus Medical Inc.), and it is also useful in observing changes over time.

4. Conclusion

In conclusion, the fever of unknown origin in this case was diagnosed based on a fundus examination. Moreover, since photographing an infant's fundus is extremely challenging, recording the fundus with a smartphone can be considered, which is relatively simple and useful for visualizing continuous changes.

Consent

Written informed consent was obtained from the parents of the patient for publication of this case report and any accompanying images.

Authors' Contributions

Daisuke Nakata, Sayaka Kakehi, and Hiroshi Okada examined the patient and collected clinical data. Daisuke Nakata drafted the manuscript. Atsuhiro Tanikawa and Yoshiaki Shimada performed manuscript editing. Masayuki Horiguchi and Yasuki Ito reviewed the manuscript. All authors read and approved the final version of the manuscript.

References

[1] E. T. Cunningham and J. E. Koehler, "Ocular bartonellosis," *American Journal of Ophthalmology*, vol. 130, no. 3, pp. 340–349, 2000.

[2] J. B. Reed, D. K. Scales, M. T. Wong, C. P. Lattuada Jr., M. J. Dolan, and I. R. Schwab, "Bartonella henselae_ neuroretinitis in cat scratch disease," *Ophthalmology*, vol. 105, no. 3, pp. 459–466, 1998.

[3] I. Ksiaa, N. Abroug, A. Mahmoud et al., "Update on Bartonella neuroretinitis," *Journal of Current Ophthalmology*, vol. 31, no. 3, pp. 254–261, 2019.

[4] Z. Habot-Wilner, O. Trivizki, M. Goldstein et al., "Cat-scratch disease: ocular manifestations and treatment outcome," *Acta Ophthalmologica*, vol. 96, no. 4, pp. e524–e532, 2018.

[5] K. Kasai, M. Mori, R. Hara, T. Miyamae, T. Imagawa, and S. Yokota, "National survey of childhood febrile illness cases with fever of unknown origin in Japan," *Pediatrics International: Official Journal of the Japan Pediatric Society*, vol. 53, no. 4, pp. 421–425, 2011.

[6] S. M. Yap, M. Saeed, P. Logan, and D. G. Healy, "Bartonella neuroretinitis (cat-scratch disease)," *Practical Neurology*, vol. 20, no. 6, pp. 505-506, 2020.

[7] N. S. Shariffudin, T. W. Min, A. Adnan, H. Hashim, and K. S. S. Teo, "A child with a rare presentation of ocular bartonellosis," *Taiwan Journal of Ophthalmology*, vol. 11, no. 3, pp. 292–295, 2021.

[8] C. H. Metz, J. Buer, N. Bornfeld, and A. Lipski, "Bilateral Bartonella henselae neuroretinitis with stellate maculopathy in a 6-year-old boy," *Infection*, vol. 40, no. 2, pp. 191–194, 2012.

[9] T. Durá-Travé, M. E. Yoldi-Petri, F. Gallinas-Victoriano, A. Lavilla-Oiz, and M. Bove-Guri, "Neuroretinitis caused by Bartonella henselae (cat-scratch disease) in a 13-year-old girl," *International Journal Of Pediatrics*, vol. 2010, Article ID 763105, 2010.

[10] E. Fleissig, F. Kim, D. K. Sigford, and C. C. Barr, "Bilateral neuroretinits and exudative retinal detachment with multifocal subretinal deposits secondary to Bartonella henselae infection," *American Journal of Ophthalmology Case Reports*, vol. 24, article 101201, 2021.

[11] R. K. Lord, V. A. Shah, A. N. San Filippo, and R. Krishna, "Novel uses of smartphones in ophthalmology," *Ophthalmology*, vol. 117, no. 6, pp. 1274–1274.e3, 2010.

[12] H. Nazari Khanamiri, A. Nakatsuka, and J. El-Annan, "Smartphone fundus photography," *Journal of Visualized Experiments*, vol. 125, no. 125, article 55958, 2017.

21

Multimodal Imaging and Macular Hyalocyte Count in a Patient with Acute Macular Neuroretinopathy

Michael J. Schatz, Oscar Otero-Marquez, Richard B. Rosen, and Deep Parikh

The New York Eye and Ear Infirmary, 310 East 14th Street, New York 10003, USA

Correspondence should be addressed to Michael J. Schatz; mschatz@nyee.edu

Academic Editor: Stephen G. Schwartz

Though rare, acute macular neuroretinopathy is a well-described clinical entity. We report for the first time a detailed analysis of macular hyalocyte count and morphology during the acute phase of acute macular neuroretinopathy. We present a case of a 19-year-old man with bilateral acute onset paracentral scotomas in the setting of an antecedent viral infection. Multimodal imaging demonstrated classic features of acute macular neuroretinopathy. Further analysis revealed increased macular hyalocyte count and an activated hyalocyte morphology during the acute phase of the disease course. Multimodal imaging not only allows for greater confidence in a diagnosis and prognosis but also helps to shed light on underlying pathophysiology. The new clinical capability of monitoring cellular behavior, such as hyalocyte count and morphology, in physiological and pathological conditions may prove useful as biomarkers of early disease activity or response to therapy.

1. Introduction

Acute macular neuroretinopathy (AMN) is a rare condition characterized by acute onset paracentral scotomas with corresponding intraretinal reddish-brown, wedge-shaped lesions that tend to point toward the fovea [1, 2]. Although no causative etiology has discovered, known risk factors include antecedent upper respiratory or gastrointestinal infection, preeclampsia, oral contraceptives, and even excessive caffeine use [1]. Most characteristically, AMN demonstrates hyporeflective petalloid parafoveal lesions on infrared reflectance photography. Optical coherence tomography (OCT) is remarkable for distortion and hyperreflectivity of the outer retinal layers and disruption of the ellipsoid zone, with preservation of the retinal pigment epithelium (RPE). These features distinguish AMN from other conditions such as paracentral acute middle maculopathy (PAMM), which demonstrate inner layer hyperreflectivity, and solar retinopathy, which often demonstrates disruption of the photoreceptors as well as the RPE [3, 4]. Over time, these lesions tend to fade, and characteristic outer retinal layer hyperreflectivity gives way to outer retinal thinning [5]. More recently, these lesions have been shown to correspond to localized choriocapillaris flow voids seen on optical coherence tomography angiography [6]. Although many patients with AMN have improvement in their paracentral scotomas, complete resolution is atypical. No intervention has been shown to be definitively beneficial in this condition.

2. Case Report

A 19-year-old man presented to the emergency department with two days of progressive bilateral blurry vision. Two days prior to his symptoms, he had fever and cough and tested positive for influenza, negative for COVID-19, and had recently taken his second dose of oseltamivir (Tamiflu). On initial examination, he had count finger vision at one foot in both eyes, but with eccentric gaze, he was able to see 20/60 in each eye. Presence of improved visual acuity in eccentric gaze prompted Amsler grid testing which revealed bilateral inferior paracentral scotomas with no metamorphopsia. The patient was unable to read Ishihara color plates. Intraocular pressure, extraocular motility, and confrontation visual field testing were full. Pupils were equal, round, and reactive, with no relative afferent pupil defect.

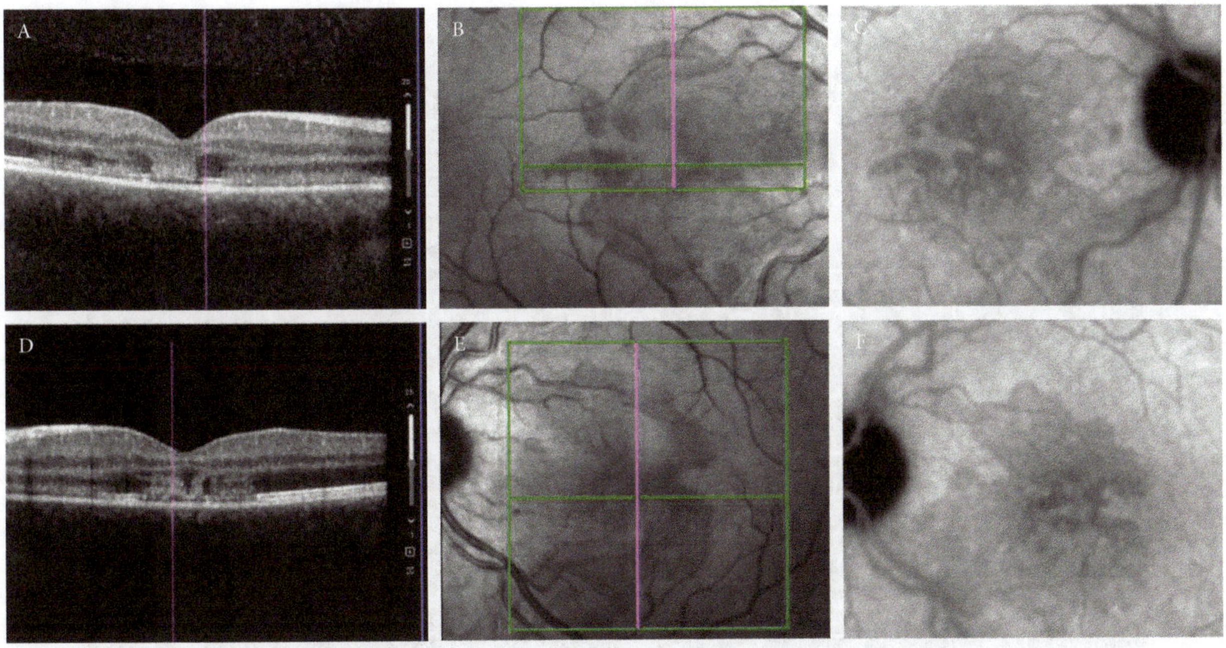

FIGURE 1: (a, d) Optical coherence tomography of the right and left eyes. Remarkable for distortion and hyperreflectivity of the outer retinal layers and disruption of the ellipsoid zone, with preservation of the retinal pigment epithelium (RPE). (b, e) Corresponding infrared reflectance photographs of the right and left eyes. Remarkable for hyporeflective macular lesions that correspond to areas of hypofluorescence seen in the indocyanine angiograms. (c, f) Late phase indocyanine green angiography of the right and left eye. Remarkable for mottled hypofluorescent macular lesions that correspond to the hypopreflective macular lesions seen on the infrared reflectance photographs.

Anterior and posterior segment exams were remarkable only for asymmetric cup to disc ratio (0.6 OD and 0.3 OS). No macular or optic nerve head edema was seen. MRI brain and orbits with and without contrast were unremarkable.

On repeat examination two days later, best corrected visual acuity with noneccentric gaze had improved to 20/25 OD and 20/70 OS. The patient reported improvement in the paracentral scotomas. Dilated fundus exam was significant for mild macular edema and subtle red-brown foveal pigmentation notably not present at the time of initial. Optical coherence tomography showed outer retinal layer hyperreflectivity with distortion of the ellipsoid layer but intact retinal pigment epithelium (RPE) (Figures 1(a) and 1(d)). Hyporeflective macular lesions were seen most clearly on the infrared reflectance photographs (Figures 1(b) and 1(e)). Fluorescein angiography and fundus autofluorescence were within normal limits; however, indocyanine green angiography (Figures 1(c) and 1(f)) showed macular hypofluorescent lesions corresponding to the lesions seen on the infrared reflectance photographs.

Optical coherence tomography angiography (OCT-A) imaging revealed choriocapillaris flow voids that roughly correspond to the lesions seen on infrared reflectance photographs (Figure 2). To assess retinal surface hyalocyte activity, a series of ten 3 × 3 mm scans centered at the fovea were acquired, registered, and averaged using a commercial spectral domain OCT system (Avanti RTVue-XR; Optovue, Fremont, CA, USA). Semiautomated macrophage identification and density measurements were performed on a 3 μm OCT-Reflectance (OCT-R) image slab located above the inner limiting membrane (ILM) surface using MATLAB (2018b; MathWorks, Natick, MA). Relative to a 35-year-old healthy control, there was a notable increased macular hyalocyte count in our patient with AMN. The morphology of the surface hyalocytes was distinctively round with few processes, consistent with an "activated" phenotype (Figure 3).

3. Discussion

Hyalocytes are the primary resident macrophages within the vitreous. They act as the first responders to neuronal injury, playing an integral role in maintaining homeostasis in the retinal microenvironment, modulating the immune response, and synthesizing extracellular matrix [7–9]. They reside adjacent to the ciliary body and along the posterior pole localized according to histopathology to within the 50 μm region above the inner limiting membrane (ILM), entangled with the collagen fibrils that compose the formed component of the vitreous cortex [10, 11].

Advances in retinal imaging have recently allowed visualization of vitreous cortex hyalocytes (VCH) in humans in vivo [12, 13]. Clinical OCT is capable of distinguishing phenotypic variation of VCH in response to changes in their activity. Under healthy conditions, hyalocytes appear primarily slender with a spindle-shaped or ramified configuration and distribute homogeneously. In retinopathic eyes, the cells transmorph into an "activated" phenotype which appears plumper with fewer, shorter processes, clustering

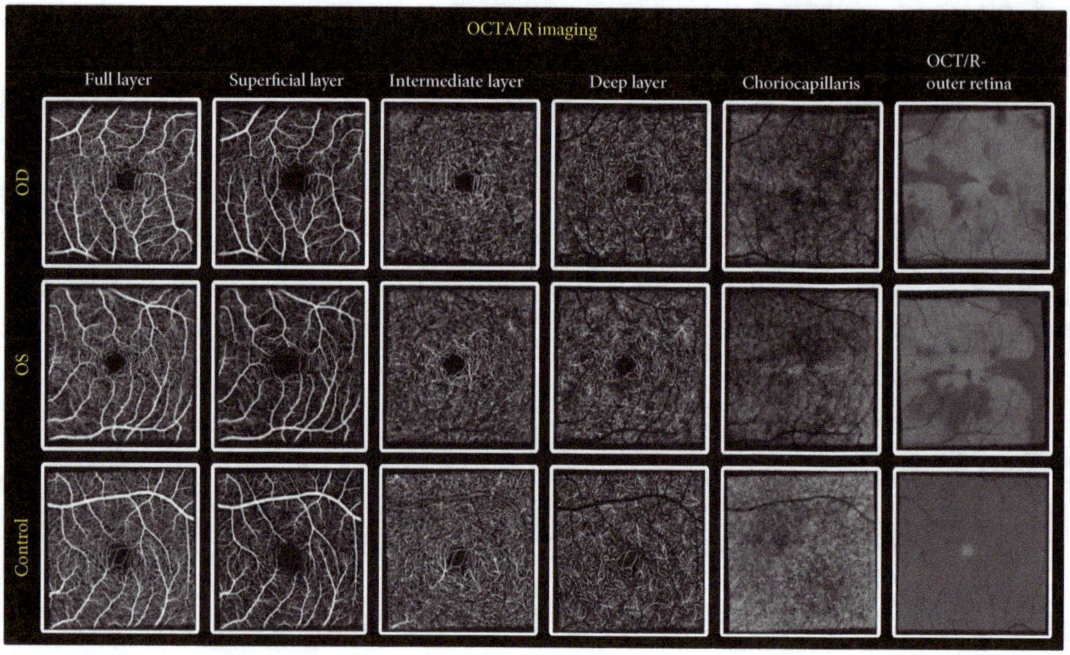

Figure 2: Optical coherence tomography angiography (OCT-A) of both eyes compared to healthy control, demonstrating choriocapillaris flow voids that roughly correspond to the overlying macular lesions seen on the infrared reflectance photographs, supporting the hypothesis that these represent areas of relative ischemia.

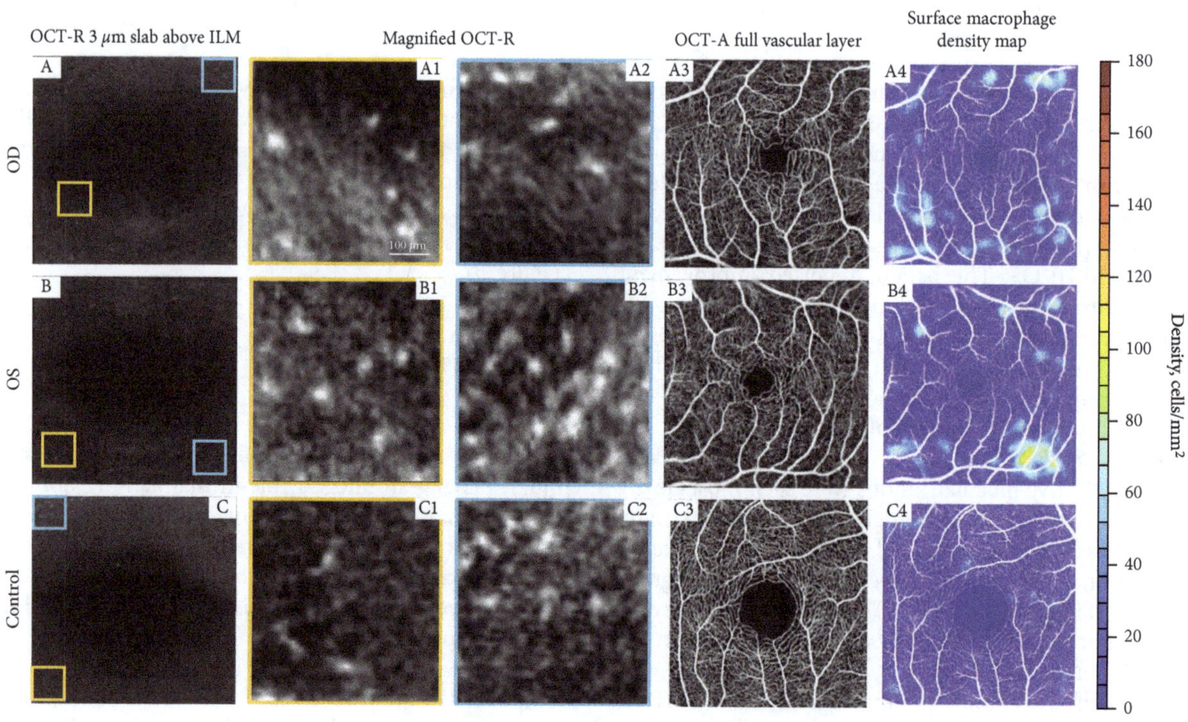

Figure 3: Surface hyalocyte distribution and morphology in right and left eye in our patient with AMN compared to 35-year-old healthy control, using en face OCT. (a–c) OCT-reflectance slab segmented 3 μm above the ILM surface shows higher density of surface macrophage cells in eyes with AMN (more apparent on A4, B4, and C4). Orange and blue outlined images correspond to two different regions of interest with magnified view of surface macrophages (A1–C2). (A1–C2) Magnified view of surface macrophages in right and left eye in our patient with AMN and a healthy control. In the eyes with AMN, the cells appear round with fewer, shortened processes, consistent with in an "activated" state. In the healthy control, there are fewer cells and they appear slender with spindle- or star-like configuration consistent with a "quiescent" state. (A3, B3, C3) OCT-A full vascular layer of right and left eye in our patient with AMN and a healthy control. (A4, B4, C4) Overlay of hyalocyte density map onto the OCT-A. Surface hyalocyte density increases in acute ischemic conditions such as AMN. Cell density: AMN eyes, OD 9.26 cells/mm^2, OS 10.38 cells/mm^2, and control eye: 2.39 cells/mm^2.

around vessels and areas of metabolic disturbance in a non-uniform spatial distribution [13, 14].

During the acute inflammatory phase, our patient demonstrated classic features of AMN consistent with descriptions in the literature: outer retinal hyperreflectivity on OCT cross-sections, parafoveal petalloid hyporeflective lesions on infrared reflectance photography, corresponding areas of hypofluorescence on ICG, and the appearance of localized choriocapillaris flow voids in OCT-A scans. In this case, we were able to image the density, distribution, and morphology of VCH during the acute phase of AMN. Compared to the healthy control presented in this paper, as well as 18 other healthy controls previously published by Castanos et al. [13], this patient with AMN demonstrated increased VCH density, clustered around areas of metabolic disturbance as indicated by choriocapillaris flow voids, and the morphologic appearance of a more active phenotype. These findings are consistent with the hypothesis that the acute release of proinflammatory and proangiogenic cytokines and chemokines in ischemic conditions results in activation of VCH which attempt to restore the immunity and homeostasis of the retinal microenvironment. As the patient's symptoms began to show signs of resolution, the patient deferred follow-up, and we were unable to document the resolution of his hyalocyte count and morphology during recovery.

Refinement of imaging strategies makes it likely that similar events in the future will be able to be studied more extensively, enabling a more complete in vivo description of the cellular transformations as they develop. Such investigations will provide greater understanding of the cellular-level events occurring and possibly suggest therapeutic approaches.

Acknowledgments

This study was supported by the National Eye Institute of the National Institutes of Health (award number R01EY027301). The content is solely the responsibility of the authors and does not necessarily represent the official views of the National Institutes of Health. Additional funding for this research was provided by the New York Eye and Ear Infirmary Foundation Grant, the Marrus Family Foundation, the Challenge Grant award from Research to Prevent Blindness, and the Jorge N. Buxton Microsurgical Foundation.

References

[1] K. V. Bhavsar, S. Lin, E. Rahimy et al., "Acute macular neuroretinopathy: a comprehensive review of the literature," *Survey of Ophthalmology*, vol. 61, no. 5, pp. 538–565, 2016.

[2] S. D. Turbeville, L. D. Cowan, and J. D. Gass, "Acute macular neuroretinopathy: a review of the literature," *Survey of Ophthalmology*, vol. 48, no. 1, pp. 1–11, 2003.

[3] E. Rahimy, L. Kuehlewein, S. R. Sadda, and D. Sarraf, "Paracentral acute middle maculopathy," *Retina*, vol. 35, no. 10, pp. 1921–1930, 2015.

[4] K. C. Chen, J. J. Jung, and A. Aizman, "High definition spectral domain optical coherence tomography findings in three patients with solar retinopathy and review of the literature," *The Open Ophthalmology Journal*, vol. 6, no. 1, pp. 29–35, 2012.

[5] A. A. Fawzi, R. R. Pappuru, D. Sarraf et al., "Acute macular NEURORETINOPATHY," *Retina*, vol. 32, no. 8, pp. 1500–1513, 2012.

[6] S. Y. Lee, J. L. Cheng, K. M. Gehrs et al., "Choroidal features of acute macular neuroretinopathy via optical coherence tomography angiography and correlation with serial multimodal imaging," *JAMA Ophthalmology*, vol. 135, no. 11, pp. 1177–1183, 2017.

[7] L. Chen, P. Yang, and A. Kijlstra, "Distribution, markers, and functions of retinal microglia," *Ocular Immunology and Inflammation*, vol. 10, no. 1, pp. 27–39, 2002.

[8] H. S. Lazarus and G. S. Hageman, "In situ characterization of the human hyalocyte," *Archives of Ophthalmology*, vol. 112, no. 10, pp. 1356–1362, 1994.

[9] A. A. Suetov and E. V. Boiko, "Hyalocytes of the vitreous body and their role in ophthalmic pathology," *Vestnik Oftalmologii*, vol. 134, no. 6, pp. 94–101, 2018.

[10] N. N. Vagaja, H. R. Chinnery, N. Binz, J. M. Kezic, E. P. Rakoczy, and P. G. McMenamin, "Changes in murine hyalocytes are valuable early indicators of ocular disease," *Investigative Ophthalmology and Visusal Science*, vol. 53, no. 3, pp. 1445–1451, 2012.

[11] H. Qiao, T. Hisatomi, K. H. Sonoda et al., "The characterisation of hyalocytes: the origin, phenotype, and turnover," *The British Journal of Ophthalmology*, vol. 89, no. 4, pp. 513–517, 2005.

[12] D. X. Hammer, A. Agrawal, R. Villanueva, O. Saeedi, and Z. Liu, "Label-free adaptive optics imaging of human retinal macrophage distribution and dynamics," *Procedings of the National Academy of Sciences of the United States of America*, vol. 117, no. 48, pp. 30661–30669, 2020.

[13] M. V. Castanos, D. B. Zhou, R. E. Linderman et al., "Imaging of macrophage-like cells in living human retina using clinical OCT," *Investigative Ophthalmology and Visual Science*, vol. 61, no. 6, 2020.

[14] J. X. Ong, P. L. Nesper, A. A. Fawzi, J. M. Wang, and J. A. Lavine, "Macrophage-like cell density is increased in proliferative diabetic retinopathy characterized by optical coherence tomography angiography," *Investigative Ophthalmology and Visual Science*, vol. 62, no. 10, 2021.

22

Iris-Occlusion of XEN Gel Stent following Ab Externo Transconjunctival Implantation Technique

Sunil Ruparelia [1] and Nir Shoham-Hazon [1,2]

[1] Faculty of Medicine, Dalhousie University, Halifax, Nova Scotia, Canada
[2] Miramichi EyeNB Centre of Excellence, Miramichi, NB, Canada

Correspondence should be addressed to Sunil Ruparelia; sn885054@dal.ca

Academic Editor: Hsin Yi Chen

The use of minimally invasive glaucoma surgery (MIGS) devices has become increasingly common for the management of elevated intraocular pressure (IOP) in the context of glaucoma. These technologies have traditionally been associated with fewer postoperative complications than conventional surgical techniques. However, we report on a rare case of transient XEN occlusion associated with pupil dilation following XEN gel stent implantation. This case highlights that in future XEN implantations, it may be preferable to position the XEN at a lesser angle to the iris to prevent such an occlusion. The use of different positionings of XEN is performed to optimize outcomes. However, it is highlighted that complications may arise in certain circumstances.

1. Introduction

Glaucomatous vision loss remains the leading cause of irreversible vision loss worldwide [1]. When topical therapy to manage intraocular pressure (IOP) fails, surgical intervention is indicated to prevent further progression of glaucomatous optic neuropathy. In recent years, minimally invasive glaucoma surgeries (MIGS) have become increasingly common in the management of uncontrolled glaucoma. Among these techniques is the XEN gel stent. The XEN gel stent is implanted beneath the conjunctiva, such that a shunt is created to drain aqueous humour from the anterior chamber of the eye into the subconjunctival space [2]. This is typically performed in an *ab interno* fashion but may also be done *ab externo* with or without dissection of the conjunctiva. These approaches have similar efficacies in terms of achieving target IOP and have similar safety profiles [3]. A major appeal of MIGS techniques is that they are typically associated with a lower complication rate than traditional surgical techniques [2]. However, we report on a rare case of transient iris-occlusion of the XEN gel stent 5 months following *ab externo* transconjunctival XEN gel stent implantation.

2. Case Presentation

A 56-year-old white male presented to the clinic for a 5-month postoperative follow-up appointment. The patient had received a superotemporal XEN gel stent implant in his left eye for management of his primary open-angle glaucoma (POAG). XEN implantation had been augmented with 0.2 mL of 0.3 mg/mL MMC, injected in an air-OVD fashion to create a pocket between the conjunctiva and Tenon's capsule.

At presentation, Snellen visual acuity was 20/60 in the left eye, and IOP was on target at 10 mmHg. However, following pupil dilation, an intraocular pressure (IOP) spike to 24 mmHg by Goldmann applanation was observed in the left eye. Other than the patient's existing diagnosis of POAG, no other ocular history or presenting symptoms were reported.

Prior to XEN gel stent surgery, pressure in the patient's left eye was 32 mmHg by Goldmann applanation on maximal tolerated medical therapy (MTMT). At that time, Snellen visual acuity in the left eye was 20/60. Following initial surgery, the patient had been discharged with a postoperative

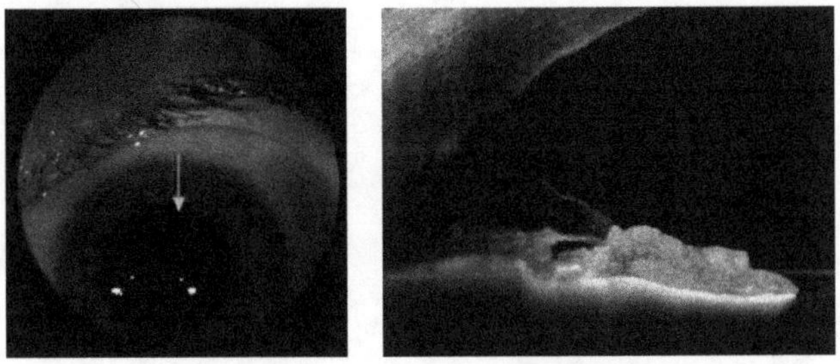

(a) (b)

Figure 1: XEN stent placement (a) and anterior segment OCT (b) showing obstruction of XEN stent lumen after pupil dilation.

drop regimen including a quinolone antibiotic for 1 week and prednisolone 1% for 2 months postoperatively. Following the procedure, IOP had remained within a range of 5-10 mmHg measured at 1-month postoperative intervals without any IOP-lowering medications. After the IOP spike to 24 mmHg with dilation, multiple challenges with dilating drops demonstrated consistent rise in the left eye IOP to 24 mmHg to 30 mmHg during dilation. An anterior chamber OCT was performed and confirmed suspected XEN stent occlusion associated with pupil dilation (Figure 1). The patient was hesitant to undergo further intervention to prevent these events. As such, an observational management approach was taken in accordance with patient preferences.

3. Discussion

The XEN stent is one of the various microinvasive glaucoma surgery (MIGS) technologies that have been introduced in recent years. Since the FDA approval of XEN in 2016, its use has become increasingly common to manage patients with elevated IOP. A major appeal of the XEN implant is that it has been associated with fewer intra- and postoperative complications than traditional surgical techniques [2]. We describe the occurrence of a rare complication following XEN gel stent implantation.

Traditionally, the XEN is placed such that the device sits approximately 35 degrees under the conjunctiva and tenon [2]. However, further innovation with XEN implantation technique has led to variations in positioning of the device. In this case, XEN gel stent implantation was performed in a transconjunctival manner, with the air-OVD technique for tenon separation. The implant was positioned such that it was perpendicular rather than parallel to the iris in the anterior chamber. This implanted angle was sufficient to occlude the XEN upon pupil dilation.

Previous studies have outlined XEN occlusion by a variety of etiologies, including blood clots and fibrous scar tissue [4, 5]. However, literature regarding iris-occlusion of XEN gel stent is sparce. When faced with iris-occlusion of the XEN gel stent, there are several treatment options that may be considered. In our case, the patient was reluctant to receive further intervention, and we elected to observe the eye to determine whether further interventions would be required. Thus, we describe a conservative observational approach to iris occlusion of XEN gel stent. Several treatment modalities for iris-occluded XEN gel stent have also been described in the current literature. One case describing management of this complication reported reoccurrence of occlusion following surgical repositioning of XEN, but successful resolution of occlusion with combined treatment with argon laser peripheral iridoplasty and low energy neodymium-doped yttrium aluminum garnet laser [6]. Another report describes successful resolution of occlusion with argon laser peripheral iridoplasty alone [7].

The use of XEN gel stent has become increasingly common in practice. With continued innovation in implantation technique, it is important for care providers to have an understanding of the presenting symptoms, available investigations and management options to potential complications which may arise.

This case outlines a unique occurrence of XEN gel stent occlusion following pupillary dilation. In future XEN implantations, it may be advantageous to position the XEN at a lesser angle to the iris to prevent such an occlusion. This would require the surgeon to place the implant more anteriorly, aiming towards the cornea and parallel to the iris when deploying the device. Although innovation in technique with different positioning of XEN is performed with the intention of optimizing outcomes, we highlight that caution should be taken when innovating an already innovative technique.

Consent

Parental consent was obtained for the preparation of this work.

Authors' Contributions

All authors attest that they meet the current ICMJE criteria for authorship.

References

[1] J. K. Parihar, "Glaucoma: The 'Black hole' of irreversible blindness," *Medical Journal, Armed Forces India*, vol. 72, no. 1, pp. 3-4, 2016.

[2] A. M. Fea, G. M. Durr, P. Marolo, L. Malinverni, M. A. Economou, and I. Ahmed, "XEN® gel stent: a comprehensive review on its use as a treatment option for refractory Glaucoma," *Clinical Ophthalmology*, vol. 14, pp. 1805–1832, 2020.

[3] N. E. Tan, N. Tracer, A. Terraciano, H. A. Parikh, J. F. Panarelli, and N. M. Radcliffe, "Comparison of safety and efficacy between ab interno and ab externo approaches to XEN gel stent placement," *Clinical Ophthalmology*, vol. 15, pp. 299–305, 2021.

[4] K. Gillmann, K. Mansouri, G. E. Bravetti, and A. Mermoud, "Chronic intraocular inflammation as a risk factor for XEN gel stent occlusion: a case of microscopic examination of a fibrin-obstructed XEN stent," *Journal of Glaucoma*, vol. 27, no. 8, pp. 739–741, 2018.

[5] N. Pinto Ferreira, L. Abegão Pinto, and C. Marques-Neves, "XEN gel stent internal ostium occlusion: ab-interno revision," *Journal of Glaucoma*, vol. 26, no. 4, pp. e150–e152, 2017.

[6] S. Rho and S. H. Lim, "Combined argon laser peripheral iridoplasty and Nd: YAG laser shock wave therapy for recurrent XEN gel stent obstruction due to iris incarceration: a case report," *Medicine (Baltimore)*, vol. 100, no. 29, article e26652, 2021.

[7] A. F. Tadrosse and A. S. Khouri, "Laser iridoplasty to treat iris-occluded XEN gel stent," *Journal of Glaucoma*, vol. 29, no. 8, pp. e91–e92, 2020.

23

Optical Coherence Tomography Angiography (OCT-A) in a Patient with Occult Retinal Dysfunction

Juliana Wons,[1] **Jana Dinges**,[1] **Matthias D. Becker**,[1,2] **and Stephan Michels**[1,3]

[1]*City Hospital Triemli, Zurich, Switzerland*
[2]*University of Heidelberg, Germany*
[3]*University of Zurich, Switzerland*

Correspondence should be addressed to Juliana Wons; juliana.wons@gmail.com

Academic Editor: Christopher G. Kiss

Multimodal imaging techniques were performed in a patient with a newly emerged visual field defect; a missing retinal lesion on fundus examination made the diagnosis challenging but infrared imaging showed a larger area of retinal abnormality temporal to the fovea. Indocyanine green angiography (IA) showed late hypofluorescence and there was mild hyperautofluorescence which is known from acute zonal occult outer retinopathy (AZOOR). Despite normal fluorescein angiography (FA) results, a perfusion loss in the outer retinal layer was detected by OCT-A. Similar OCT-A findings were recently described in patients with acute macular neuroretinopathy (AMN). *Methods.* The methods included FA and IA, spectral domain optical coherence tomography (SD-OCT), near infrared imaging, and autofluorescence imaging (AF), as well as OCT-A. *Patient.* A 36-year-old patient who suffered from acute symptoms of photopsia and scotoma on her left eye. She had an influenza-like illness two weeks earlier. The scotoma could be verified by visual field testing. *Results.* The affected retinal zone showed mild fading of external limiting membrane (ELM) and a disorganisation of the ellipsoid zone (EZ) on SD-OCT. OCT-A revealed a large area of reduced perfusion in the outer retinal vascular layer. *Conclusion.* OCT-A can help to detect reduced capillary network in patients with visual field defects and no visible fundus changes. This case seems to have features of different occult retinal disorders such as AZOOR and AMN.

1. Introduction

AZOOR was initially described by Gass in 1992 as an outer retinal dysfunction that affects young Caucasian patients, more often women than men [1, 2]. Photopsia and visual field defects are the main symptoms [2]. The dysfunction can be uni- or bilateral [2]. Some patients suffer from an initial episode of flu like symptoms. Only slight or no fundus changes are detectable [3].

Until now it remains unclear if the retinal lesions progress due to an autoimmune process, idiopathic, or due to a viral affection [2]. In some cases a mild periphlebitis in the affected area is described [3]. After the initial phase, sometimes mild fundus changes like pigment shift or a slight chorioretinal scaring as well as a bonespicule-like pigmentation can be observed [2]. OCT images show often initially fading of the ellipsoid zone (EZ), potentially due to higher reflectivity of the outer nuclear layer (ONL), and show loss of photoreceptor outer segments during the course of disease [3]. Fluorescein angiography is usually normal at the onset of a lesion. Over time with degenerative changes at the level of the RPE, an early FA hyperfluorescence can be detected.

AMN was initially described by Bos and Deutman in 1975 [4]. They described cases of patients with red and wedge-shaped paracentral lesions [4]. The apices of these lesions often point towards the fovea. Patients suffer from acute paracentral scotoma; visual acuity is mostly normal or mildly reduced. The symptoms can occur uni- or bilateral. While fundus examination often shows only mild or sometimes even no fundal changes, the lesions are well visualised by red-free or infrared imaging, typically as dark or grey regions with well-demarcated margins [5]. Patients are more often young and female; a number of supposed triggers have been reported, such as flu-like illness, fever, oral contraceptives, and some sympathomimetics [5]. The defect remains stable or can occasionally recover [5].

Before standard use of OCT in ophthalmic diagnostics, AMN was rarely diagnosed. OCT imaging shows wedge

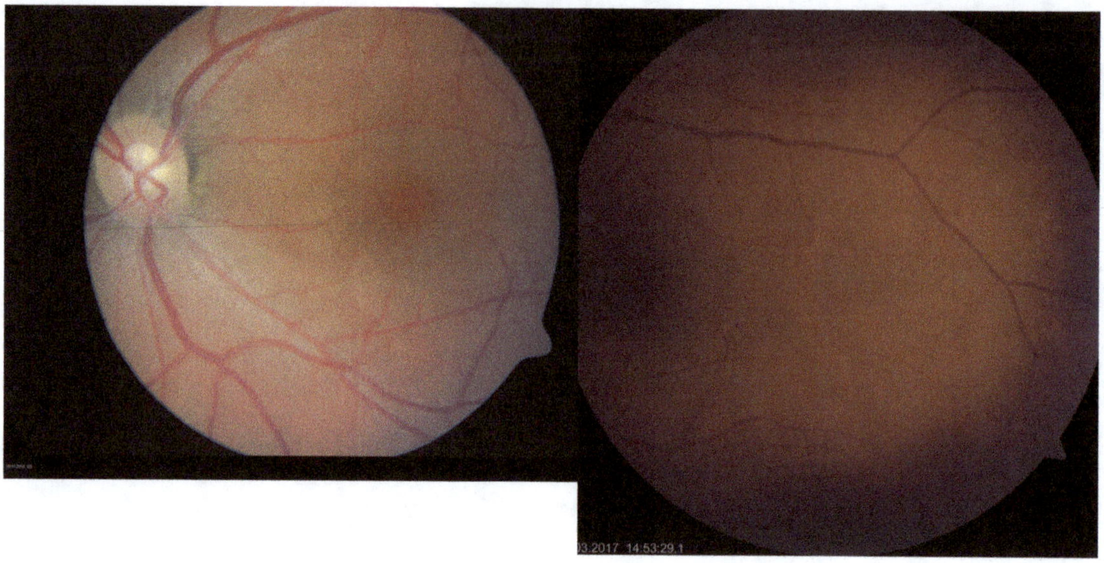

FIGURE 1: Color fundus photography of the left eye.

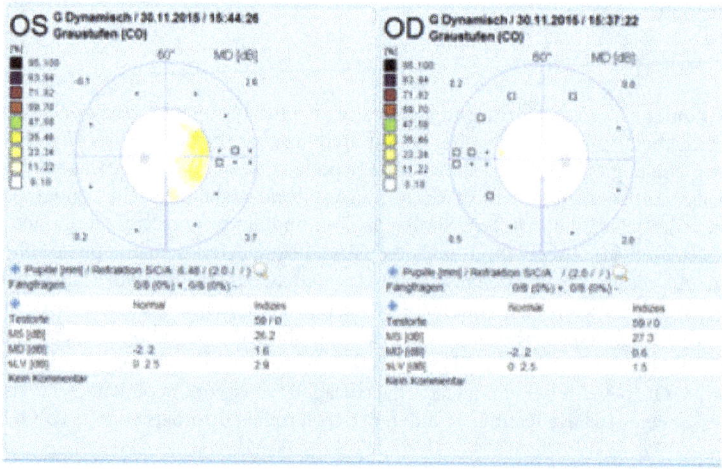

FIGURE 2: Octopus perimetry confirms the nasal defect on the left eye.

shaped hyperreflectivity in the outer nuclear layer or a fading EZ in patients with AMN [6]. Studies using OCT-angiography have revealed an ischemia in the deep retinal plexus as a pathogenic mechanism [7, 8].

2. Case Report

A 36-year-old female had photopsia on her left eye for ten days. Furthermore, she noticed a dark spot on the nasal side of the left eye. Two weeks earlier, she had suffered from influenza-like symptoms. There was no history of previous general or eye disease, neither operations nor treatments.

3. Results

The BCVA was 20/20 on both eyes, normal eye pressure, and no signs of inflammation in the anterior chamber. There was no vitreous haze or vitreous destruction. The fundus examination showed no obvious pathology (Figure 1). The scotoma was confirmed by using 30° perimetry (Figure 2). Blood tests for uveitis were negative, and screening for rheumatic diseases showed normal findings. An electroretinogram revealed reduced receptor potentials in the impaired retinal zone on the left eye corresponding to the visual defect (Figure 3). The near infrared image showed a significant demarcation line temporal to the fovea, and there was a fading of the EZ on the SD-OCT (Spectralis®; Heidelberg Engineering GmbH, Heidelberg, Germany) image (Figure 4). The autofluorescence (AF) imaging (Figure 5) showed very mild focal hyperautofluorescence superotemporally to the fovea. FA revealed normal retinal perfusion, there was no sign of ischemia, no leakage, nor hyperfluorescence. However, ICG revealed an area of hypofluorescence temporal to the fovea (Figure 6). This region correlates to the scotoma on the

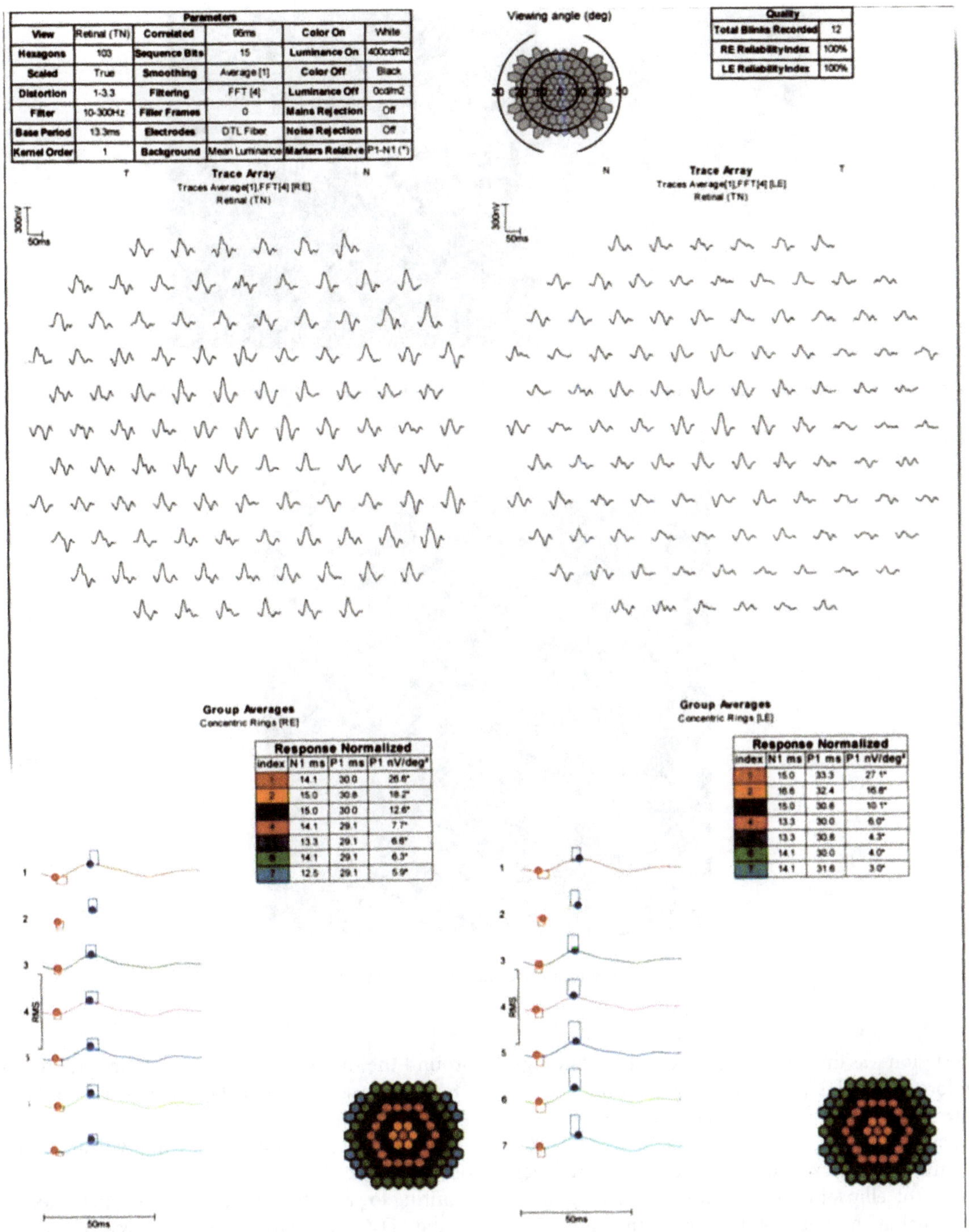

FIGURE 3: Multifocal ERG with reduced response signal in the area of the temporal retina on the left eye.

left eye. No pathologic changes were found in the right eye (Figure 7.).

OCT angiography (OCT-A) was performed using the Topcon, DRI OCT Triton/Swept source OCT-A. The affected area of the left eye was demarcated and changes in the density of the retinal capillaries were demonstrated (Figure 8). These changes were only in the deep retinal vascular layer.

4. Discussion

Comparable findings in OCT-A were recently described in several cases of patients with AMN [7–9]. But only one article mentioned changes on OCT-A in AZOOR. Pichi et al. describe reduced deep capillary flow on OCT-A in an inactive peripapillary lesion of a patient with AZOOR [10]. In our case, the first OCT-A was performed several months after the

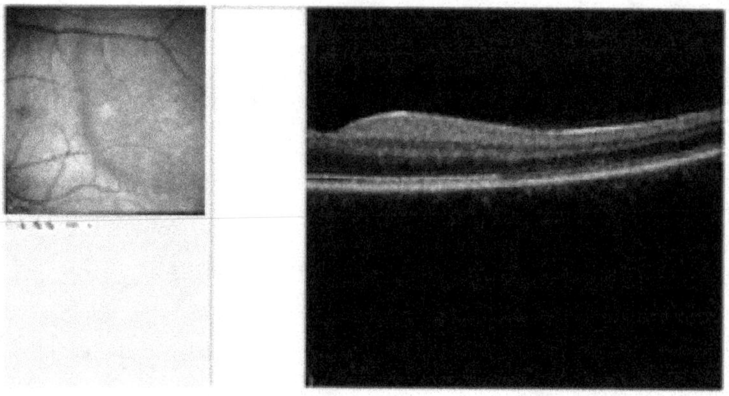

FIGURE 4: Optical coherence tomography showing fading of the ellipsoid zone and infrared imaging indicating affected zone.

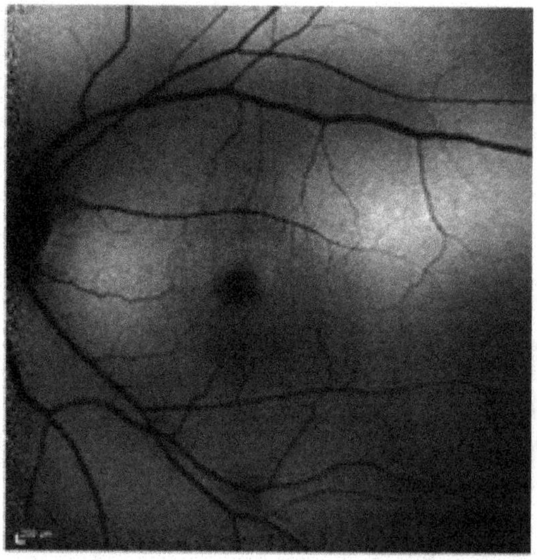

FIGURE 5: Autofluorescence image of the left eye.

first visit, the lesion was inactive at that time and our findings would therefore be conclusive with the other article.

There are several findings that would fit to the diagnosis of AZOOR, such as hypofluorescence in late phase of ICG, thinning of the outer plexiform layer, outer nuclear layer and disruption of ellipsoid zone. Fluorescein angiography is usually normal at the onset of a lesion, with subsequent degenerative changes at the level of the RPE. AZOOR shows loss of photoreceptor outer segments, beginning with abnormalities in the ellipsoid line. In the course of disease early FA hyperfluorescence from depigmentation of the RPE produce a window defect [11]. We followed the patient over more than 2 years and the lesion did not change neither in SD-OCT, nor in FA.

Often there are no changes on infrared imaging in AZOOR. This patient has changes on near infrared, a feature that is often a hallmark of AMN. The ellipsoid line and outer segments are affected in AMN and also the deep retinal capillaries. Most AZOOR patients show affection of the peripapillary zone and only rarely does it spare the area around the disc but affect an area temporal to the macula. The multifocal ERG can show reduced amplitudes both in AZOOR and in AMN.

Some features in this case are not typical for the diagnosis of AMN either. There were no classical wedge shaped lesions pointing towards the macula and no hyperreflective changes in the SD-OCT. However, the demarcated area in the near infrared image and the ischemia in the outer retinal layer are consistent with AMN [6, 9].

In appearance of newer imaging techniques making diagnosis by OCT and OCT-A is in discussion. Some authors claim that there might be the risk of determining diseases on a fragile basis where technical artefacts may lead to false interpretations. Otherwise, the modern imaging methods may help us to improve our current classification of retinal diseases.

The pathology of the AZOOR complex is still under debate. Anti-retinal bodies could play, according to a recent publication, a key role leading to the damage of the retinal area in AZOOR [12]. A dysfunction in the blood-retina

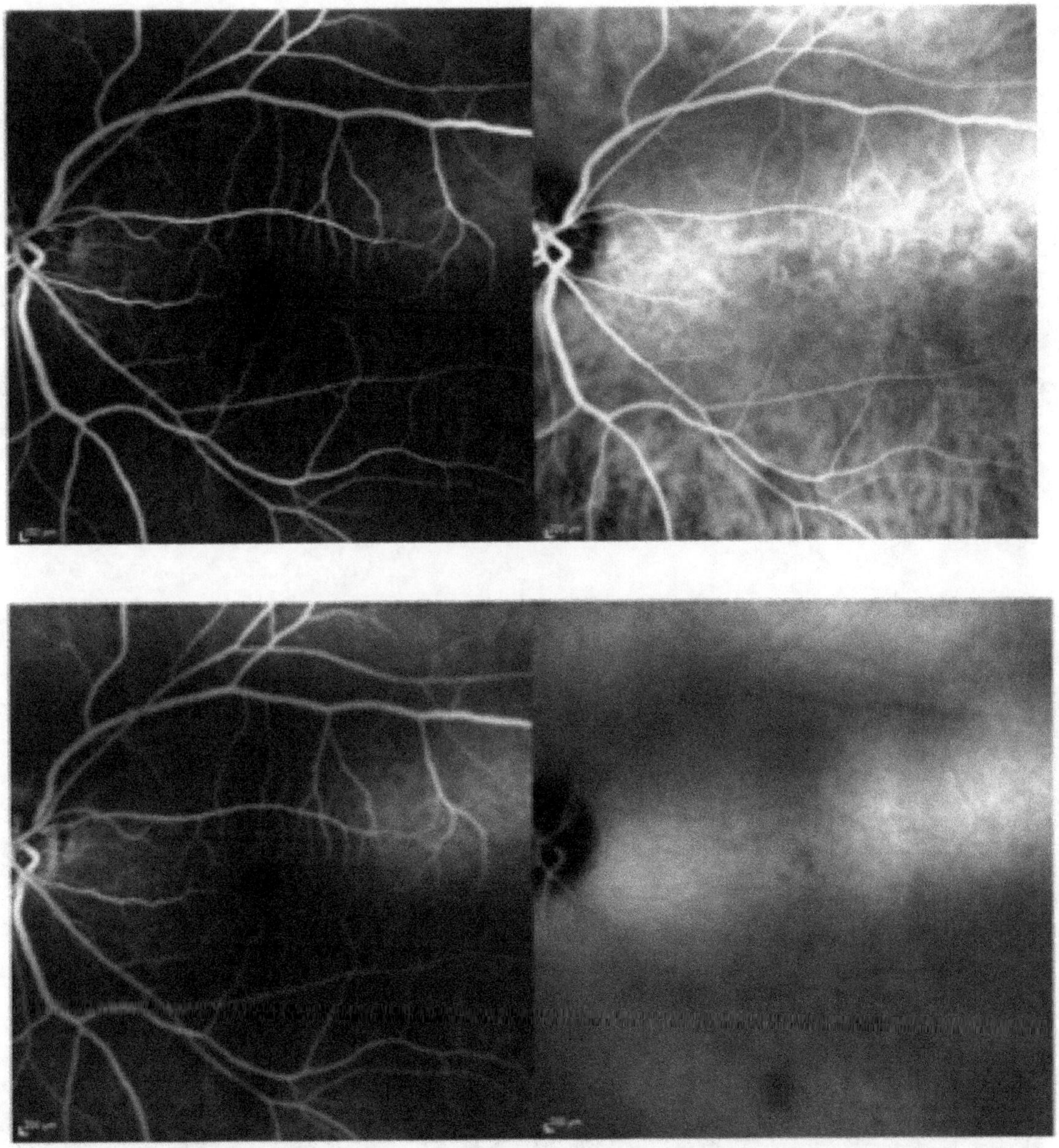

FIGURE 6: On the left early and late fluorescein (FA), and on the right early and late indocyanine green (IA) angiography. Late IA reveals a hypofluorescent area temporal to the fovea.

barrier due to inflammation or autoimmune process could be involved in the pathogenic process [12]. The current challenge, as discussed by Mrejen et al., is the lack of consistency regarding the definition of the disease and the clinical findings [11]. An advantage in the challenge of finding the diagnosis of this relatively rare disease can be achieved through modern multimodal imaging techniques.

5. Conclusion

OCT-A identifies retinal ischemic diseases on clinically undetectable fundus lesions.

The changes in the perfusion of the deep retinal capillaries indicated by OCT-A in this young female patient with visual field defect helped to establish the diagnosis of an outer retinal dysfunction, combining features of AZOOR and AMN. A better understanding of the pathophysiology in these rare occult retinal diseases may be achieved by increasing use of OCT-A.

Disclosure

The present address of Juliana Wons is Berner Augenklinik am Lindenhofspital, Bern, Switzerland. The present address of Jana Dinges is Eye Clinic Hoechst, Frankfurt, Germany.

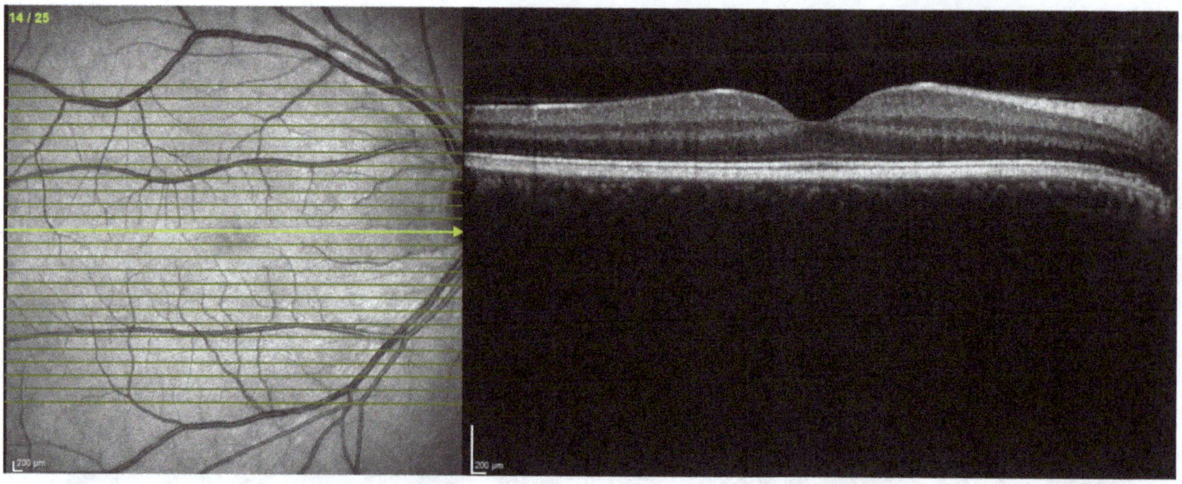

FIGURE 7: Optical coherence tomography and infrared imaging of the right eye.

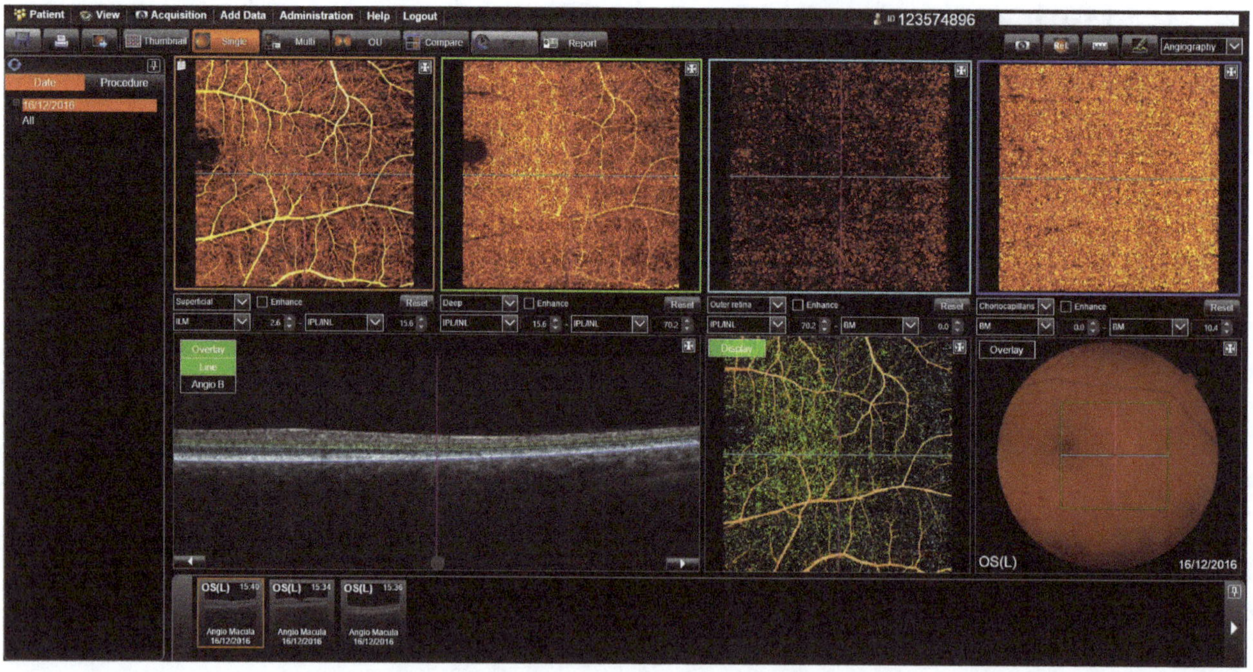

FIGURE 8: Optical coherence tomography angiography (OCTA) shows a rarefication of the deep retinal capillaries. Superficial retinal capillaries and choroidal circulation do not seem to be affected.

Acknowledgments

The study was supported by the Werner H. Spross Foundation (Zurich, Switzerland).

References

[1] J. D. Gass, "Acute zonal occult outer retinopathy," *Journal of Clinical Neuro-Ophthalmology*, vol. 13, pp. 79–97, 1993.

[2] J. D. Gass, A. Agarwal, and I. U. Scott, "Acute zonal occult outer retinopathy: a long-term follow-up study," *American Journal of Ophthalmology*, vol. 134, no. 3, pp. 329–339, 2002.

[3] Y. Takai, S. Ishiko, H. Kagokawa, K. Fukui, A. Takahashi, and A. Yoshida, "Morphological study of acute zonal occult outer retinopathy (AZOOR) by multiplanar optical coherence tomography," *Acta Ophthalmologica*, vol. 87, no. 4, pp. 408–418, 2009.

[4] P. J. M. Bos and A. F. Deutman, "Acute macular neuroretinopathy," *American Journal of Ophthalmology*, vol. 80, no. 4, pp. 573–584, 1975.

[5] K. V. Bhavsar, S. Lin, E. Rahimy et al., "Acute macular neuroretinopathy: A comprehensive review of the literature," *Survey of Ophthalmology*, vol. 61, no. 5, pp. 538–565, 2016.

[6] K. Hufendiek, M. Gamulescu, K. Hufendiek, H. Helbig, and D. Märker, "Classification and characterization of acute macular neuroretinopathy with spectral domain optical coherence tomography," *International Ophthalmology*, vol. 38, no. 6, pp. 2403–2416, 2018.

[7] E. Rahimy and D. Sarraf, "Paracentral acute middle maculopathy spectral-domain optical coherence tomography feature of deep capillary ischemia," *Current Opinion in Ophthalmology*, vol. 25, no. 3, pp. 207–212, 2014.

[8] J. Nemiroff, D. Sarraf, J. P. Davila, and D. Rodger, "Optical coherence tomography angiography of acute macular neuroretinopathy reveals deeo capillary ischemia," *Retinal Cases & Brief Reports*, vol. 12, pp. S12–S15, 2018.

[9] P. E. Pecen, A. G. Smith, J. P. Ehlers et al., "Optical coherence tomography angiography of acute macular neuroretinopathy/paracentral acute middle maculopathy," *JAMA Ophthalmology*, vol. 133, no. 12, pp. 1478–1480, 2015.

[10] F. Pichi, D. Sarraf, M. Morara, S. Mazumdar, P. Neri, and V. Gupta, "Pearls and pitfalls of optical coherence tomography angiography in the multmodal evaluation of uveitis," *Journal of Ophthalmic Inflammation and Infection*, vol. 7, no. 1, 2017.

[11] S. Mrejen, S. Khan, R. Gallego-Pinazo, L. M. Jampol, and L. A. Yannuzzi, "Acute zonal occult outer retinopathy: a classification based on multimodal imaging," *JAMA Ophthalmology*, vol. 132, no. 9, pp. 1089–1098, 2014.

[12] C. X. Qian, A. Wang, D. L. DeMill et al., "Prevalence of antiretinal antibodies in Acute Zonal Occult Outer Retinopathy (AZOOR): a comprehensive review of 25 cases," *American Journal of Ophthalmology*, vol. 176, pp. 210–218, 2017.

24

Case Series of Brittle Cornea Syndrome

Taher Eleiwa ,[1,2] Mariam Raheem,[1] Nimesh A. Patel,[1] Audina M. Berrocal,[1] Alana Grajewski,[1] and Mohamed Abou Shousha [1]

[1]*Bascom Palmer Eye Institute, Miller School of Medicine, University of Miami, Miami, FL, USA*
[2]*Department of Ophthalmology, Faculty of Medicine, Benha University, Benha, Egypt*

Correspondence should be addressed to Mohamed Abou Shousha; mshousha@med.miami.edu

Academic Editor: Sandra M. Johnson

Purpose. This case series demonstrate diagnostic features, treatment options, and challenges for Brittle Cornea Syndrome. *Observations.* Three cases presented with bluish sclera and extremely thin cornea. Genetic workup was performed and confirmed the diagnosis of Brittle Cornea Syndrome, a rare autosomal recessive disorder characterized by corneal thinning and blue sclera. Case 1 was a 4-year-old boy who developed cataract and glaucoma after undergoing right tectonic penetrating keratoplasty (PK) secondary to a spontaneous corneal rupture. Glaucoma was controlled medically. Later, the kid underwent right transcorneal lensectomy and vitrectomy with synechiolysis. After 6 weeks, he sustained graft dehiscence that was repaired using onlay patch graft. Case 2 was a 7-year-old boy who underwent PK in the right eye, then a pericardial patch graft in the left eye following spontaneous corneal rupture. Glaucoma in both eyes was controlled medically. Case 3 was the 2-year-old sister of the 2nd case. She had a pachymetry of 238 μm OD and 254 μm OS. In the 3 cases, parents were instructed to take protective measures for both eyes and to continue with follow-up visits. Also, they were instructed to have regular screenings for late-onset hearing loss, dental abnormalities, and bone deformities. *Conclusions.* Long-term follow-up of children diagnosed with Brittle Cornea Syndrome is paramount to minimize the morbidity of corneal rupture and late-onset extraocular conditions.

1. Introduction

Brittle Cornea Syndrome is an autosomal recessive disorder that is characterized by corneal thinning and blue sclera [1]. This places the patient at an increased risk of spontaneous rupture or rupture due to minor trauma. Due to the severity of the corneoscleral thinning, surgical repair and postoperative management pose extra challenges. Here, we present clinical outcomes of 3 cases with Brittle Cornea Syndrome.

2. Findings

2.1. Case 1. A 4-year-old Indian boy was brought by his parents to Bascom Palmer Eye Institute three months after having a penetrating keratoplasty (PK) done in his right eye. Three months earlier, the patient had rubbed his right eye while eating. Initially, the patient was seen by his pediatrician and was started on topical antibiotics. The patient returned with white discharge from the right eye. The patient was referred to an ophthalmologist and immediately sent him to the Emergency Room where he was admitted and had a PK for right perforated cornea.

Upon initial examination, the patient had bluish sclera bilaterally (Figure 1). The patient's visual acuity was light perception in the right eye and fix and follow in the left eye. The graft was large and clear (Figure 1(a)). The patient had history of glaucoma in the right eye that was treated medically.

Examination under anesthesia revealed that the patient's IOP in the right eye was 34 mmHg and 14 mmHg in the left eye. The Retinoscopy in the right eye revealed $-6.00 + 3.00 \times 180$ and $-3.00 + 1.00 \times 90$ in the left eye. In the right eye, the corneal diameters were 11.5 mm horizontally and 12.0 mm vertically. In the left eye, the corneal diameters were 11.0 mm horizontally and 11.0 mm vertically. The anterior segment exam of the right eye showed peripheral anterior

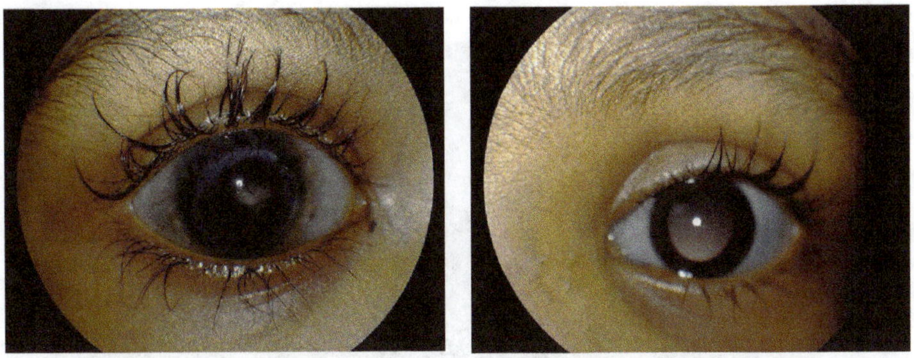

(a) (b)

Figure 1: Slit-lamp photography showing bilateral blue sclera in the right (a) and left (b) eye. Corneal graft in the right eye (1a) is large and clear with intact sutures.

synechiae, intact corneal graft sutures, and no signs of graft rejection. Anterior segment exam of the left eye revealed clear, thin cornea, and optically empty anterior chamber. The cup/disc ratio of the right eye was 0.9 and 0.5 in the left eye. B-scan revealed a posterior staphyloma in the left eye. The axial length was 25.5 mm in the right eye and 23.7 mm in the left eye. An anterior segment OCT was obtained while patient was under anesthesia (Figure 2). The thinnest point of the left cornea determined by the OCT was 237 μm.

There was a concern for Osteogenesis Imperfecta (type I) indicated by thin corneas and bilateral bluish sclera. The patient was sent for genetic analysis. The geneticist noted that the mother and father were first cousins and both had bluish sclera, but were otherwise healthy. Physical findings included dolichocephaly, a prominent forehead, and increased joint flexibility. A buccal sample was collected and tested for 49 different genes, including the ZNF469. The ZNF469 gene showed a homozygous mutation from the patient's buccal samples, confirming the diagnosis of Brittle Cornea Syndrome.

On follow up, the patient was found to have a secondary cataract in his right eye with inferior posterior synechiae and a fibrotic capsule adhered to the iris. The corneal graft was clear with intact sutures (Figure 3). Two months later, the patient underwent a transcorneal lensectomy (through the donor cornea), limited vitrectomy without lifting the hyaloid, synechiolysis, and removal of iris membrane in the right eye (Figure 4, supplementary video (available here)). This was indicated because the cataract was visually significant and presented difficulty when trying to examine the fundus. One day after surgery, the VA was counting fingers and improved to 20/200 2 weeks later. The VA in the left eye was 20/80 without correction. Patient's IOP is well controlled on medications. Unfortunately, 6 weeks after the procedure, the patient presented with a 3-clock hour dehiscence (from the area of the original cornea) of the corneal graft superonasally with no uveal prolapse. The patient underwent repair with a corneal patch graft (Figure 5).

2.2. Case 2 and 3: A Case of Two Siblings of Consanguineous Parents. A 7-year-old boy presented with parents and his 2-year-old sister for evaluation of Brittle Cornea Syndrome, which was confirmed by genetic testing and presented for a second opinion. The 7-year-old boy underwent a PK following spontaneous rupture of the right cornea when the patient was 4 years old. One year later, he underwent a pericardial patch graft following a spontaneous rupture of the left eye which has since fallen and scarred. On examination, the patient had a corneal graft which was vascularized and had inferonasal secondary lipid keratopathy in the right eye (Figure 6). In the left eye, patient's superior cornea was clear, and there was an inferior vascularized leukoma adherent (Figure 6). The patient's 2-year-old sister had no previous surgeries. Both patients had bluish sclera bilaterally (Figure 7). Table 1 summarizes the clinical characteristics in both patients. The patient's parents were instructed to take protective measures for both children and to continue with follow-up visits. Parents were also instructed to have regular screenings for hearing loss, dental abnormalities, and bone deformities during development.

3. Discussion

Brittle Cornea Syndrome is an autosomal recessive syndrome that affects connective tissues. Type I is diagnosed through the identification of mutation in the ZNF469 gene which encodes the transcription regulator that participate in pathways regulating extracellular matrix and collagen synthesis [2]. This results in severe thinning of the cornea and prevents proper development of the anterior chamber and creates a high risk of spontaneous corneal rupture [3]. Type II results from a mutation of PRDM 5. The exact phenotype of the type II mutation is unclear.

Spontaneous rupture or rupture following a minor trauma is a significant risk in patients with Brittle Cornea Syndrome. At glance, there can be a concern for potential child abuse. In our patients, there was no evidence of child abuse. Parents were compliant with all medical instructions as well as office visits and were attentive about their children's progress.

In this series, two out of three cases had corneal perforations. In patients diagnosed with Brittle Cornea Syndrome, precautions are taken in order to prevent ruptures such as polycarbonate goggles and close monitoring of symptoms [4]. Wound repair after rupture can result in further tissue

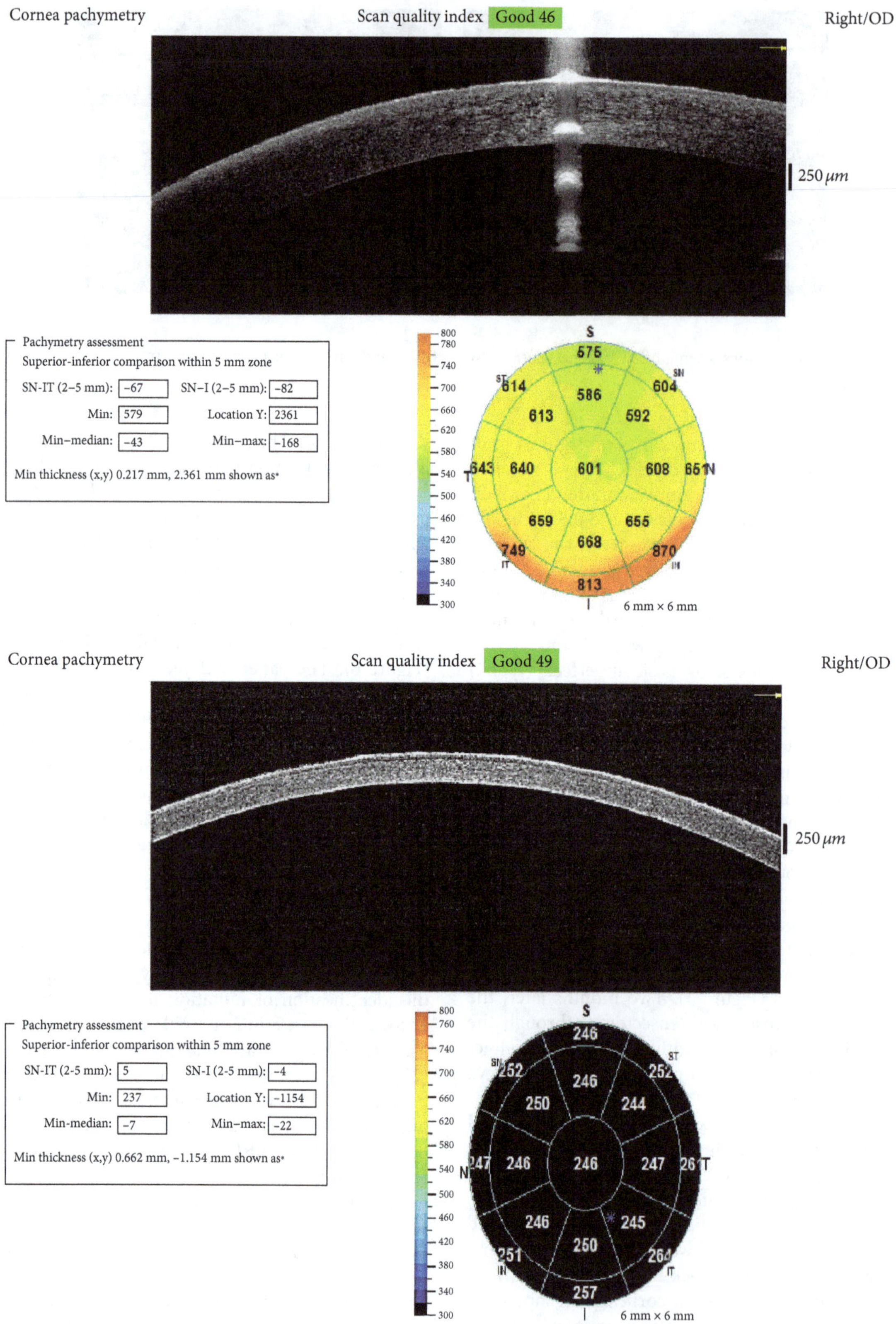

Figure 2: Anterior segment OCT showing corneal thickness maps of both eyes. The right cornea graft has a minimal thickness of 579 μm versus 237 μm in the left eye with Brittle Cornea.

loss. Additionally, sutures that are implanted during a primary keratoplasty have an increased risk of cheese-wiring due to the thin cornea, and there is a risk of overriding due to mismatch between graft and host thickness, both of which could result in increased risk of postoperative infection and leakage [5].

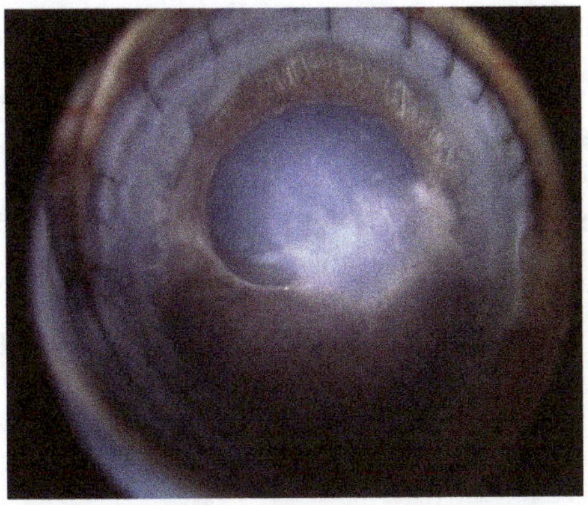

FIGURE 3: Demonstration of cataract and inferior posterior synechiae of the right eye. The corneal graft is clear with intact sutures.

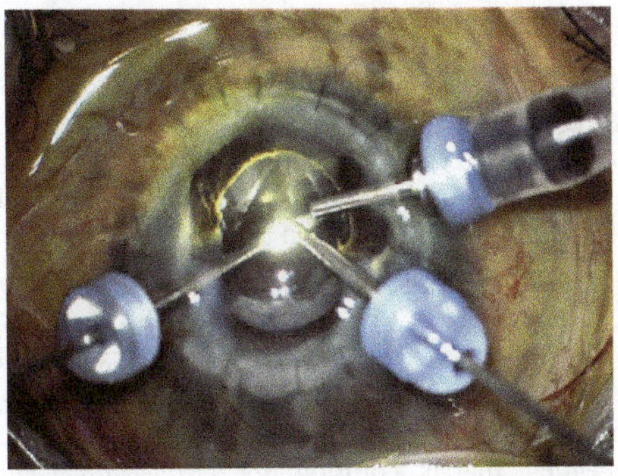

FIGURE 4: Screenshot captured during the cataract removal surgery demonstrating the transcorneal placement of the trocars 0.5 mm anterior to the graft-host junction.

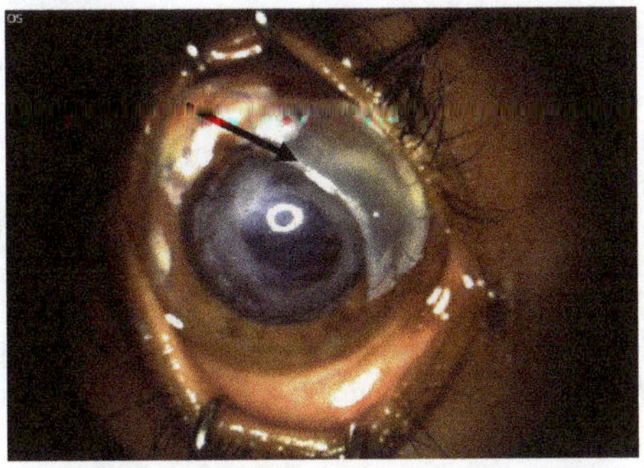

FIGURE 5: Slit-lamp photography of the right eye showing a superonasal corneal patch graft (arrow).

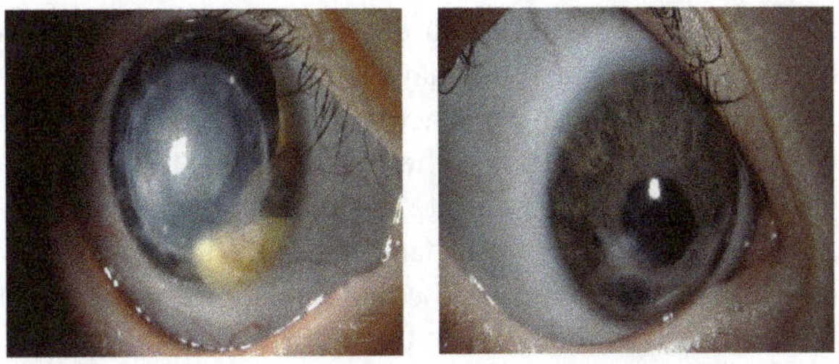

(a) (b)

FIGURE 6: Slit-lamp photography showing vascularized corneal graft with inferonasal secondary lipid keratopathy in the right eye (a) and inferior vascularized leukoma adherent in the left eye.

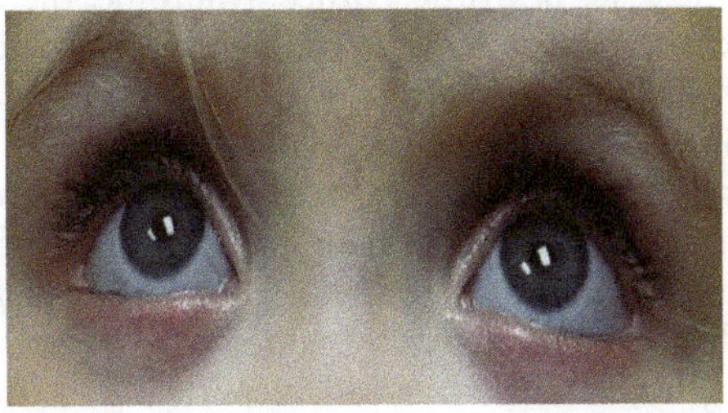

FIGURE 7: External photography showing blue sclera on a 2-year-old girl with Brittle Cornea Syndrome.

TABLE 1: Clinical features of case 2 and case 3.

	Case 2	Case 3
Age	7 years	2 years
Gender	Male	Female
Gene	ZNF469	ZNF469
Presenting visual acuity	OD: counting fingers OS: 20/70 cc	OD: 20/70 cc OS: 20/60 cc
IOP	OD: 16 mmHg OS: 15 mmHg	OD: 16 mmHg OS: 14 mmHg
Minimal corneal thickness	OD: 366 μm OS: 232 μm	OD: 238 μm OS: 254 μm
Refraction	OD: +12.00 OS: $-14.00/+4.75 \times 085$	OD: $-9.25/+4.25 \times 090$ OS: $-9.25/+4.50 \times 090$
Surgical history	OD: penetrating keratoplasty OS: pericardial patch graft	None
Medications	OU: timolol 0.5% bid	OU: timolol 0.5% bid

The impaired collagen integrity with Brittle Cornea Syndrome provided a challenge in the surgical approach and incision placement for the lensectomy and vitrectomy in case 1. On inspection under anesthesia, there was severe host circumferential limbal and scleral thinning. The concern with utilizing conventional limbal wounds was the possible inability to reapproximate the compromised tissues [5]. The approach taken was to place the trocars through the donor keratoplasty tissue, 0.5 mm anterior to the graft-host junction (Supplementary video). This allowed for adequate access for lensectomy, anterior chamber stability, and uncomplicated closure. To the authors' knowledge, there are no prior reports on lensectomy or the use of trocar placement through donor tissue in brittle cornea syndrome. There was dehiscence of the graft 6 weeks later. It is possible that surgical manipulation further wreaked the zone of attachment. Again, the integrity of the tissue provided a challenge for repair and a patch graft was needed. The choroidals resolved and the retina remained attached. The problem is that the original cornea continues to suffer from progressive weakness.

The issues with potential wound leak add to the well-established risks of keratoplasty in pediatric patients. Pediatric patients have a greater risk of postoperative inflammatory reaction and increased fibrin deposition [6]. 20-50% of patients under 5 years old have graft failure attributed to the increased inflammatory activity of patients in this age group [7]. Overall, patients who receive grafts under 4 years of age have a 65% survival rate in the first year [8]. Patients aged 5-12 have an increased chance of graft survival [9]. Postoperative steroid should be used cautiously in patients with brittle cornea syndrome due to the negative effects of steroids on collagen synthesis as well as the risk of secondary glaucoma development [10]. The management of comorbidities also becomes complicated by the graft. About 56% of grafts in pediatric eyes that underwent removal of cataract, IOL implantation, or YAG laser capsulotomy had failed [9].

In some cases of Brittle Cornea Syndrome, there is progressive corneal thinning which may result in the development of keratoglobus or keratoconus. As a result, corneal cross-linking using a modified method in order to account for the thin cornea has been tried as a treatment in pediatric patients [11]. It is worth mentioning that corneal perforations after corneal cross-linking for keratoconus in a woman harboring potentially pathogenic variants in the ZNF469 gene have been recently reported [12]. Additionally, in a case of a monocular patient due to previous rupture and severe corneal ectasia in the seeing eye may have an onlay corneoscleral graft [13]. Five out of six corneas that had surgery for tectonic support placement had successful visual improvement [14].

Glaucoma is the leading cause of irreversible blindness postkeratoplasty [15] and is a leading cause of graft failure [10]. Glaucoma management in pediatric patients is challenging due to the lack of cooperation of these patients. However, effective management is necessary in order to prevent visual loss and prevent damage to the cornea and optic nerve [16]. Also, glaucoma after corneal graft surgery can potentially lead to visual loss and graft failure [17]. The risk of developing glaucoma after a penetrating keratoplasty ranges from 5.5-31% in the early postoperative period and can be as high as 17-35% in the late postoperative period [18]. Patients with peripheral anterior synechiae are at high risk for developing glaucoma [18]. Additionally, in a retrospective study on patients with fragile corneas, it was found that 50% of pediatric patients developed glaucoma after penetrating keratoplasty [19]. In the meantime, it has been credibly proven that corneal thickness exerts an influence on the accuracy of applanation tonometry by about 1 mmHg per 25 microns corneal thickness change [20]. Therefore, IOP measurements have to be corrected in the setting of Brittle Cornea Syndrome.

The decision making for glaucoma management with the thinning present is complex. The absence of reliable sclera poses difficulties in suturing of a plate for a glaucoma drainage implant. An option could be posterior plate location and a pars plana location of the tube at the time of lensectomy and vitrectomy. Also, the use of fibrin glue to secure the plate to the sclera as a substitute for the sutures has been reported [21–23]. Another approach, if topical pharmacotherapy is not successful, is cyclophotocoagulation with adjusted energy parameters [24]. This could again be achieved transsclerally or with an endoscopic technique at the time of the lensectomy.

4. Conclusion

Patients with Brittle Cornea Syndrome require close monitoring, use of protective polycarbonate lenses, and appropriate lifestyle modifications in order to prevent ocular rupture. High-risk patients may require prophylactic corneal cross-linking or corneoscleral grafts. Surgical management in these cases can provide unique challenges due to impaired wound healing. Early diagnosis and continuous care with a multidisciplinary approach, including glaucoma management, are essential in order to prevent vision loss.

Disclosure

All authors attest that they meet the current ICMJE criteria for authorship.

References

[1] J. Swierkowska and M. Gajecka, "Genetic factors influencing the reduction of central corneal thickness in disorders affecting the eye," *Ophthalmic Genetics*, vol. 38, no. 6, pp. 501–510, 2017.

[2] M. Rohrbach, H. L. Spencer, L. F. Porter et al., "ZNF469 frequently mutated in the brittle cornea syndrome (BCS) is a single exon gene possibly regulating the expression of several extracellular matrix components," *Molecular Genetics and Metabolism*, vol. 109, no. 3, pp. 289–295, 2013.

[3] Q. Wan, J. Tang, Y. Han, Q. Xiao, and Y. Deng, "Brittle cornea syndrome: a case report and review of the literature," *BMC Ophthalmology*, vol. 18, no. 1, p. 252, 2018.

[4] E. M. M. Burkitt Wright, L. F. Porter, H. L. Spencer et al., "Brittle cornea syndrome: recognition, molecular diagnosis and management," *Orphanet Journal of Rare Diseases*, vol. 8, no. 1, article 68, 2013.

[5] R. Natarajan, G. Y. Shah, S. K. Rao, and P. Padamanabhan, "Penetrating keratoplasty as a globe-saving procedure in fragile cornea," *Cornea*, vol. 22, no. 2, pp. 164-165, 2003.

[6] B. Bachmann, G. Avgitidou, S. Siebelmann, and C. Cursiefen, "Pediatric corneal surgery and corneal transplantation," *Der Ophthalmologe*, vol. 112, no. 2, pp. 110–117, 2015.

[7] D. Trief, M. C. Marquezan, C. J. Rapuano, and C. R. Prescott, "Pediatric corneal transplants," *Current Opinion in Ophthalmology*, vol. 28, no. 5, pp. 477–484, 2017.

[8] ACGS, *The Australian Corneal Graft Registry*, Flinder's Medical Centre, Australia, 2012, The Australian Corneal Graft Registry.

[9] M. T. Lowe, M. C. Keane, D. J. Coster, and K. A. Williams, "The outcome of corneal transplantation in infants, children, and adolescents," *Ophthalmology*, vol. 118, no. 3, pp. 492–497, 2011.

[10] E. Jamerson, A. Elhusseiny, R. ElSheikh, T. Eleiwa, and Y. El Sayed, "Role of matrix metalloproteinase 9 in ocular surface disorders," *Eye & Contact Lens: Science & Clinical Practice*, vol. 46, pp. S57–S63, 2020.

[11] C. Kaufmann, G. Schubiger, and M. A. Thiel, "Corneal cross-linking for brittle cornea syndrome," *Cornea*, vol. 34, no. 10, pp. 1326–1328, 2015.

[12] W. Zhang, J. B. Margines, D. S. Jacobs et al., "Corneal perforation after corneal cross-linking in keratoconus associated with potentially pathogenic *ZNF469* mutations," *Cornea*, vol. 38, no. 8, pp. 1033–1039, 2019.

[13] K. Muthusamy and S. Tuft, "Use of an onlay corneal lamellar graft for brittle cornea syndrome," *BMJ Case Reports*, vol. 2018, 2018.

[14] J. A. Cameron, J. B. Cotter, J. M. Risco, and H. Alvarez, "Epikeratoplasty for keratoglobus associated with blue sclera," *Ophthalmology*, vol. 98, no. 4, pp. 446–452, 1991.

[15] R. I. Haddadin and J. Chodosh, "Corneal transplantation and glaucoma," *Seminars in Ophthalmology*, vol. 29, no. 5-6, pp. 380–396, 2014.

[16] A. M. Elhusseiny, Y. M. El Sayed, R. H. El Sheikh, G. I. Gawdat, and H. M. Elhilali, "Circumferential Schlemm's canal surgery in adult and pediatric glaucoma," *Current Eye Research*, vol. 44, no. 12, pp. 1281–1290, 2019.

[17] V. Maurino and F. Aiello, "Glaucoma risks in advanced corneal surgery," *Progress in Brain Research*, vol. 221, pp. 271–295, 2015.

[18] H. L. Kornmann and S. J. Gedde, "Glaucoma management after corneal transplantation surgeries," *Current Opinion in Ophthalmology*, vol. 27, no. 2, pp. 132–139, 2016.

[19] V. M. Rathi, S. I. Murthy, B. Bagga, M. Taneja, S. Chaurasia, and V. S. Sangwan, "Keratoglobus: an experience at a tertiary eye care center in India," *Indian Journal of Ophthalmology*, vol. 63, no. 3, pp. 233–238, 2015.

[20] A. Esmael, Y. M. Ismail, A. M. Elhusseiny, A. E. Fayed, and H. M. Elhilali, "Agreement profiles for rebound and applanation tonometry in normal and glaucomatous children," *European Journal of Ophthalmology*, vol. 29, no. 4, pp. 379–385, 2019.

[21] M. Y. Kahook and R. J. Noecker, "Fibrin glue-assisted glaucoma drainage device surgery," *The British Journal of Ophthalmology*, vol. 90, no. 12, pp. 1486–1489, 2006.

[22] N. S. Choudhari, A. Neog, A. Sharma et al., "Our experience of fibrin sealant-assisted implantation of Ahmed glaucoma valve," *Indian Journal of Ophthalmology*, vol. 61, no. 1, p. 23, 2013.

[23] J. D. Harvey, R. L. Gross, and B. D. McMillan, "Novel use of fibrin sealant for scleral suture free placement of a glaucoma drainage device in advanced scleral thinning," *American Journal of Ophthalmology Case Reports*, vol. 9, pp. 7–9, 2018.

[24] D. J. Palmer, J. Cohen, E. Torczynski, and T. A. Deutsch, "Transscleral diode laser cyclophotocoagulation on autopsy eyes with abnormally thinned sclera," *Ophthalmic Surgery and Lasers*, vol. 28, no. 6, pp. 495–500, 1997.

25

Streptococcus mitis/oralis Corneal Ulcer in a Patient with Severe Rheumatoid Arthritis: An Unusual Route

Mustafa Jaffry[1] and Mark Lister[2]

[1]Rutgers New Jersey Medical School, Newark NJ, USA
[2]New York Medical College, Valhalla, New York, USA

Correspondence should be addressed to Mustafa Jaffry; mj502@njms.rutgers.edu

Academic Editor: Kamal Kishore

Purpose. To report a case of Streptococcus mitis oralis (*S. mitis/oralis*) corneal ulcer in a patient with a possible preventable cause. *Methods.* Cultures were obtained from a 64-year-old woman with a 3.5 mm × 5 mm corneal ulcer with hypopyon in the left eye. *Results.* Culture reports demonstrated the growth of S. *mitis/oralis*, a commensal organism of the oral flora. Fortified vancomycin 5% eye drops were started, and the patient was counseled on the rarity of the bacteria as an etiology of corneal ulcers. On the return visit, the patient, who works in a doctor's office, volunteered information that the preservative free artificial tear vials that she used were difficult to open because of her hand deformity due to rheumatoid arthritis; thus, she had to bite the vials open. *Conclusions.* S. *mitis/oralis* is an organism commonly found in the mouth but is rarely found in the eye. We report a unique case of an immunocompromised patient with rheumatoid arthritis, severe dry eye, and a history of multiple episodes of keratolysis, who developed a corneal ulcer from a rare pathogen, with a plausible and preventable route of infection.

1. Introduction

Streptococcus mitis (*S. mitis*) is an alpha-hemolytic gram-positive coccus and belongs to the group of viridans streptococci. Streptococcus oralis (*S. oralis*) belongs to the mitis group of bacteria, and direct speciation is often difficult in clinical settings. Usually isolated as part of the oral flora of the mouth, *S. mitis/oralis* is known to have a low virulence but can be opportunistic and cause severe infections such as endocarditis, meningitis, and bacteremia [1]. Corneal ulcers due to *S. mitis/oralis* have only rarely been described in the literature, limited to a few case reports in a variety of contexts. Herein, we report a unique case of corneal ulcer caused by *S. mitis/oralis* in an immunocompromised patient with severe rheumatoid arthritis (RA).

2. Case Report

A 64-year-old woman with a long history of RA and severe ulnar deviation of both hands presented with a central corneal ulcer in a previous corneal transplant of the left eye. She had a long history of multiple episodes of keratolysis in both eyes secondary to severe dry eye and RA. Throughout the course of her disease she had been on oral prednisone, methotrexate, hydroxychloroquine, intravenous immunoglobulin, and multiple immunosuppressants. Punctal plugs were placed in all 4 lids. The patient had a history of corneal melt in right eye initially, which resolved with oral steroids but resulted in significant scarring. Subsequently, she developed keratolysis in the left eye, which resulted in perforation and required a corneal patch graft that had difficulty healing. The patch graft continued to struggle with reepithelialization, even after multiple amniotic membranes were placed. The patient then developed a suspected fungal infection in the left cornea and underwent a full-thickness corneal transplant. Fungal cultures were not performed. Two months later, after natamycin therapy, there were no signs of residual fungus.

At this time, the patient underwent retinal surgery for retinal detachment in the left eye. Two weeks later, the patient developed a corneal ulcer with hypopyon in the same eye. Fortified vancomycin 5% was started every half hour.

Cultures were taken and demonstrated moderate growth of *Streptococcus mitis/oralis*. Susceptibility testing was not performed, as is usual, because this is a commensal organism of the oral flora. The patient had no recent dental procedures and was counseled and alerted that this is an unusual bacterium that infects the eye and is commonly found in the mouth. Two days later, the hypopyon had decreased, and the ulcer was smaller. On follow up, 2 days after this, the hypopyon had decreased considerably and the patient, who works in a doctor's office, volunteered information on how she thought she may have gotten this infection. The patient reported "Since my hands are so deformed from the arthritis, I am unable to open the vials of preservative-free artificial tears. So, I have been biting off the tops of the vials, so I could insert the tears." We concurred that oral bacteria from her mouth could have contaminated the vials before drop application. On follow-up, the corneal ulcer had quickly resolved.

3. Discussion

Corneal ulcers due to *S. mitis/oralis* represent a diagnostic challenge because of their rarity and have infrequently been described in the literature. In addition to the mouth, *S. mitis/oralis* can be found on the skin, gastrointestinal tract, and female genital tract. Rahman et al. studied microbial contamination in preservative-free eye drops in multidose containers and found significant growth in 8 out of 95 bottles tested. It was observed that *Staph aureus* was the most common contaminant [2]. Preservative-free artificial tears, which this patient used, came in single-use vials, an advantage of which, reduces the risk of contamination with multidose containers. Nevertheless, this patient's method of opening the bottle likely served as a route of infection. Although this patient had prior retinal detachment surgery, which could be another possible route for *S. mitis/oralis*, those complications usually lead to endophthalmitis and not corneal infection [3]. Our patient, prior to the corneal ulcer caused by *S. mitis/oralis*, also had suspected fungal keratitis, highlighting the vulnerability of the patient's cornea and the likely presence of epithelial defects. Although corneal ulcers caused by *S. mitis/oralis* are rare, some cases have been reported in the literature. It is conceivable that the immunocompromised state, along with the multiple ocular morbidities present in the patient, allowed for normally low virulence bacteria to cause a devastating infection. Khan et al. described a case of *S. mitis/oralis* causing a corneal ulcer after transplantation and reported that this was likely due to a reduction in local immunity after the surgery, opening the way for an opportunistic infection [4]. In another report, Hsiao et al. described a patient with recurrent corneal ulcers and a corneal culture that grew *S. mitis/oralis*. Topical vancomycin and ceftriaxone were administered, and the ulceration gradually resolved after amniotic membrane placement [5].

Rheumatoid corneal melt or keratolysis is the most severe complication of peripheral ulcerative keratitis (PUK), a rare form of ocular inflammation associated with rheumatoid arthritis (RA). PUK that results in perforation, caused by RA has been reported to have an incidence of 0.234 per million per year [6]. Corneal melt refers to the severe corneal stromal thinning that leads to perforation and is associated with abrupt loss of vision. PUK is described as inflammation of the limbal area of the cornea and is characterized by collagen destruction, infiltration, and vascular changes [7]. The current understanding of the pathogenesis of corneal melt as a consequence of PUK is unknown, but is thought to be autoimmune mediated inflammation, which results in unstable corneal epithelia, leading to vulnerability and a greater risk of infection as evidenced in this patient. The patient's severe RA was also demonstrated by the deformation of her hands bilaterally with ulnar deviation. This led to a difficulty in opening vials for preservative-free artificial tears, potentially contaminating the tear solution and infecting the eye.

In our case, fortified vancomycin was sufficient to resolve the infection with *S. mitis/oralis*, which agrees with the prior literature that has treated this pathogen [8]. Clinicians should be aware that biting bottles may be a method by which some patients cope with their disability. In this case report, we describe a patient with a corneal ulcer caused by *S. mitis* that was successfully resolved with antibiotics. We stress the importance of educating patients on sterile methods for applying eye drops, to avoid contamination. We also emphasize the importance of counseling patients and following up on how they may use their eye drops, especially in the elderly and those with physical difficulty. We advocate for the development of vials that are easier to use for patients with RA or other deforming arthropathies. This unique case highlights the importance of having accessible tear vials available to patients who cannot open them in the conventional way. With careful observation, close follow-up and open communication, immunocompromised patients at risk of opportunistic ocular infections can be protected. Anecdotally, cases of ocular infections caused by *S. mitis/oralis* have been increasing. A possible hypothesis for this could be widespread mask use, with contaminating fomites of oral bacteria from an individual's breath moving up from the mask and infecting the eye, which has been recently suggested [9]. However, no studies have yet been done to explore this.

Consent

An informed consent to publish this case was provided by the patient.

References

[1] J. Mitchell, "Streptococcus mitis: walking the line between commensalism and pathogenesis," *Molecular Oral Microbiology*, vol. 26, no. 2, pp. 89–98, 2011.

[2] M. Q. Rahman, D. Tejwani, J. A. Wilson, I. Butcher, and K. Ramaesh, "Microbial contamination of preservative free eye drops in multiple application containers," *The British Journal of Ophthalmology*, vol. 90, no. 2, pp. 139–141, 2006.

[3] J. K. Chung and S. J. Lee, "Streptococcus mitis/oralis endophthalmitis management without phakic intraocular lens removal in patient with iris-fixated phakic intraocular lens implantation," *BMC Ophthalmology*, vol. 14, no. 1, p. 92, 2014.

[4] I. D. Khan, A. Sati, S. Arif et al., "Streptococcus mitis/oralis corneal ulcer after corneal transplantation," *Basic & Clinical Medicine*, vol. 5, pp. 8–10, 2016.

[5] F. C. Hsiao, Y. J. Meir, L. K. Yeh et al., *Amniotic membrane transplantation in a patient with impending perforated corneal ulcer caused by Streptococcus mitis: a case report*, Research Square, 2019.

[6] H. M. Timlin, H. N. Hall, B. Foot, and P. Koay, "Corneal perforation from peripheral ulcerative keratopathy in patients with rheumatoid arthritis: epidemiological findings of the British ophthalmological surveillance unit," *The British Journal of Ophthalmology*, vol. 102, no. 9, pp. 1298–1302, 2018.

[7] Y. Cao, W. Zhang, J. Wu, H. Zhang, and H. Zhou, "Peripheral ulcerative keratitis associated with autoimmune disease: pathogenesis and treatment," *Journal of Ophthalmology*, vol. 2017, Article ID 7298026, 12 pages, 2017.

[8] V. J. Hsu, J. Affeldt, and C. Blanton, "Streptococcus mitis corneal ulcer," *Investigative Ophthalmology & Visual Science*, vol. 46, no. 13, p. 2632, 2005.

[9] M. Soleimani, A. Masoumi, H. Farrokhpour, M. Keykhaei, H. Zeidabadinejad, and S. A. Tabatabaei, "Increased rate of infectious keratitis after PRK in the COVID-19 era: the possible role of face masks," *Journal of Refractive Surgery*, vol. 38, no. 2, pp. 78–81, 2022.

Retinal Surface Macrophage Changes in Thyroid Eye Disease before and after Treatment with Teprotumumab

Oscar Otero-Marquez,[1] **Mona Fayad**,[1,2] **Alexander Pinhas**,[1] **Toco Y. P. Chui**,[1,2] **Richard B. Rosen**,[1,2] **and Harsha S. Reddy**[1,2]

[1]*Department of Ophthalmology, New York Eye and Ear Infirmary of Mount Sinai, 310 E 14th St, New York, NY 10003, USA*
[2]*Icahn School of Medicine at Mount Sinai, 1 Gustave L. Levy Pl, New York, NY 10029, USA*

Correspondence should be addressed to Harsha S. Reddy; hreddy@nyee.edu

Academic Editor: Stephen G. Schwartz

Retinal surface macrophages play key roles in the regulation of immune response, maintenance of vitreous clarity, and tissue repair. We examined the variation of parafoveal surface macrophages in a thyroid eye disease (TED) patient before and after treatment with teprotumumab (Tepezza, Horizon therapeutics). Pre- and posttreatment parafoveal surface macrophages were imaged using clinical *en face* OCT, and their density was assessed using a novel cell density mapping technique. Pretreatment, surface macrophage cell density was high. Macrophages had a nonuniform spatial distribution, and their appearance was round with few protrusions, consistent with an "activated" state. Posttreatment, cell density decreased. The macrophages were regularly spaced and had a ramified appearance and filopodia-like processes, consistent with a "quiescent" state. Surface macrophage density decreased as the Clinical Activity Score (CAS) decreased with teprotumumab treatment, suggesting a potential association of these cells with an underlying intraocular and retinal inflammatory process previously not described in TED.

1. Introduction

Thyroid eye disease (TED) is an autoimmune disease characterized by orbital inflammation followed by tissue remodeling and fibrosis. It is most commonly associated with Graves' disease; however, its causes are incompletely understood [1]. The insulin-like growth factor I receptor (IGF-IR), which is overexpressed by orbital fibroblasts and B and T cells in Graves' disease and TED, seems to play a key role [2]. Teprotumumab, a recently FDA-approved monoclonal antibody, targets and blocks IGF-1R and inhibits fibroblast activation via the IGF-1R/TSHR signaling complex. It has been shown to reduce proptosis, improve motility, and reduce Clinical Activity Scores (CAS) [3].

TED has been classically described as an extraocular disease; however, in some patients with active disease, intraocular findings such as optic nerve edema secondary can be seen. TED may have a component of intraocular inflammation, and evaluating intraocular biomarkers of inflammation could be a potential tool to effectively monitor the disease. One potential biomarker involves monitoring the activity of retinal surface macrophages, such as microglia and hyalocytes. These cells are the primary resident immune cells in the posterior chamber and play key roles in homeostasis and neuroprotection. They act as the first responders to neural injury and change their morphology and density in response to damage or external threats [4, 5].

Human retinal surface macrophages have previously been evaluated in healthy subjects and patients with retinopathies and glaucoma [6–8]. To the best of our knowledge, this imaging method has not yet been applied in TED. In this case report, we examine key characteristics of parafoveal surface macrophage cells in a patient with TED, before and after treatment with teprotumumab, including spatial distribution and cell morphology. In addition, we present a semiautomated cell density mapping technique

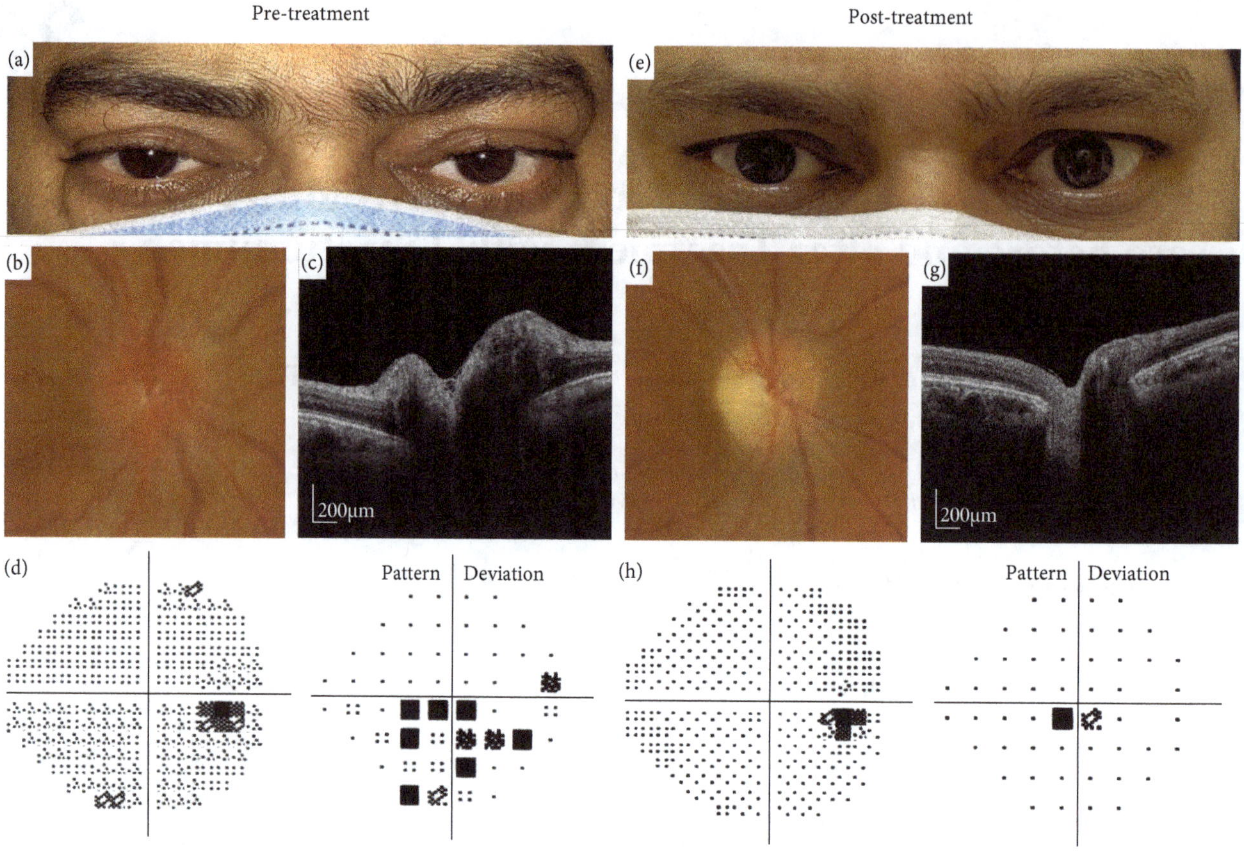

Figure 1: Pre- and post-teprotumumab evaluation of a patient with thyroid eye disease. (a) and (e) External photos show improvement in orbital congestion after treatment. (b) and (f) Right eye, color fundus pictures show improvement in ONH edema and less congestive vasculature. (c) and (g) Right eye, OCT-scans of the ONH show less edema after treatment. RFNL thickness decreased from 209 μm to 107 μm. (d) and (h) Right eye, central 24-2 Humphrey visual field (HVF). HVF prior to treatment showed central and inferior visual field defects. HVF after 5 infusions of teprotumumab with significant improvement in visual defects.

that allows easy visualization and interpretation of cell distribution, with a potential for clinicians to better grade the severity of disease activity and measure treatment effect. This case was HIPAA compliant with protection of any identifiable information and adhered to the tenets of the Declaration of Helsinki.

2. Case Presentation

A 45-year-old male with history of Graves' disease and long-term TED on methimazole 20 mg/day and prednisolone 50 mg/day presented with worsening vision and light sensitivity. His visual acuity was 20/25 in both eyes. Physical examination revealed bilateral proptosis with Hertel's exophthalmometry readings of 24 mm (right) and 22 mm (left), eyelid edema, conjunctival injection, chemosis (Figure 1(a)), and intraocular pressures of 21 mmHg in his right eye and 20 mmHg in his left eye. His CAS was 3/7. Fundus examination revealed bilateral optic nerve head (ONH) edema (Figure 1(b)). OCT scan (DRI OCT Triton plus, Topcon Corp, Tokyo, Japan) of the posterior pole evidenced bilateral ONH edema, more severe in the right eye (Figure 1(c)). RFNL thickness was 209 μm in the right eye and 137 μm in the left eye. Visual field defects were identified (Figure 1(d)). In the figures, only the right eye is shown. Treatment with teprotumumab was initiated.

To assess retinal surface macrophages, ten 3×3 mm scans centered at the fovea were acquired (Avanti RTVue-XR; Optovue, Fremont, CA, USA) and averaged pre- and posttreatment (after the 5th infusion).

Semiautomated macrophage identification was performed on a 3 μm OCT-reflectance (OCT-R) slab located above the inner limiting membrane (ILM) surface using MATLAB (2018b; MathWorks, Natick, MA) (Figures 2(a) and 2(d)). The OCT angiography (OCT-A) full vascular slab located between the ILM and 9 μm below the posterior boundary of the OPL was used for FAZ delineation and capillary density measurements of the entire OCT-A scan (Figures 2(b) and 2(e)).

Surface macrophage density maps were generated in both visits to allow for easy visualization and rapid interpretation of cell distribution across the 3×3 mm scan area (Figures 2(c) and 2(f)). Pretreatment, surface macrophage cell density was higher. Macrophages had a nonuniform spatial distribution, and their appearance was round with few protrusions, consistent with an "activated" state (Figures 3(b) and 3(c)).

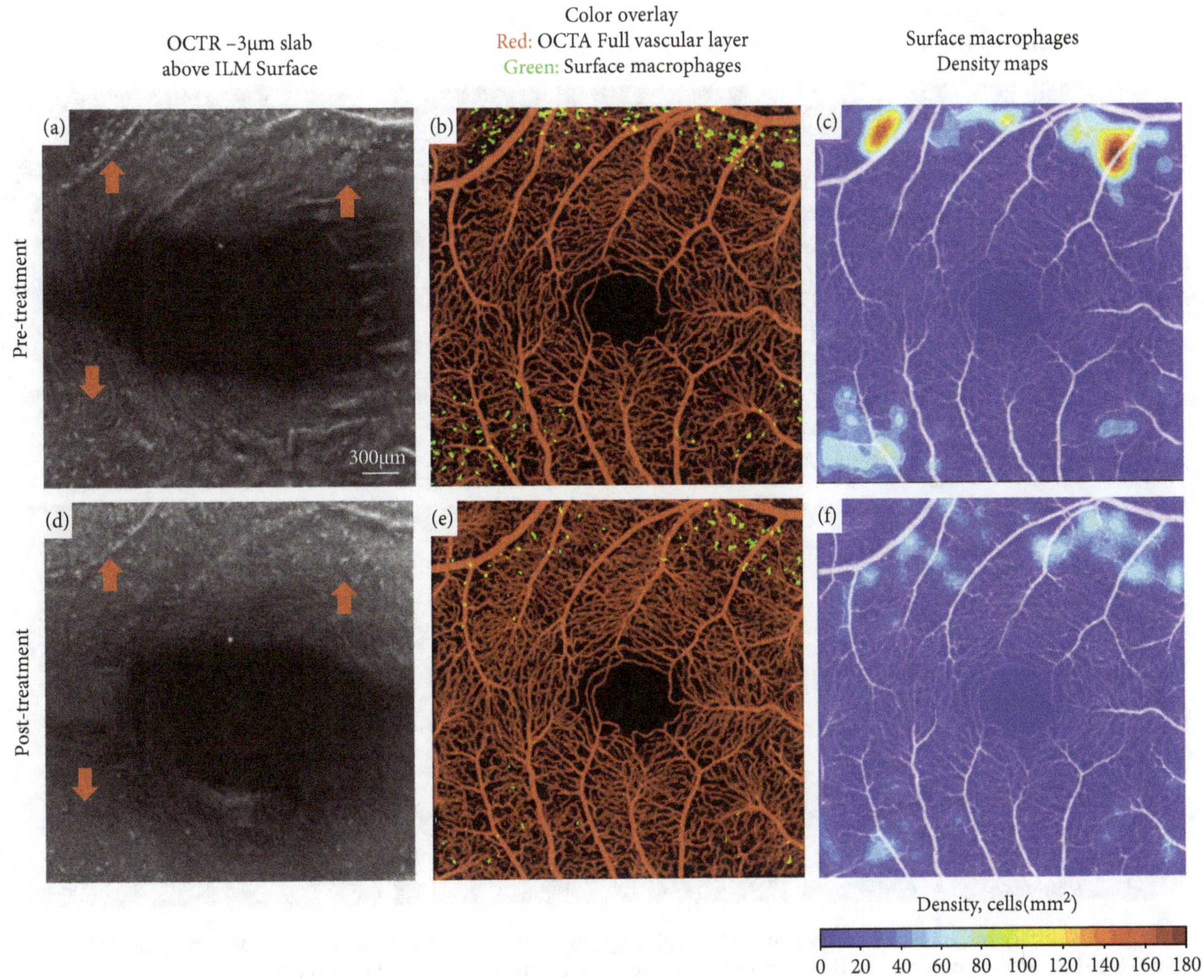

FIGURE 2: Right eye. In vivo imaging of parafoveal surface macrophages and the underlying microvasculature pre- (top row) and post-teprotumumab treatment (bottom row), using clinical OCT. (a) and (d) OCT-R slab located 3 μm above the ILM surface shows the presence of macrophages. Red arrows indicate the presence of surface macrophages where significant differences in cell density and/or morphology can be seen. (b) and (e) Overlay of surface macrophages and corresponding OCT-A full vascular layer. (c) and (f) Overlay of macrophage density map and OCT-A. Surface macrophage density decreased as the inflammatory burden decreased with teprotumumab treatment.

Posttreatment, orbital congestion and ONH edema improved significantly (Figures 1(e)–1(g)). The light sensitivity resolved, and his vision returned to baseline (20/20 OU). Hertel's exophthalmometry readings decreased to 21 mm (right) and 20.5 mm (left), IOPs remained stable, and his CAS improved to 0/7. RFNL thickness decreased to 107 μm in the right eye and 109 μm in the left eye. Visual field defects resolved as well (Figure 1(h)). Fewer surface macrophages were seen (Figure 3(e)). Cell density decreased from 9.10 to 6.55 cells/mm^2 in the right eye and from 5.75 to 3.35 cells/mm^2 in the left eye. The macrophages were regularly spaced and had a ramified appearance consistent with a "quiescent" state (Figure 3(f)). No significant change in capillary density was observed between the pre- and posttreatment imaging sessions. Of note, ten 4.5 mm × 4.5 mm scans centered at the ONH were also acquired pre- and posttreatment. However, surface macrophage evaluation at the initial presentation was not possible due to edema and retinal folds around the ONH which made cell identification nonviable and comparison between visits not feasible.

3. Discussion

In the retina, as in the rest of the CNS, microglia and related macrophage-like cells, such as hyalocytes, act as sentinels, playing key roles in homeostasis, neuroprotection, regulation of immune response, and tissue repair [4, 5]. Until recently, studies of surface macrophages were predominantly performed ex vivo or in animal models using staining and confocal imaging modalities. Nowadays, advances in noninvasive retinal imaging have enabled the visualization of retinal components at a cellular level in humans using clinical optical coherence tomography (OCT) and adaptive optics-OCT (AO-OCT) [6–8]. These investigations have visualized dynamic cells at the vitreoretinal interface with a ramified morphology and mobile soma and processes, consistent with the appearance of macrophages.

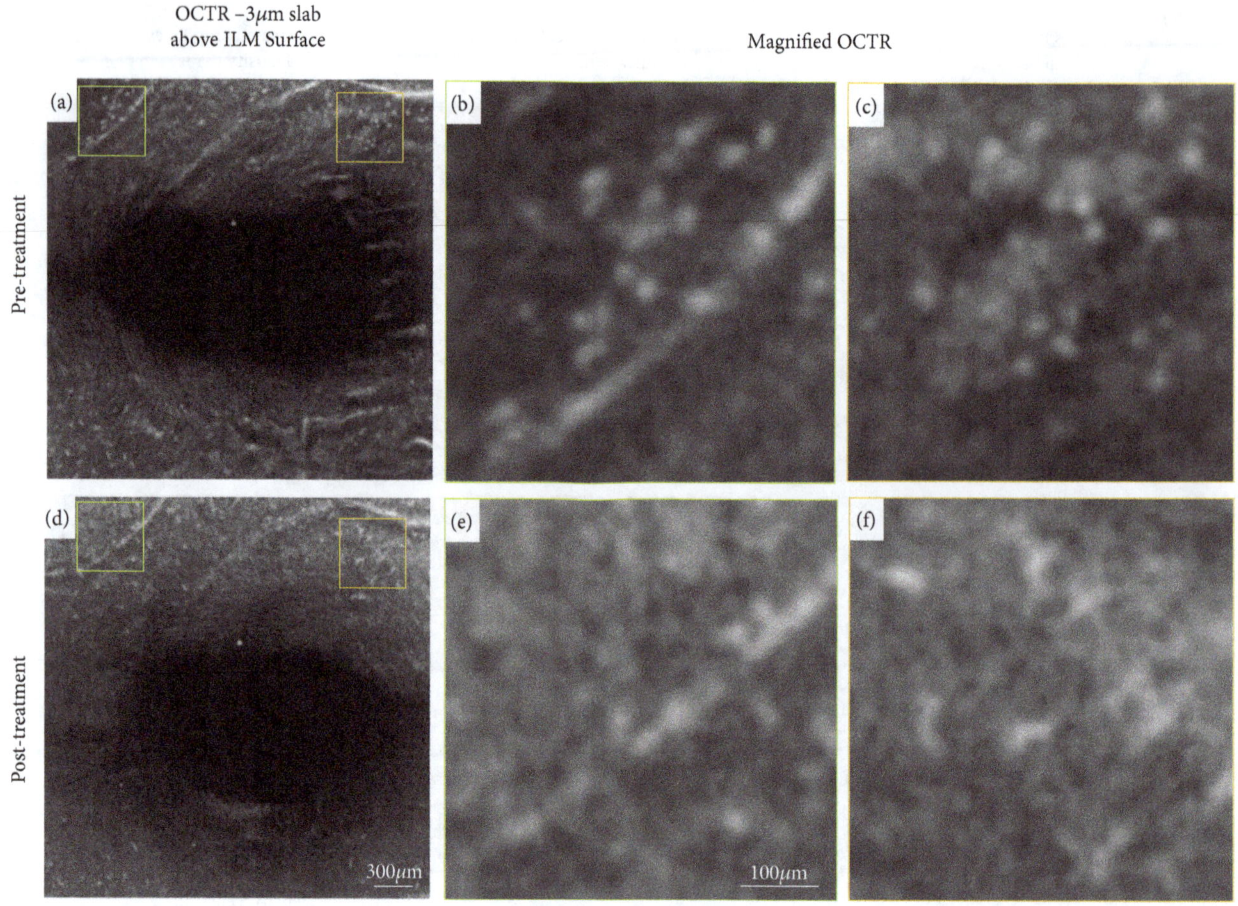

Figure 3: Right eye, surface macrophages distribution and morphology pre- (top row) and post-teprotumumab treatment (bottom row). (a) and (d) OCT-R slab located 3 μm above the ILM surface (green and orange outline correspond to two different regions of interest). (b) and (c) Pretreatment, the cells looked plump with fewer protrusions, clustering around large vessels and areas of metabolic stress. Posttreatment, (e) fewer cells were visible and (f) appeared slender with spindle- or star-like configuration and with a uniform spatial distribution.

Prior research has shown that these immune cells assume a variety of conformational shapes to fulfill these functions and are broadly active in two different phenotypes, depending on whether they serve a neuroprotective or a neurotoxic role [9]. In the neurotoxic or "activated" state, microglia and related macrophage-like cell processes shorten, and their cell bodies change into an amoeboid state with plumper cell bodies, as they proliferate and migrate to the site of injury or disease, releasing inflammatory factors and becoming highly phagocytic [6]. In the neuroprotective phenotype or "quiescent" state, these cells are characterized by spindle cell bodies and ramified filopodia-like processes that constantly probe the local environment, releasing anti-inflammatory and neurotrophic factors [10].

In our patient, before treatment with teprotumumab, we observed a higher density of surface macrophage cells. In addition, these cells were round in appearance, with a non-uniform spatial distribution, and appeared to cluster around vessels and regions of metabolic stress, compatible with the neurotoxic "activated" state previously described in the literature. Posttreatment, as orbital congestion and ONH edema improved, surface macrophage cell density decreased. The distribution and appearance of parafoveal macrophages also changed with treatment. Surface macrophages became more regularly spaced and changed their morphology to a slender and ramified appearance, compatible with the neuroprotective "quiescent" state.

Our findings are consistent with the notion that TED is a systemic inflammatory disease that affects not only the periorbital tissues but the eye itself. In TED, orbital fibroblasts express IGF-1R at higher levels and secrete proinflammatory cytokines such as interleukin-1β (IL-1β), IL-1α, IL-6, IL-8, macrophage chemoattractant protein-1 (MCP-1), and transforming growth factor-β (TGF-β) to perpetuate orbital inflammation [11]. In addition, a recent study by Spadaro et al. [12] provides compelling evidence that macrophages in an activated state secrete IGF-1 and express IGF1-R suggesting an auto or paracrine role of this growth factor in macrophage function, and thus, a possible activation and proliferation of retinal surface macrophages in TED. Another possibility is that an ischemic etiology may be causing the intraocular inflammatory response [11, 13]. IGF-1R and TGF-β are well known to induce hypertrophic and proliferative responses in vascular smooth cells, thereby leading to an increase in wall thickness, decreased perfused luminal areas, potentially resulting in subclinical ischemia in TED. Although we did not find a significant change in capillary and noncapillary densities after teprotumumab treatment, minimal changes in vessel thickness after treatment could be correlated with resolution of subclinical ischemia and less activation of surface macrophages. These findings should be interpreted with caution, and further observational studies are needed to confirm whether the reduction of inflammation alone is responsible for the surface macrophages changes or mediated by teprotumumab directly.

In conclusion, clinical OCT is capable of imaging parafoveal surface macrophages in patients with TED, and is able to monitor changes in distribution and morphology and quantify changes in cell density with treatment. Our results suggest a potential association of the presence of "activated" macrophages with an underlying intraocular and retinal inflammatory process previously not described in TED. Furthermore, our results suggest the potential clinical utility in monitoring these cells to assess disease activity and response to treatment.

Acknowledgments

This report was supported by the National Eye Institute of the National Institutes of Health under award number R01EY027301. Additional funding for this research was provided by the New York Eye and Ear Infirmary Foundation Grant, the Marrus Family Foundation, the Challenge Grant award from Research to Prevent Blindness, and the Jorge N. Buxton Microsurgical Foundation.

References

[1] T. J. Smith and L. Hegedüs, "Graves' disease," *The New England Journal of Medicine*, vol. 375, no. 16, pp. 1552–1565, 2016.

[2] J. Pritchard, R. Han, N. Horst, W. W. Cruikshank, and T. J. Smith, "Immunoglobulin activation of T cell chemoattractant expression in fibroblasts from patients with Graves' disease is mediated through the insulin-like growth factor I receptor pathway," *Journal of Immunology*, vol. 170, no. 12, pp. 6348–6354, 2003.

[3] R. S. Douglas, G. J. Kahaly, A. Patel et al., "Teprotumumab for the treatment of active thyroid eye disease," *The New England Journal of Medicine*, vol. 382, no. 4, pp. 341–352, 2020.

[4] L. Chen, P. Yang, and A. Kijlstra, "Distribution, markers, and functions of retinal microglia," *Ocular Immunology and Inflammation*, vol. 10, no. 1, pp. 27–39, 2002.

[5] H. S. Lazarus and G. S. Hageman, "In situ characterization of the human hyalocyte," *Archives of Ophthalmology*, vol. 112, no. 10, pp. 1356–1362, 1994.

[6] M. V. Castanos, D. B. Zhou, R. E. Linderman et al., "Imaging of macrophage-like cells in living human retina using clinical OCT," *Investigative Ophthalmology and Visual Science*, vol. 61, no. 6, 2020.

[7] D. X. Hammer, A. Agrawal, R. Villanueva, O. Saeedi, and Z. Liu, "Label-free adaptive optics imaging of human retinal macrophage distribution and dynamics," *Proceedings of the National Academy of Sciences of the United States of America*, vol. 117, no. 48, pp. 30661–30669, 2020.

[8] J. X. Ong, P. L. Nesper, A. A. Fawzi, J. M. Wang, and J. A. Lavine, "Macrophage-like cell density is increased in proliferative diabetic retinopathy characterized by optical coherence tomography angiography," *Investigative Ophthalmology and Visual Science*, vol. 62, no. 10, p. 2, 2021.

[9] A. I. Ramirez, R. de Hoz, E. Salobrar-Garcia et al., "The role of microglia in retinal neurodegeneration: Alzheimer's disease, Parkinson, and glaucoma," *Frontiers in Aging Neuroscience*, vol. 9, 2017.

[10] L. Todd, I. Palazzo, L. Suarez et al., "Reactive microglia and IL1β/IL-1R1-signaling mediate neuroprotection in excitotoxin-damaged mouse retina," *Journal of Neuroinflammation*, vol. 16, no. 1, 2019.

[11] J. J. Khong, A. A. McNab, P. R. Ebeling, J. E. Craig, and D. Selva, "Pathogenesis of thyroid eye disease: review and update on molecular mechanisms," *The British Journal of Ophthalmology*, vol. 100, no. 1, pp. 142–150, 2016.

[12] O. Spadaro, C. D. Camell, L. Bosurgi et al., "IGF1 shapes macrophage activation in response to immunometabolic challenge," *Cell Reports*, vol. 19, no. 2, pp. 225–234, 2017.

[13] A. Bouallegue, G. Vardatsikos, and A. K. Srivastava, "Role of insulin-like growth factor 1 receptor and c-Src in endothelin-1- and angiotensin II-induced PKB phosphorylation, and hypertrophic and proliferative responses in vascular smooth muscle cellsThis article is one of a selection of papers published in a special issue on Advances in Cardiovascular Research," *Canadian Journal of Physiology and Pharmacology*, vol. 87, no. 12, pp. 1009–1018, 2009.

27

Unprompted Closure of Spontaneous Macular Hole Secondary to Retained Subfoveal Perfluorocarbon Liquid

Hamouda Hamdy Ghoraba,[1,2] Hashem Hamouda Ghoraba,[2] and Adel Galal Zaky[3]

[1]*Ophthalmology Department, Faculty of Medicine, Tanta University, Tanta, Egypt*
[2]*Magrabi Eye Hospital, Tanta, Egypt*
[3]*Ophthalmology Department, Faculty of Medicine, Menoufia University, Shibin el Kom, Egypt*

Correspondence should be addressed to Adel Galal Zaky; adelzaky12@gmail.com

Academic Editor: Stephen G. Schwartz

Purpose. To report unprompted closure of spontaneous macular hole secondary to inadvertent subfoveal perfluorocarbon liquid (PFCL) after vitrectomy surgery. *Observations.* We present a case of a retained large single subfoveal PFCL droplet following vitrectomy and silicone oil injection for subtotal rhegmatogenous retinal detachment that showed spontaneous release 3 weeks postoperatively, with subsequent development of full thickness macular hole (FTMH) which completely closed later on after silicone oil removal without internal limiting membrane peeling with marvelous anatomic and visual improvement after spontaneous closure of MH. *Conclusions.* Different fates of subfoveal PFCL droplets may happen. Spontaneous release of subfoveal PFCL without surgical interference has rarely been reported.

1. Introduction

The unique chemical and physical properties of perfluorocarbon liquid (PFCL) have enabled internal displacement of subretinal fluid and stabilization of mobile retina, transforming the surgical approach of complex retinal detachments repair. Despite these advantages, the use of PFCL may be complicated by inadvertent retention of PFCL droplets in the subretinal space [1]. Subfoveal PFCL may be visually significant, and prompt surgical removal or displacement is indicated according to the visual prognosis [1]. While peripheral subretinal PFCL can often be observed, migration of peripherally located droplets towards the fovea is well recognized, although the mechanisms of migration remain unknown [2]. Spontaneous resolution of subfoveal PFCL without surgical evacuation or displacement has rarely been described [3]. We present a case of a retained large single subfoveal PFCL droplet that spontaneously resolved in out of classic manner.

2. Case Report

A male patient, 52 years old, presented with subtotal rhegmatogenous retinal detachment with single large upper equatorial break (10-12 o' clock) with macula off in the left eye with visual acuity of hand movement. He underwent pars plana vitrectomy (PPV) and silicone oil injection. Transconjunctival 23 gauge 3-port PPV technique using the EVA surgical system (Dutch Ophthalmic Research Center (DORC), Zuidland, Netherlands) and a noncontact wide-angle viewing system BIOM (binocular indirect ophthalmoscope; Oculus, Wetzlar, Germany) were used. Posterior vitreous detachment was created using aspiration by a vitreous cutter with triamcinolone. PFCL was used to stabilize the posterior pole, and the vitreous base was shaved 360 degrees as safe as possible without lensectomy using high-speed vitreous cut rates (8000-9000 cuts/min) and low vacuum settings (100-150 mmHg). Conventional internal limiting membrane (ILM) peeling was performed after

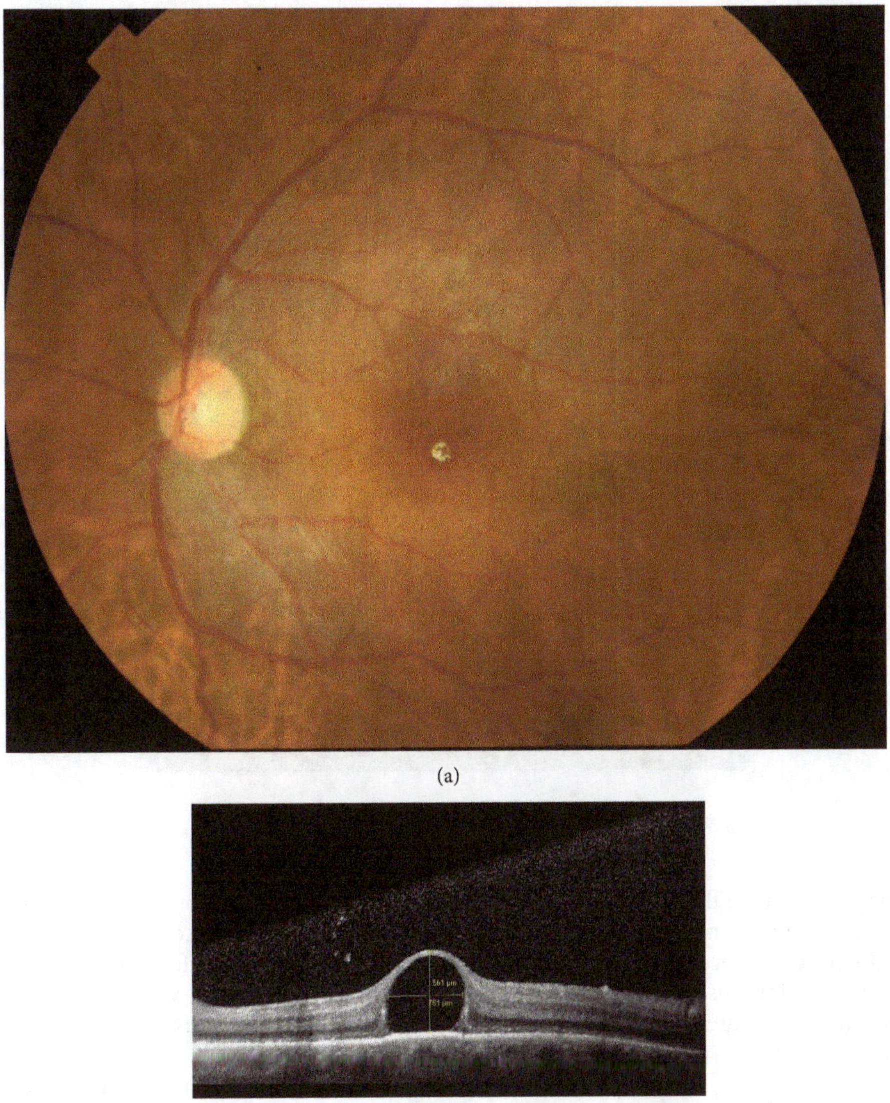

(a)

(b)

FIGURE 1: (a) Colored fundus photography showing subfoveal PFCL droplet. (b) OCT showing 'Ω sign.

injection of brilliant blue dye (ILM Blue; DORC International, Zuidland, Netherlands) under PFCL. Subretinal fluid was drained anteriorly through the original break with the assistance of PFCL by injection with 23-gauge dual bore cannula (MedOne Surgical, Sarasota, USA) keeping the injection within the single PFCL bubble to avoid "satellite" bubbles followed by air-PFC exchange. Endolaser photocoagulation was performed around identifiable retinal tear. Silicon-air exchange using silicon oil 5000 centistokes was performed. On postoperative day 1 and then at postoperative week 1, the patient had counting finger vision with retinal attachment under silicone oil, but a subfoveal PFCL droplet was noted on ophthalmoscopy (Figure 1(a)) and confirmed with optical coherence tomography (OCT) imaging, which revealed a focal area of severely thinned retinal tissue overlying the droplet with omega sign (Figure 1(b)). After 2 weeks, visual acuity (VA) improved to 0.1, and the patient complained of metamorphopsia. The decision was made to aspirate PFCL by 41-gauge cannula after 1 week. The patient came at the time, but he complained of marked drop of vision with central scotoma; VA was counting fingers 2 meters. Fundus examination showed development of full thickness macular hole with disappearance of PFCL droplet which was confirmed by OCT (Figure 2). We preferred to follow the patient, and after 4 months from original surgery, he underwent phacoemulsification with intraocular lens implantation, and silicone oil removal (SOR) without any further ILM peeling techniques or free ILM flap and subretinal or intravitreal PFCL was never identified. In the 1st day and 1st week post, SOR fundus examination showed attached retina with FTMH, and VA was 0.05. On postoperative 3rd week, he noted improvement in his vision 3 days before the visit. By examination, VA was 0.4, and ophthalmoscopy was performed, demonstrating closure of MH. OCT performed that day revealed a restored foveal depression. Without any surgical intervention, these architectural changes improved over the subsequent months, with restoration of the ellipsoid zone at the fovea (Figure 3). VA improved to 0.7 after 3 months of SOR.

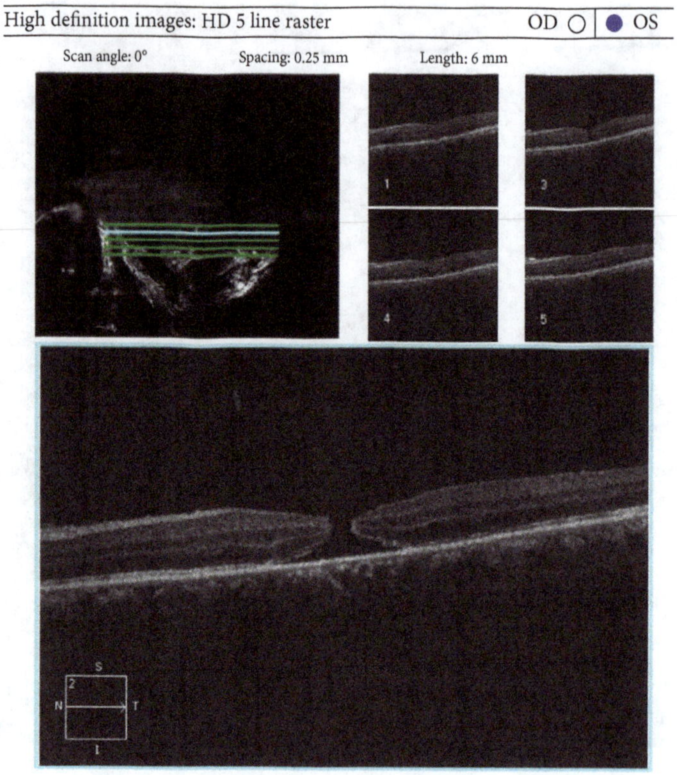

Figure 2: OCT showing development of FTMH.

The study was approved by the Ethical Committee of the Magrabi Eye Hospital Foundation, and the patient was fully informed regarding the technique of the surgery, including the potential risks and complications, and signed a written informed consent document before surgery. This study followed the tenets and guidelines of the Declaration of Helsinki.

3. Discussion

Few complications have been associated with use of PFCLs. The most common is postoperative residual PFCL in vitreous cavity or in the anterior chamber. Subretinal retention of PFCL has been reported, and it has the most significant ocular toxicity. Inadvertent postoperative retention of PFCL occurs in approximately 1% to 7% of eyes. Multiple studies have shown that even with highly purified PFCLs, retinal toxicity occurs after just a few days of intravitreal PFCL exposure and an even shorter period for subretinal PFCL [2].

In this report, we demonstrate a case of spontaneous resolution of subfoveal PFCL. Examination of the posterior and peripheral retina just revealed FTMH without any subretinal PFCL droplets following release. We hypothesize that the surface tension of the PFCL droplet resulted in tangential forces that created a defect at the fovea which may be weakened by ILM peeling which was done in 1ry surgery. PFCL droplet is more likely to be spontaneously released, because the force acting to confine them in a normal retina might be disturbed [4]. We suggest that the PFCL droplet extruded through this retinal defect into the vitreous cavity, where it remained undetected, but was subsequently removed during SOR or may be allocated inferiorly at ciliary body. The possibility of retinal hole formation due to chronic subretinal PFCL retention with a very thin overlying retina has been reported in the literature.

Ghoraba et al. [5] revealed spontaneous formation of MHs in 2 patients. In those 2 patients, subfoveal PFCL droplets disappeared. Tanabu et al. [4] reported a case of MH secondary to subfoveal PFCL that subsequently closed after its spontaneous resolution. This happened after doing a vitrectomy for traumatic retinal detachment. They postulated that the retinal structure in the macula was fragile. Thus, subretinal PFCL droplets were likely to discharge more easily. Also, they explained that the eyes in which the ILM has already become detached or removed PFCL droplets are more likely to be spontaneously discharged.

In other studies, a large PFCL bubbles spontaneously migrated from the fovea in a downward direction or a subretinal PFCL droplet subsequently disappeared from the central fovea, resulting in improvement of the retinal structure [6]. Also, Oellers et al. [7] postulated that the PFCL droplet discharged through a transient hole created in the thinned retina overlying the droplet spontaneously, which later on closed leaving the macula flat and atrophic.

OCT was important especially for the follow-up of the patients and the differential diagnosis of retained subretinal fluid, subretinal SO, sticky SO, and subretinal PFCL because of their differences in viscosity, density, and surface tension. Entrapped PFCL bubble has distinct border, and retina adapts to the shape of Greek letter 'Ω; thus, the angle

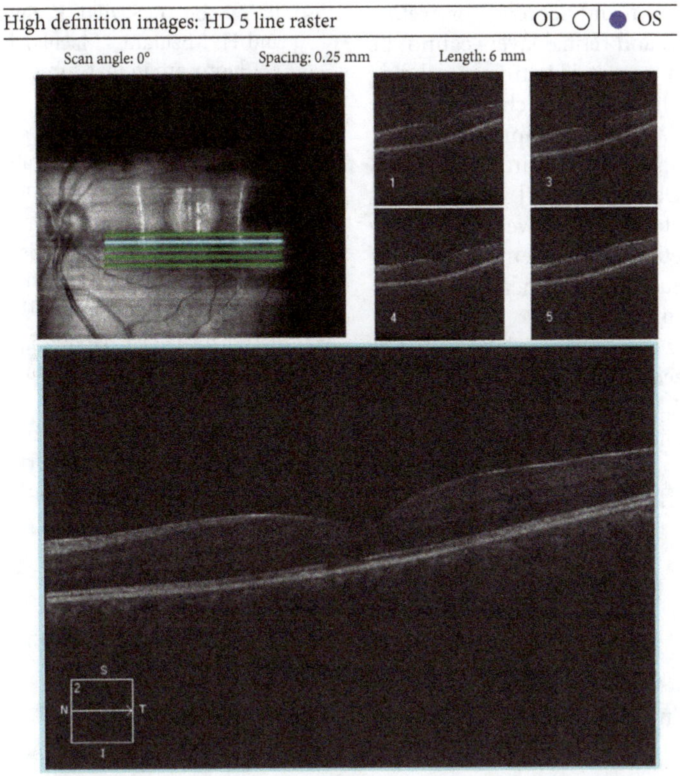

(a)

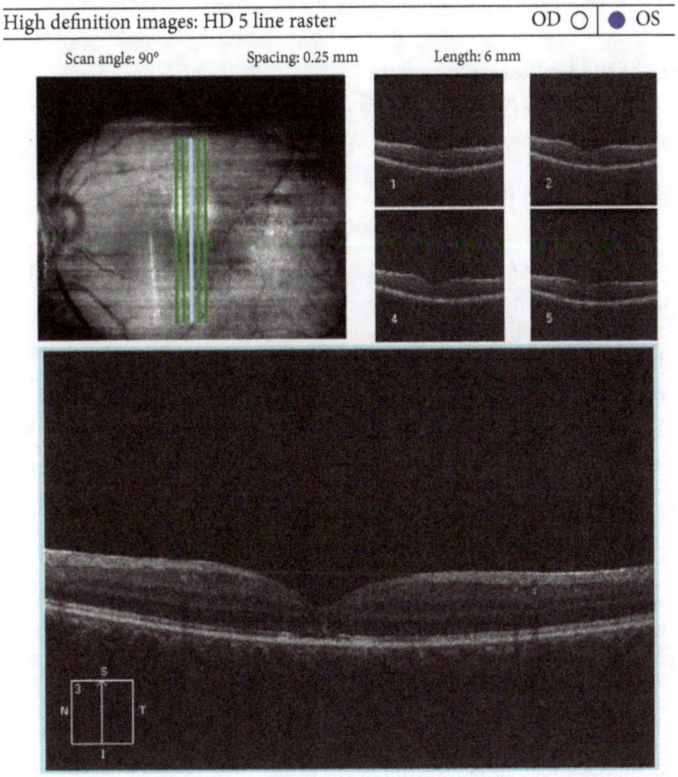

(b)

FIGURE 3: OCT horizontal and vertical HD raster scan showing closure of MH with improvement of microarchitecture of the retina.

between retinal pigment epithelium and neurosensory retina at base of PFCL bubble is acute, and retinal layers cannot be identified above PFCL droplet as whole retina was being squeezed with hyperreflective shadow at the choroid [5].

As regards VA, it was dramatically improved in our patient after release PFCL droplet and closure of MH and reached 0.7. This agrees with Oellers et al. [7] who reported in their case VA improvement to 20/70 at 6 weeks following oil removal, with sustained retinal attachment, absence of any retained PFCL, and continued improvement of the retinal contour and microarchitecture.

The mechanism of this rare event is scarcely reported in literature, and poorly recognized as different behaviors and scenarios of submacular PFCL droplets may occur [8]. In the future, improved understanding of the mechanisms of spontaneous resolution may enable the development of non-surgical or minimal invasive techniques to remove subfoveal PFCL.

Consent

Written consent to publish this case has not been obtained. This report does not contain any personal identifying information.

Disclosure

A preprint has previously been published in Research Square platform (https://www.researchsquare.com/article/rs-1514998/v1).

Authors' Contributions

H.G and A.Z conceptualized the idea. A.Z and H.H.G designed the study. H.G and A.Z recruited the case for the study and performed surgeries and clinical follow-up examinations. H.G performed fundus photography and OCT examination and its analysis. A.Z and H.H.G drafted the manuscript. H.G revised manuscript. All authors approved the final manuscript.

References

[1] K. J. Blinder, "Use of perfluorocarbon liquids," in *Vitreoretinal Surgical Techniques*, G. A. Peyman, S. A. Meffert, M. D. Conway, and F. Chou, Eds., pp. 173–191, Martin Dunitz, London, UK, 2001.

[2] S. Meffert and G. A. Peyman, "Intraoperative complications of perfluoroperhydrophenanthrene: subretinal perfluorocarbon, retinal slippage and residual perfluorocarbon. Vitreon Study Group," *Canadian Journal of Ophthalmology*, vol. 34, no. 5, pp. 272–280, 1999.

[3] M. Shulman, Y. J. Sepah, S. Chang, G. W. Abrams, D. V. do, and Q. D. Nguyen, "Management of retained subretinal perfluorocarbon liquid," *Ophthalmic Surgery, Lasers & Imaging Retina*, vol. 44, no. 6, pp. 577–583, 2013.

[4] R. Tanabu, Y. Suzuki, K. Suzuki, S. Takahashi, M. Nakazawa, and H. Mizutani, "Macular hole caused by retained subfoveal perfluorocarbon that subsequently closed after its spontaneous resolution: a case report," *Ophthalmol Ther.*, vol. 6, no. 2, pp. 381–384, 2017.

[5] H. H. Ghoraba, H. H. Ghoraba, M. A. Heikal et al., "Submacular perfluorocarbon liquid: long-term follow-up," *International Ophthalmology*, vol. 40, no. 5, pp. 1209–1219, 2020.

[6] C. A. Toth, E. W. Schneider, and F. A. Folgar, "Spontaneous peripheral migration of subfoveal perfluorocarbon," *Retina*, vol. 34, no. 11, pp. 2315-2316, 2014.

[7] P. Oellers, L. D. Charkoudian, and P. Hahn, "Spontaneous resolution of subfoveal perfluorocarbon," *Clinical Ophthalmology*, vol. 9, pp. 517–519, 2015.

[8] H. H. Ghoraba, H. H. Ghoraba, and A. G. Zaky, "Unusual behavior of subfoveal perfluorcarbon liquid," https://www.researchsquare.com/article/rs-1514998/v1.

28

RPE65 c.393T>A, p.(Asn131Lys): Novel Sequence Variant Detected

Mirjana Bjeloš,[1,2,3] **Mladen Bušić**,[1,2,3] **Ana Ćurić**,[1,3] **Damir Bosnar**,[1,2,3] **Borna Šarić**,[1] **Leon Marković**,[1,3] **Biljana Kuzmanović Elabjer**,[1,2,3] **and Benedict Rak**[1]

[1]*Department of Ophthalmology, Reference Center of the Ministry of Health of the Republic of Croatia for Pediatric Ophthalmology and Strabismus, University Hospital "Sveti Duh", Zagreb, Croatia*
[2]*Faculty of Medicine, Josip Juraj Strossmayer University of Osijek, Osijek, Croatia*
[3]*Faculty of Dental Medicine and Health Osijek, Josip Juraj Strossmayer University of Osijek, Osijek, Croatia*

Correspondence should be addressed to Mladen Bušić; mbusic@kbsd.hr

Academic Editor: Benedetto Falsini

Background. Leber congenital amaurosis (LCA) is a monogenic, but genetically heterogenous disease, and at least 27 genes are implicated. This case report is aimed at providing evidence to link the novel variant *RPE65* c.393T>A, p.(Asn131Lys), variant of uncertain significance (VUS), to clinical phenotype and to set the ground for objective assignment of pathogenicity confidence. *Case Presentation.* A case report of a female patient with LCA who manifested with nystagmus, night blindness, profound visual deficiency, and peripheral involvement of the retina consistent with *RPE65* dystrophy. A thorough clinical examination, diagnostic evaluation, and genetic testing were performed. The patient was a compound heterozygote in *trans* form: *RPE65* c.304G>T, p.(Glu102*) pathogenic, and *RPE65* c.393T>A, p.(Asn131Lys), VUS. The latter variant is absent in healthy controls and is considered harmful on in silico prediction. *Conclusions.* We conclude that *RPE65* c.393T>A, p.(Asn131Lys) contributed to the pathologic phenotype, demonstrating its significance clearly in the case presented, and should be reclassified according to the criteria of evidence as likely pathogenic. This being the case, patients with this specific variant are likely candidates for genetic treatment.

1. Introduction

Leber congenital amaurosis (LCA) is one of the most common causes of blindness in children with incidence of 2 to 3 per 100 000 newborns [1], characterized by early and severe visual loss occurring usually before the age of 1 year, nystagmus, sluggish or almost absent pupillary reflexes, and reduced or flattened electroretinogram (ERG) [2].

LCA is a monogenic, but genetically heterogeneous disease, and around 27 genes are implicated [3] and inherited in an autosomal recessive manner, except for *IMPDH1* linked to dominant transmission and *CRX* known to cause either dominant or recessive disease [2, 3]. Among the known disease-causing genes, *RPE65* mutations were first identified with the prevalence ranging from 1.7% to 16% in LCA cohorts in the United States, Canada, Saudi Arabia, Asia, and India, with most cases occurring in Western populations [4].

RPE65 protein (GenBank accession No. NP000320.1) is an isomerase preferentially expressed in the retinal pigment epithelium (RPE) [4]. It is of utmost importance to define the molecular diagnosis of the patients with LCA due to existing targeted therapeutic option: voretigene neparvovec (Luxturna®, Novartis, Basel, Switzerland). The prevalence of *RPE65* variants in LCA patients has been estimated to 6-8% [5, 6].

This is the first report of the novel variant c.393T>A, p.(Asn131Lys), variant of uncertain significance (VUS), RP, LCA, autosomal recessive. This case report is aimed at providing evidence to link the variant to clinical phenotype and to provide the ground for objective assignment of pathogenicity confidence.

2. Case Presentation

A 66-year-old female with inherited retinal dystrophy (IRD) was referred to our clinic in June 2021 for clinical examination and genetic testing. Since infancy, her parents noticed that her eyes are "flickering" and she could not see well in the dark or find toys on the floor in the dark room. Her visual performance was sufficient to enable attendance at regular elementary school until the 7th grade (13 years), when her visual acuity further declined, and was thus enrolled in the Center for the Education of the Blind. At the age of 16, a more pronounced decline in visual acuity ensued, progressively worsening over the years. Her mother and father were healthy, as well as 12 siblings. She has 3 healthy children and 2 healthy grandchildren.

At clinical examination, at 1355 lux of room illumination, her visual acuity (VA) measured 1.0 logMAR binocularly at distance (tested on 3 m) and 1.1 logMAR at near (tested on 40 cm). Right eye (RE) measured 1.5 logMAR on 1 m and 30 cm, while left eye (LE) measured 1.0 logMAR distance (tested on 3 m) and 1.1 logMAR near (tested on 40 cm). She could not perform CSV-1000 contrast sensitivity testing or standardized color vision tests. Tested with A4 colored papers, the patient was able to discriminate red, orange, green, and blue colors clearly, while purple color could not be distinguished from blue. Octopus® (Haag-Streit Inc, Mason (OH), USA) static G1 perimetry evidenced markedly reduced retinal sensitivity within the central 30°: mean deviation measured 26.5 dB on the RE and 26.2 dB on the LE, while mean sensitivity measured 0.0 dB and 0.3 dB, respectively. MAIA microperimetry (iCare Finland Oy, Vantaa, Finland) was attempted, but the patient failed to fixate the test badge with either eye due to low VA and nystagmus. Central foveal thickness analysed by optical coherence tomography (HRA+ OCT Spectralis®, Heidelberg Engineering, Heidelberg, Germany) measured 258 and 251 microns in the RE and LE, respectively.

Optos® California (Optos Inc, Marlborough, MA, USA) ultra-widefield imaging depicted pale and waxy optic nerve head with clear boundaries and area of atrophy peripapillary. The macula was mostly atrophic; however, wider areas without atrophy larger than 3-disc diameter were present bilaterally. Diffuse patches of paving-stone degeneration, drusen-like retinal deposits, bone spicule-like pigmentary clumping, and attenuated retinal vessels were observed at the mid- and far periphery (Figure 1). Fundus autofluorescence was absent (Figure 2).

Electrophysiological testing (Roland Consult RETI-port/scan 21, Roland Consult Stasche & Finger GmbH–German Engineering, Brandenburg an der Havel, Germany) according to ISCEV standards was further performed. Full-field ERG bilaterally depicted barely detectable scotopic and photopic responses. Retinoscopy in cycloplegia did not detect significant refractive error: RE: +1.50/−0.50 × 50°, and LE: +1.50/−0.50 × 120°.

The patient's buccal swab was collected for genetic testing for mutations in the *RPE65* gene and sent to Blueprint Genetics Laboratory, Espoo, Finland.

The Blueprint Genetics Retinal Dystrophy Panel (version 6, 2020, Feb 22) Plus sequence analysis and copy number variation analysis identified a heterozygous nonsense variant *RPE65* c.304G>T, p.(Glu102∗) and a heterozygous missense variant *RPE65* c.393T>A, p.(Asn131Lys) [7]. The Next-Generation Sequencing data indicated that these variants were on different parental alleles (in *trans*) in this patient.

3. Discussion

3.1. RPE65 c.304G>T, p.(Glu102∗). This pathological variant is linked to LCA type 2 phenotype [8]. Clinical features of the disease include the following: blindness, cataract, decreased light- and dark-adapted ERG amplitude, fundus atrophy, keratoconus, photophobia, RP, and reduced VA [3, 9]. In the Genome Aggregation Database [10], a large reference population database ($n > 120{,}000$ exomes and >15,000 genomes) which is aimed at excluding individuals with severe pediatric disease, 9 individuals heterozygous for the variant and no homozygotes were found in the dataset [10]. The variant is a cause of a premature stop codon in exon 4 (of 14 total exons) and leads to loss of normal protein function, either through protein truncation or nonsense-mediated mRNA decay [8]. The *RPE65* c.304G>T, p.(Glu102∗) has been reported in a homozygous state in two siblings with LCA [11] and together with c.271C>T, p.(Arg91Trp) in two patients with autosomal-recessive *RPE65*-related IRD [12].

3.2. RPE65 c.393T>A, p.(Asn131Lys). This missense variant predicts asparagine (uncharged polar, hydrophilic) and lysine (basic) substitution resulting in changes in charge. This variant is absent in gnomAD [10]. The mutation targets high evolutionary conserved nucleotide in the carotenoid oxygenase domain of the protein. Grantham score of 94 affirms moderate physicochemical difference between asparagine and lysine. Muttaster, PolyPhen, and Sift in silico tools predict this alteration to be disease causing, possibly damaging, and deleterious. To the best of our knowledge, this variant has not been described in the medical literature or reported in disease-related variation databases such as ClinVar or HGMD [8, 13]. The variant is found in *trans* with another pathogenic variant in a patient with *RPE65* specific phenotype (Figure 2). Maternity and paternity segregation analysis could not have been performed to exclude/confirm de novo event as both unaffected parents were deceased.

There are currently more than 230 known variants in *RPE65* annotated as disease-causing in the HGMD Professional variant database (version 2021.1) [13]. Approximately 60% of the variants are explicitly missense variants, while 40% are truncating variants (i.e., nonsense, frameshift, variants affecting splicing, and gross deletions) [9]. The loss of *RPE65* gene function involves various mechanisms including a lower expression level of RPE65 protein, loss of catalytic activity, or rapid degradation of the protein [14, 15].

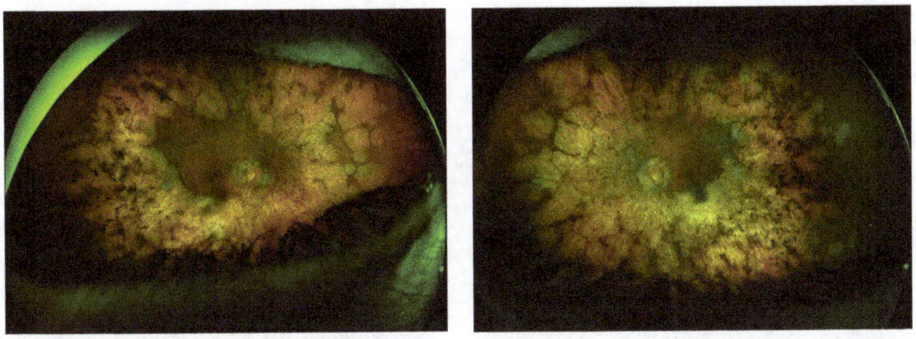

(a) (b)

Figure 1: ultra-widefield fundus photos of the (a) right eye and the (b) left eye showing pale and waxy optic nerve head with clear boundaries and area of atrophy peripapillary, paving-stone degeneration, drusen-like retinal deposits, bone spicule-like pigmentary clumping, and attenuated retinal vessels at mid- and far periphery.

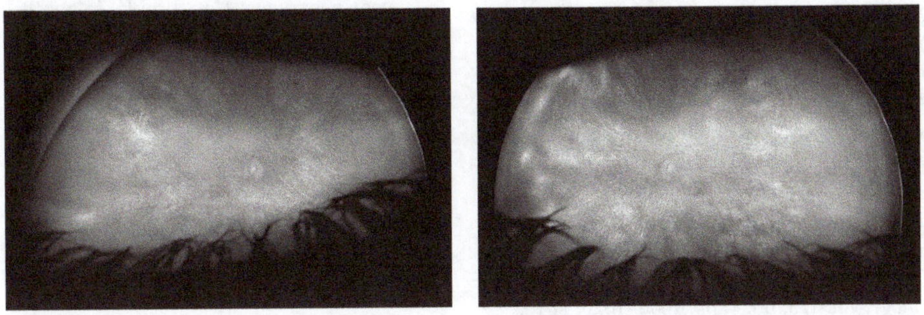

(a) (b)

Figure 2: Fundus autofluorescence photos of the (a) right eye and the (b) left eye. Pale fundi and absence of RPE autofluorescence. Chorioretinal atrophy reveals the hyperautofluorescent attributes of the sclera.

Although termed VUS, *RPE65* c.393T>A, p.(Asn131Lys) is (a) absent in population databases and (b) detected *in trans* with a pathogenic variant, representing moderate evidence of pathogenicity [16]. Moreover, the following determinants, (a) multiple computational evidence (Muttaster, PolyPhen, and Sift in-silico tools) supports its deleterious effect, affecting a highly conserved amino acid in the carotenoid oxygenase domain of the protein, (b) the variant is present in the *RPE65* in which missense variants are a common mechanism of disease and benign missense variation occur at a low rate, and (b) patient phenotype is highly specific for a disease with a single genetic etiology (Figure 2), conform with the supporting pathogenic criteria [16]. In general, combining 2 moderate and ≥2 supporting criteria the variant *RPE65* c.393T>A, p.(Asn131Lys) could be reclassified as likely pathogenic [16].

Our patient is a compound heterozygote in *trans* form and manifests disease with all characteristics typical for the *RPE65* gene mutation [17]. Therefore, we conclude that the variant *RPE65* c.393T>A, p.(Asn131Lys) contributed to the pathologic phenotype, demonstrating its significance clearly in the case presented, and should be reclassified according to the criteria of evidence as likely pathogenic.

This being the case, patients with this specific variant in homozygous or compound heterozygous form would be likely candidates for genetic treatment based on recombinant adeno-associated virus vector providing a working *RPE65* gene to act in place of a mutated *RPE65* gene [18].

Consent

Written informed consent was obtained from the patient for publication of this case report and any accompanying images.

Authors' Contributions

M.B., M.Bu., and A.Ć. designed the study; M.B. and A.Ć. provided screening of potentially eligible studies and extracted and analysed data; M.B., M.Bu., A.Ć., D.B., B.Š., L.M., B.K.E., and B.R. analysed and interpreted data; M.B., M.Bu., and A.Ć. wrote the manuscript; M.B., M.Bu., A.Ć., D.B., B.Š., and L.M. identified the patient; M.B., A.Ć., D.B., B.Š., L.M., and B.R. examined the patient and characterized the clinical features of the disease; M.B., M.Bu., and A.Ć. conceived the study; M.B., M.Bu., D.B., B.Š., and B.K.E. supervised the study. All authors approved the final version of the manuscript and agreed to be accountable for all aspects of the work in ensuring that questions related to the accuracy or integrity of any part of the work are appropriately investigated and resolved.

References

[1] "National Library of Medicine: MedlinePlus Genetics," February 2022, https://medlineplus.gov/genetics/condition/leber-congenital-amaurosis/.

[2] C. Jakobsson, I. S. Othman, F. L. Munier, D. F. Schorderet, and H. Abouzeid, "Cone-rod dystrophy caused by a novel homozygous RPE65 mutation in Leber congenital amaurosis," *Klinische Monatsblätter für Augenheilkunde*, vol. 231, no. 4, pp. 405–410, 2014.

[3] "National Organisation for Rare Disorders (NORD): Rare Disease Database," February 2022, https://rarediseases.org/rare-diseases/leber-congenital-amaurosis/.

[4] G. Mo, Q. Ding, Z. Chen et al., "A novel mutation in the RPE65 gene causing Leber congenital amaurosis and its transcriptional expression in vitro," *PLoS One*, vol. 9, no. 11, 2014.

[5] D. C. Chung, M. Bertelsen, B. Lorenz et al., "The natural history of inherited retinal dystrophy due to biallelic mutations in the RPE65 gene," *American Journal of Ophthalmology*, vol. 199, pp. 58–70, 2019.

[6] R. G. Weleber, M. E. Pennesi, D. J. Wilson et al., "Results at 2 years after gene therapy for RPE65-deficient Leber congenital amaurosis and severe early-childhood-onset retinal dystrophy," *Ophthalmology*, vol. 123, no. 7, pp. 1606–1620, 2016.

[7] "Blueprint Genetics: Retinal Dystrophy Panel," February 2022, https://blueprintgenetics.com/tests/panels/ophthalmology/retinal-dystrophy-panel/.

[8] ClinVar, *National Center for Biotechnology Information*, U.S. National Library of Medicine, Bethesda, 2021, https://www.ncbi.nlm.nih.gov/clinvar/variation/98863/.

[9] R. B. Hufnagel, Z. M. Ahmed, Z. M. Correa, and R. A. Sisk, "Gene therapy for Leber congenital amaurosis: advances and future directions," *Graefe's Archive for Clinical and Experimental Ophthalmology*, vol. 250, no. 8, pp. 1117–1128, 2012.

[10] "Genome Aggregation Database (gnom AD). gnomAD Production Team at the Broad Institute," February 2022, https://gnomad.broadinstitute.org/gene/ENSG00000116745?dataset=gnomad_r2_1.Accessed.

[11] "National Center for Biotechnology Information, U.S. National Library of Medicine: MedGen," February 2022, https://www.ncbi.nlm.nih.gov/medgen/C1859844/.

[12] S. R. Dharmaraj, E. R. Silva, A. L. Pina et al., "Mutational analysis and clinical correlation in Leber congenital amaurosis," *Ophthalmic Genetics*, vol. 21, no. 3, pp. 135–150, 2000.

[13] "The Human Gene Mutation Database at the Institute of Medical Genetics in Cardiff: HGMD®," February 2022, http://www.hgmd.cf.ac.uk/ac/index.php.

[14] T. M. Redmond, E. Poliakov, S. Yu, J. Y. Tsai, Z. Lu, and S. Gentleman, "Mutation of key residues of RPE65 abolishes its enzymatic role as isomerohydrolase in the visual cycle," *Proceedings of the National Academy of Sciences of the United States of America*, vol. 102, no. 38, pp. 13658–13663, 2005.

[15] Y. Chen, G. Moiseyev, Y. Takahashi, and J. X. Ma, "Impacts of two point mutations of RPE65 from Leber's congenital amaurosis on the stability, subcellular localization and isomerohydrolase activity of RPE65," *FEBS Letters*, vol. 580, no. 17, pp. 4200–4204, 2006.

[16] S. Richards, N. Aziz, S. Bale et al., "Standards and guidelines for the interpretation of sequence variants: a joint consensus recommendation of the American College of Medical Genetics and Genomics and the Association for Molecular Pathology," *Genetics in Medicine*, vol. 17, no. 5, pp. 405–424, 2015.

[17] S. Hanein, I. Perrault, S. Gerber et al., "Leber congenital amaurosis: comprehensive survey of the genetic heterogeneity, refinement of the clinical definition, and genotype-phenotype correlations as a strategy for molecular diagnosis," *Human Mutation*, vol. 23, no. 4, pp. 306–317, 2004.

[18] German Society of Ophthalmology (Deutsche Ophthalmologische Gesellschaft, DOG), German Retina Society e. V. (Retinologische Gesellschaft e. V., RG), and Professional Association of German Ophthalmologists (Berufsverband der Augenärzte Deutschlands e. V., BVA), "Statement of the DOG, the RG, and the BVA on the therapeutic use of voretigene neparvovec (Luxturna™) in ophthalmology. English version: January 2019," *Ophthalmologe*, vol. 117, no. S1, pp. 16–24, 2020.

29

Successful Management of Infectious Crystalline Keratopathy with Intrastromal Antibiotic Injections

Luis Martinez-Velazquez, Kevin K. Ma, Neal S. Patel, and Zhonghui Katie Luo

Massachusetts Eye and Ear Infirmary, 243 Charles St, Boston, MA 02114, USA

Correspondence should be addressed to Luis Martinez-Velazquez; luis_martinezvelazquez@meei.harvard.edu

Academic Editor: Hiroshi Eguchi

Purpose. To report the successful treatment of a case of presumed infectious crystalline keratopathy with repeated intrastromal antibiotic injections in a cornea graft in the setting of severe ocular graft-vs.-host-disease (GVHD). *Observations.* A 62-year-old man with a history of ocular GVHD and tectonic penetrating keratoplasty (PK) for corneal melt from herpes zoster keratopathy developed presumed infectious crystalline keratopathy (ICK) in the corneal graft. Given the patient's complicated ocular history, chronic immunosuppression and new cardiac comorbidities, a therapeutic PK would most likely fail. Efforts were then directed to rescue the graft with minimally invasive approaches. Two separate intrastromal injections of cefuroxime and moxifloxacin successfully treated his ICK. *Conclusions and Importance.* This case supports a role for repeated intrastromal antibiotic injections in patients with ICK refractory to topical antibiotic therapy, which might eliminate the need for therapeutic PK and preserve vision.

1. Introduction

Infectious crystalline keratopathy (ICK) is an indolent infective keratitis characterized by fine branch-like crystalline opacities in the anterior corneal stroma accompanied by minimal inflammation [1, 2]. Identification of the causative pathogens is often not possible given that cultures from corneal scrapings are often too superficial to reach the causative organisms, which are commonly located deep in the anterior stroma [2]. Gram-positive bacteria, in particular *Streptococcus mitis*, appear to be the most common causative organism among published reports of ICK with a positive corneal culture [2]. However, there have also been reports of ICK caused by gram-negative bacteria, fungus, or *Acanthamoeba* [3, 4].

ICK has been classically described in patients with topical immunosuppression following a penetrating keratoplasty (PK) and is notoriously difficult to treat [1, 5]. ICK has also been described in patients treated with immunosuppressive agents for other ocular or systemic conditions including Stevens-Johnson syndrome, and chronic graft-vs.-host disease (GVHD) [6, 7]. Although local or systemic immunosuppression often precedes ICK, this condition has been linked to neurotrophic corneal diseases such as herpetic keratitis, denervation after corneal surgery (PK [2, 8], laser-assisted *in situ* keratomileusis (LASIK) [9]), or even after long-term topical anesthetic use [10] in the absence of immunosuppression. Initial treatment usually consists of topical broad spectrum fortified antibiotics. These can then be refined based on microorganism sensitivities if a successful culture is obtained. Many cases require corneal transplantation if they are refractive to topical therapy.

Our case report describes the successful treatment of presumed ICK with two sequential sessions of intrastromal antibiotic injections in a patient that had previously undergone tectonic PK for corneal melt from herpes zoster keratopathy and ocular GVHD following allogeneic hematopoietic stem cell transplantation (allo-HSCT). This treatment modality successfully prevented progression of the infection and preserved his baseline best corrected visual acuity (BCVA) after twenty-three months from initial diagnosis, without requiring a repeat PK following failed topical antibiotics treatment.

2. Case Report

A 62-year-old man with a complex ocular history presented to our ophthalmology clinic with blurry vision of the right eye for 2 days. His ophthalmic history was notable for herpes zoster virus (VZV) keratitis of the right eye, ocular GVHD in both eyes and a tectonic PK in his right eye PK following an urgent presentation for a descemetocele. Under the emergency circumstance of his initial presentation to our service, corneal sensation was not checked before his PK. He was fitted with scleral lenses (Boston Sight) in both eyes to improve his vision and support his fragile ocular surface. Figure 1 outlines a timeline of his ophthalmic disease course. His chronic GVHD also involved multiple organ systems including his eyes, lungs, mouth mucosa, skin, liver, and soft tissues, which was classified as "moderate" based on the 2014 NIH consensus [11, 12].

Seven days prior to the onset of his blurry vision, he was hospitalized at an intensive care unit for pericardial effusion and new atrial fibrillation in the setting of a chronic systemic GVHD flare-up. Following his allo-HSCT, he had always required multiple systemic immunosuppression therapies for chronic GVHD management. After a recent hospital admission, his oral prednisone was increased from 10 mg daily to 50 mg daily. He was concurrently taking tacrolimus 2 mg daily, topical betamethasone (0.05%) ointment for his skin, undergoing extracorporeal photopheresis twice a week, and receiving monthly intravenous immunoglobulin (IVIG) infusions. His prophylactic treatment includes valacyclovir 1 g daily and trimethropim-sulfamethaxozole 400-80 mg daily. He was also on topical ocular immunosuppression including non-preserved prednisolone acetate 1% twice a day in the right eye and loteprednol 0.5% gel once a day in the left eye chronically in addition to frequent lubrication with nonpreserved artificial tears. His puncti were all occluded with silicone punctual plugs. He wore his scleral lenses daily in both eyes for 12 to 14 hours per day.

The ocular exam was notable for a decrease in vision in his scleral lens from 20/30 to 20/40, intraocular pressures of 14 mm Hg and rare cell in the anterior chamber in the right eye. His left eye had a stable vision in scleral lens of 20/25, intraocular pressure of 22 mm Hg with no new findings. Examination of the right cornea (Figure 2(a)) demonstrated a stable preexisting triangular 1.5 mm anterior stromal haze paracentrally and a new crystalline pattern of branching thin structures in the anterior stroma centrally, and keratic precipitates in the endothelium (Figure 2(b)). The left cornea was clear. Confocal microscopy revealed hyperreflective needle-like structures located in the mid stroma at approximately 195 μm consistent with crystalline keratopathy, but nonspecific for an individual pathogen (Figure 2(c)). The central corneal epithelium was scraped and cultured, but unfortunately did not identify the causative organism. Fortified nonpreserved ceftazidime (50 mg/mL) and moxifloxacin (5 mg/mL) drops were started every hour as empiric therapy for gram-positive organisms. The likelihood of a gram-positive organism was reinforced when on further history; the patient reported that he was with his grandchild who had strep throat a few days prior to onset of symptoms (Figure 1).

One week after initial presentation, we found a stable appearance of the branch-like lesions, slight improvement of the epi-defect, and persistent anterior chamber inflammation despite the resolution of the keratic precipitates. To control the infection as early as possible, the patient was brought to the operating room for intrastromal and intracameral antibiotic injections. Given his systemic comorbidities, only topical lidocaine (3.5%) gel was used for anesthesia. Under the operating microscope, we injected 0.1 mL of 1 mg/0.1 mL nonpreserved cefuroxime intrastromally through a 30-gauge needle to the branch lesions, and 0.1 mL of 0.5 mg/0.1 mL moxifloxacin (Apotex pharmaceuticals) intracamerally using a 30-gauge irrigator. The moxifloxacin is commercially available and was aliquoted by our inpatient pharmacy under sterile conditions for use in the operating room. One hundred microliters of aqueous humor were collected from the anterior chamber for culture, which resulted negative for bacteria or fungi. The patient resumed wear of his scleral lens two days after the intrastromal injection to protect his ocular surface.

Five weeks after the initial presentation and while on continued topical antibiotics, the patient reported subjectively worse vision, which was measured in his scleral lens at 20/30-2. On examination, the "branch-like" lesions were slightly larger in size and clearly invaded a deeper layer in the stroma with increased central stromal haze. While the first intrastromal injection of cefuroxime only transiently stalled but failed to control his ICK, other treatment options did not seem more promising at the time. Notably, the patient was not medically stable for surgery given his cardiac status with persistent atrial fibrillation, pericardial, and pleural effusion. Therefore, we administered a second round of intrastromal injections as previously described consisting of non-preserved 0.1 mL of 0.5 mg/0.1 mL moxifloxacin and 0.06 mL of 1 mg/0.1 mL cefuroxime injected through a 30-gauge needle in a circular pattern surrounding the "branches". We settled on these volumes after reaching an appropriate degree of stromal edema, and with the intention to reduce the risk of a Descemet's membrane detachment. This sequence created a higher concentration centrally and kept the needle tracks away from the visual axis (Figure 3). We discontinued topical antimicrobials following the procedure, and two days later, the patient resumed his scleral lens wear in the right eye.

Five weeks after the second round of intrastromal injections, the patient reported subjective improvement in his right eye vision, which was measured in the same scleral lens at 20/25, despite the residual needle tracks adjacent to his visual axis. Twenty-three months after his intrastromal injections, he continues doing well with a stable vision of 20/25 in the right eye while wearing his current scleral lens. The appearance of the branch like structures was mostly stable with slightly less defined borders without any further

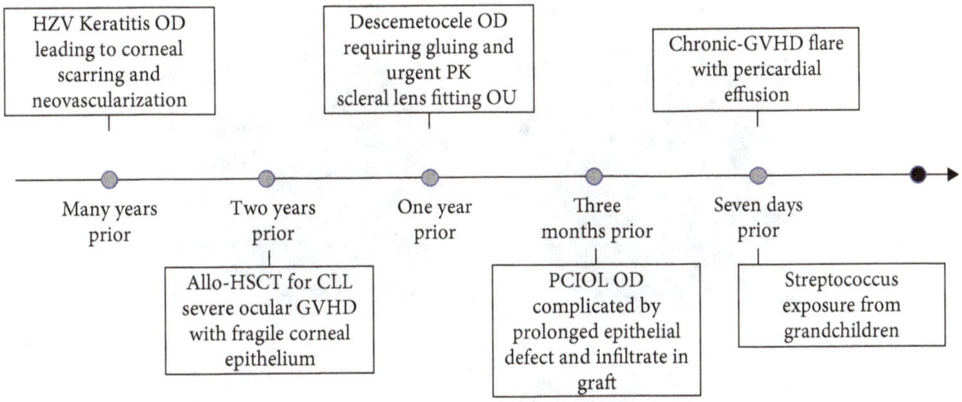

Figure 1: Timeline of history of present illness. Graphical representation of the ocular and systemic disease course for this patient.

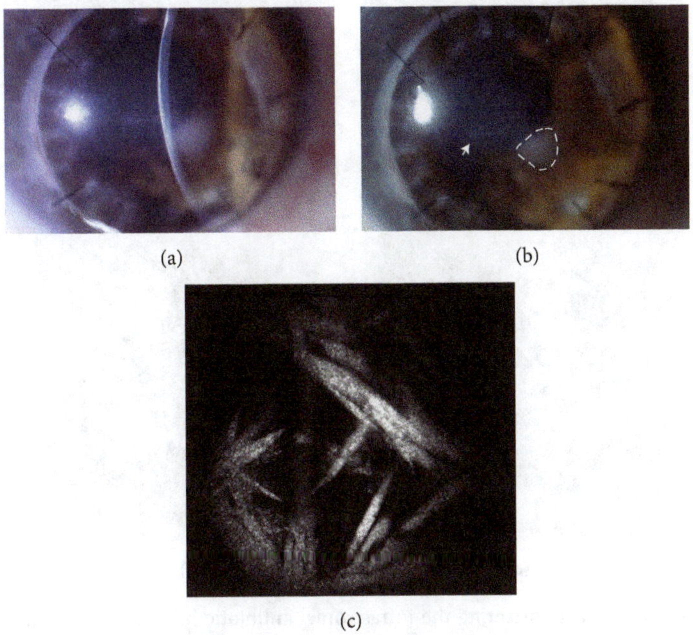

Figure 2: Slit-lamp photograph of the right eye at initial presentation. (a) A slit-beam photograph centered over the new crystalline pattern of branching thin structures in the anterior stroma. (b) A wide-beam photograph demonstrating the branch-like structures in the anterior stroma of the central visual axis (arrowhead), and nasally, a preexisting triangular anterior stromal scar (dashed outline). (c) Confocal microscopy revealed mid-stromal (195 μm deep) highly reflective needle-like structures consistent with crystalline keratopathy, but not specific for an individual pathogen.

increase in size (Figure 4). His left eye did stably well throughout the whole disease course.

3. Discussion

ICK is an indolent infectious keratitis characterized by fine branch-like crystalline opacities commonly found in the anterior stroma [1, 2]. Initial inoculation occurs through an epithelial defect, and the microorganisms are then able to proliferate through the space between the lamellar planes of the stroma and the crisscrossing cell bodies of the keratocytes. Immunosuppression enables the crystalline appearance of this condition by suppressing the inflammatory reaction and infiltration of immune cells and edema seen in other types of infectious keratitis.

Cases of ICK may be asymptomatic or present with some of the symptoms of keratitis including decreased visual acuity, photophobia, and pain. The degree of conjunctival injection and adjacent inflammation is usually lower than in other forms of keratitis due to the indolent nature of the infection and the common association with long-term use of topical corticosteroids [13].

Our patient was immunosuppressed through multiple mechanisms including systemic and topical steroids to address complications of his GVHD secondary to his allo-HSCT. Post-transplantation patients suffer from severe immune deficiency due to thymic damage, and secondary to pharmacologic immunosuppressive agents used for GVHD prophylaxis [14]. Ocular GVHD affects more than 50% of these patients reducing their quality of life significantly through ocular

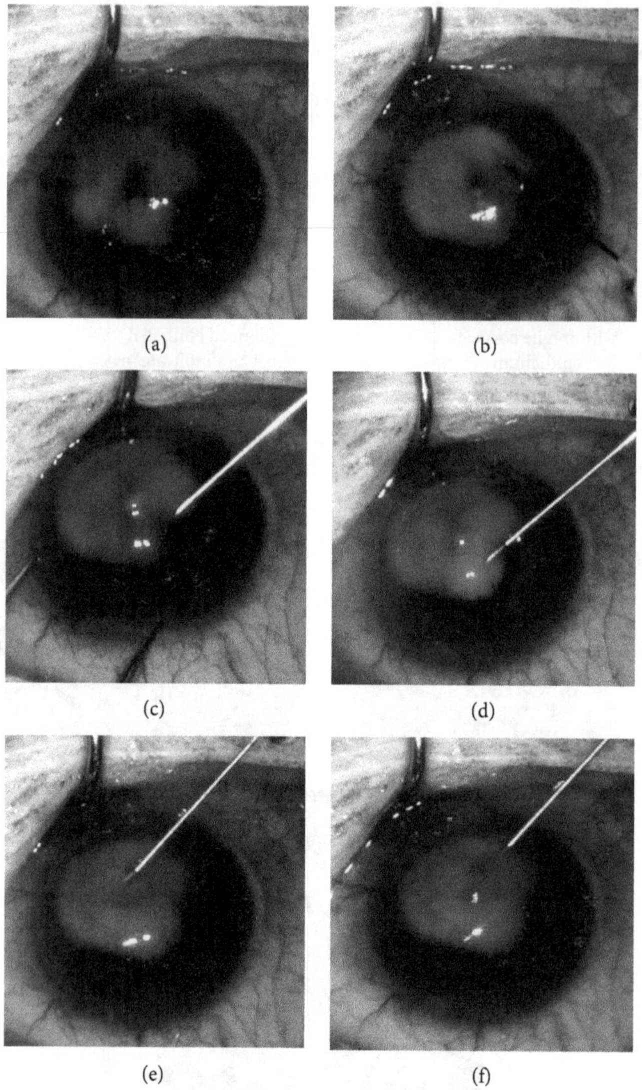

FIGURE 3: Image series from surgical video demonstrating the intrastromal antibiotic injections through a 30-gauge needle. The injections were made in a circular pattern surrounding the crystalline deposits, achieving a higher concentration centrally and keeping the needle tracks away from the visual axis (image progression from (a) to (f)). Full video available here in https://www.dropbox.com/s/x0gbutn8d64a5sd/Video1.mp4?dl=0.

manifestations ranging from irritation, poor vision to nonhealing epithelial defects, corneal melt, intractable pain, and irreversible vision loss [15]. Treatment for moderate to severe chronic GVHD in general requires systemic and topical immunosuppression such as steroids and calcineurin inhibitors, which increases the risk of infections and impairs healing.

ICK has also been previously linked to neurotrophic corneal diseases such as herpetic keratitis, denervation after corneal surgery (PK [2, 8], laser-assisted *in situ* keratomileusis (LASIK) [9]), or even after long-term topical anesthetic use [10] in the absence of immunosuppression. Neurotrophic conditions are associated with delays in corneal wound healing [16] which provide an opportunity for the initial seeding of the cornea by a pathogen. Our patient initially presented to our care in the setting of a descemetocele requiring urgent PK; therefore, as previously mentioned corneal sensation was not checked prior to the PK or subsequently after the PK. Nevertheless, a degree of neurotrophic keratitis is presumed given expected denervation from the PK and his prior history of herpetic keratitis.

Many of the microbial species that cause ICK form biofilms, which limit the effectiveness of topical antimicrobials. Meisler and colleagues reported a case of ICK in which they cultured *Streptococcus viridans* and measured a minimum inhibitory concentration for antibiotic treatment four times greater than what was required to treat this species in other contexts [5]. It was later proposed that this was due to the protective effects of a biofilm [2]. Historically, PK is often required to remove the infected corneal tissue, or to restore vision in cases with severe corneal scarring despite successful treatment of the infection. However, our patient's unique medical and ocular history rendered him a poor candidate for repeat PK.

Intrastromal injections of antibiotics have been suggested to treat ICK refractory to topical antimicrobials. Khan and colleagues reported successfully treating ICK caused by

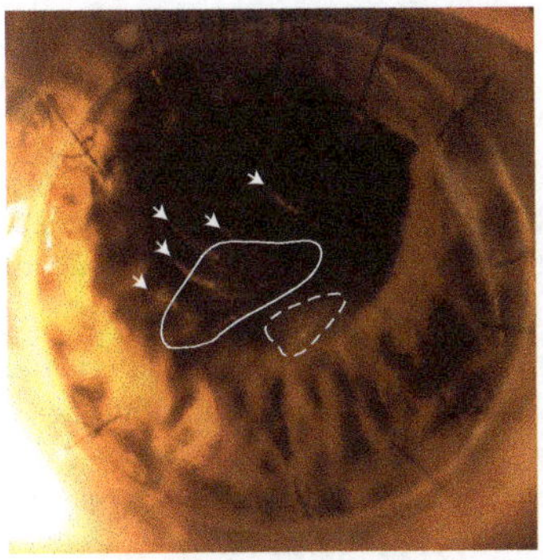

FIGURE 4: Slit-lamp photograph of the right eye 23 months after initial presentation. The "branch-like" infiltrates were still visible centrally (solid outline). Multiple linear needle tracks from the intrastromal injections were in the paracentral cornea stroma (arrowheads). The triangular 1.5 mm anterior stromal haze was stable in appearance (dashed outline).

Streptococcus mitis and *Streptococcus parasanguinis* with intrastromal injection of cefuroxime [17]. There have also been reports of successful intrastromal amphotericin B and voriconazole to treat fungal keratitis [18, 19]. Injections into the anterior stroma have the advantage of delivering higher concentrations of antimicrobials directly where the microorganisms are located and overcome the barrier set by biofilms. While we considered injecting voriconazole due to its effectiveness for treating fungal cases, we decided to focus initial therapy on agents that would cover gram positive organisms given that they are the most frequent cause of crystalline keratopathy. This focus was important to minimize the total volume of antimicrobials injected to the stroma to avoid possible complications such a Descemet's membrane detachment.

Corneal biopsies have been used with success to identify the causative microbe in atypical cases of crystalline keratopathy [20]. This approach should be given fair consideration when adjusting the antimicrobial therapy in a treatment refractory case. Our patient, however, had a deep (~195 μm per confocal) and central lesion. A corneal biopsy would have certainly caused a large epithelial defect and risk delayed healing or scarring. The decision to proceed with empiric antimicrobial therapy was based on maximizing the chances of saving the corneal graft given that he was a poor surgical candidate for a PK.

Our case report is unique in that it demonstrates therapeutic success of treatment of ICK by sequential intrastromal antibiotic injections in an immunocompromised patient with ocular GVHD. The first intrastromal injection of 0.1 mL of 1 mg/0.1 mL cefuroxime only stalled the progression of ICK for a few weeks, showcasing the role of biofilms in antimicrobial treatment resistance. The second intrastromal injection of 0.1 mL of 0.5 mg/0.1 mL moxifloxacin and 0.06 mL of 1 mg/0.1 mL cefuroxime delivered a high concentration of two antibiotics simultaneously, which likely reached the bactericidal level and eradicated the organism. After the second intrastromal injection, the patient did not require additional antimicrobial therapies and has maintained good visual acuity at the most recent 2-year follow-up. The interbranch spaces remained clear without any further increase in the number or size of the branches for two years, indicating that the injections were an effective treatment.

There are no current guidelines for the selection of antibiotic agents, concentration, or injection volume for such unconventional treatment. We chose the nonpreserved preparations of moxifloxacin and cefuroxime, at higher concentrations than previously reported [8]. The concentrations were chosen because they have been routinely used for intracameral injection in cataract surgeries world-wide [21]. We limited the delivered volume of the antibiotics (only 0.06 mL of cefuroxime was injected) to avoid a Descemet's membrane detachment from the significant stromal edema created by the injections. We also aimed to place our needle-tracks outside of the visual-axis. Within one to two days after each intrastromal injection, the patient was able to resume wear of his scleral lens, which provided him with essential surface protection and sharper vision. Merely two weeks after the second injection, the patient regained 20/40 vision in his scleral lens, which would have been impossible had he undergone a repeat PK. To date, more than two years after the intrastromal injections, there were no signs of endothelial dysfunction or other signs of corneal toxicity. Our case indicated the more concentrated stromal injections were well tolerated by the endothelium of a corneal graft. The prominence of the needle-tracks has reduced with time, and while they are not affecting his vision, they are still visible on examination.

4. Conclusions

This novel strategy expands our treatment options for ICK intractable to topical antibiotics. We propose that this treatment can be considered before a therapeutic PK and/or in patients with high risk of graft failure. Future controlled trials are needed to determine the treatment efficacy of this approach in comparison to therapeutic PK.

Consent

The patient verbally consented to publication of the case report. Furthermore, this report does not contain any personal information that could be used to identify this patient.

Authors' Contributions

All authors attest that they have met the current ICMJE criteria for Authorship. Senior author: Zhonghui Katie Luo.

Acknowledgments

We are grateful for Dr. Deborah S. Jacob's assistance in reviewing and interpreting the confocal micrographs included in this case report.

References

[1] M. S. Gorovoy, G. A. Stern, C. I. Hood, and C. Allen, "Intrastromal Noninflammatory Bacterial Colonization of a Corneal Graft," *Archives of Ophthalmology*, vol. 101, no. 11, pp. 1749–1752, 1983.

[2] A. J. Porter, G. A. Lee, and A. S. Jun, "Infectious crystalline keratopathy," *Survey of Ophthalmology*, vol. 63, no. 4, pp. 480–499, 2018.

[3] R. M. Davis, R. P. Schroeder, J. J. Rowsey, H. G. Jensen, and R. C. Tripathi, "Acanthamoeba Keratitis and Infectious Crystalline Keratopathy," *Archives of Ophthalmology*, vol. 105, no. 11, pp. 1524–1527, 1987.

[4] T. T. Khater, D. B. Jones, and K. R. Wilhelmus, "Infectious crystalline keratopathy caused by gram-negative bacteria," *American Journal of Ophthalmology*, vol. 124, no. 1, pp. 19–23, 1997.

[5] D. M. Meisler, R. H. Langston, T. J. Naab, A. A. Aaby, J. T. McMahon, and R. R. Tubbs, "Infectious crystalline keratopathy," *American Journal of Ophthalmology*, vol. 97, no. 3, pp. 337–343, 1984.

[6] B. Bostancı and A. Y. Aydın, "Unusual course of crystalline keratopathy in a patient with graft-versus-host disease," *Turkish Journal of Ophthalmology*, vol. 47, no. 6, pp. 344–347, 2017.

[7] H. S. Uy, Q. D. Nguyen, M. L. Durand, B. Paton, and C. S. Foster, "Infectious crystalline keratopathy and endophthalmitis secondary to _mycobacterium abscessus_ in a monocular patient with Stevens-Johnson syndrome," *American Journal of Ophthalmology*, vol. 127, no. 2, pp. 209-210, 1999.

[8] A. Matsumoto, Y. Sano, K. Nishida, N. Yokoi, J. Hara, and S. Kinoshita, "A case of infectious crystalline keratopathy occurring long after penetrating keratoplasty," *Cornea*, vol. 17, no. 1, pp. 119–122, 1998.

[9] P. Garg, A. K. Bansal, S. Sharma, and G. K. Vemuganti, "Bilateral infectious keratitis after laser in situ keratomileusis: a case report and review of the literature," *Ophthalmology*, vol. 108, no. 1, pp. 121–125, 2001.

[10] J. C. Kintner, H. E. Grossniklaus, J. H. Lass, and G. Jacobs, "Infectious crystalline keratopathy associated with topical anesthetic abuse," *Cornea*, vol. 9, no. 1, pp. 77–80, 1990.

[11] M. H. Jagasia, H. T. Greinix, M. Arora et al., "National institutes of health consensus development project on criteria for clinical trials in chronic graft-versus-host disease: i. the 2014 diagnosis and staging working group report," *Biology of Blood and Marrow Transplantation*, vol. 21, no. 3, pp. 389–401.e1, 2015.

[12] S. J. Lee, "Classification systems for chronic graft-versus-host disease," *Blood*, vol. 129, no. 1, pp. 30–37, 2017.

[13] M. S. Sridhar, S. Sharma, P. Garg, and G. N. Rao, "Epithelial infectious crystalline keratopathy," *American Journal of Ophthalmology*, vol. 131, no. 2, pp. 255–257, 2001.

[14] G. Socie and J. Ritz, "Current issues in chronic graft-versus-host disease," *Blood*, vol. 124, no. 3, pp. 374–384, 2014.

[15] Y. Inamoto, N. Valdés-Sanz, Y. Ogawa et al., "Ocular graft-versus-host disease after hematopoietic cell transplantation: expert review from the late effects and quality of life working committee of the CIBMTR and transplant complications working party of the EBMT," *Bone Marrow Transplantation*, vol. 54, no. 5, pp. 662–673, 2019.

[16] K. Araki, Y. Ohashi, S. Kinoshita, K. Hayashi, Y. Kuwayama, and Y. Tano, "Epithelial wound healing in the denervated cornea," *Current Eye Research*, vol. 13, no. 3, pp. 203–211, 1994.

[17] I. J. Khan, S. Hamada, and S. Rauz, "Infectious crystalline keratopathy treated with intrastromal antibiotics," *Cornea*, vol. 29, no. 10, pp. 1186–1188, 2010.

[18] E. Garcia-Valenzuela and C. D. Song, "Intracorneal Injection of Amphothericin B for Recurrent Fungal Keratitis and Endophthalmitis," *Archives of Ophthalmology*, vol. 123, no. 12, p. 1721, 2005.

[19] G. Prakash, N. Sharma, M. Goel, J. S. Titiyal, and R. B. Vajpayee, "Evaluation of intrastromal injection of voriconazole as a therapeutic adjunctive for the management of deep recalcitrant fungal keratitis," *American Journal of Ophthalmology*, vol. 146, no. 1, pp. 56–59, 2008.

[20] A. Huck, L. E. Moore, B. K. Firestone, R. L. Siatkowski, and K. M. Riaz, "Diagnostic Utility of CDC DPDx for an Atypical Presentation of Infectious Crystalline Keratopathy-Like Infiltrate Secondary to Microsporidia," *Cornea*, vol. 41, no. 1, pp. 109–112, 2022.

[21] A. Grzybowski, P. Brona, L. Zeman, and M. W. Stewart, "Commonly used intracameral antibiotics for endophthalmitis prophylaxis: a literature review," *Survey of Ophthalmology*, vol. 66, no. 1, pp. 98–108, 2021.

30

Novel Mutations in the *MKKS*, *BBS7* and *ALMS1* Genes in Iranian Children with Clinically Suspected Bardet–Biedl Syndrome

Roghayeh Dehghan,[1] **Mahdiyeh Behnam**,[2] **Mansoor Salehi**,[1,3,4] **and Roya Kelishadi**[5]

[1]*Department of Genetics and Molecular Biology, School of Medicine, Isfahan University of Medical Science, Isfahan, Iran*
[2]*Cellular, Molecular and Genetics Research Center, Isfahan University of Medical Sciences, Isfahan, Iran*
[3]*Pediatric Inherited Diseases Research Center, Research Institute for Primordial Prevention of Non-Communicable Disease, Isfahan University of Medical Sciences, Isfahan, Iran*
[4]*Child Growth and Development Research Center, Research Institute for Primordial Prevention of Non-Communicable Disease, Isfahan University of Medical Sciences, Isfahan, Iran*
[5]*Department of Pediatrics, Child Growth and Development Research Center, Research Institute for Primordial Prevention of Non-Communicable Disease, Isfahan University of Medical Sciences, Isfahan, Iran*

Correspondence should be addressed to Mansoor Salehi; m.salehii@med.mui.ac.ir

Academic Editor: Takaaki Hayashi

Bardet–Biedl syndrome is a rare autosomal recessive form of syndromic obesity which is characterized by retinal degeneration, obesity, polydactyly, cognitive impairment, and renal and urogenital anomalies. In this study, we used whole exome sequencing (WES) to investigate the underlying mutations in four Iranian children from consanguineous families with a clinical diagnosis of Bardet–Biedl syndrome (BBS). In three out of four children, we identified one previously reported frameshifting variant in the *BBS12* gene (c.265-266delTT, p.L89fs) and two novel nonsense variants in *MKKS* (c.1196T>G, p.L399X) and *BBS7* genes (c.1636C>T, p.Q546X). In the other child, no mutations were detected in known genes for BBS. However, we identified a novel variant in the *ALMS1* gene (c.10996delC, p.Q3666fs) indicative of Alström syndrome. All variants were interpreted as pathogenic according to American College of Medical Genetics and Genomics (ACMG) guidelines and confirmed through Sanger sequencing. In conclusion, our results not only expand the spectrum of mutations in BBS and *ALMS1* genes but also accentuate the importance of genetic testing for differentiating BBS from Alström syndrome.

1. Introduction

Bardet–Biedl syndrome (BBS) is an autosomal recessive (AR) ciliopathy characterized by six primary diagnostic features: retinal degeneration, obesity, polydactyly, cognitive impairment, and renal and urogenital anomalies. In addition, BBS has a wide array of secondary features, among which the typical ones are developmental delay, behavioral abnormalities, speech delay, orthodontic anomalies, brachydactyly/syndactyly, ataxia/poor conditioning, liver disease, craniofacial dysmorphism, Hirschsprung's disease, anosmia, cataract, and nystagmus. The clinical diagnosis is usually prompted by the presence of either four primary features or three primary and two secondary features [1–3]. Thus far, approximately a total of 25 causative genes have been identified for BBS that can explain the molecular causes in about 80% of affected families [3–5]. Most of these genes are related to the formation and/or function of cilia.

Therefore, many clinical features of BBS overlap with those of other ciliopathies such as Alström syndrome, Meckel-Gruber syndrome, and Joubert syndrome [6].

Whole-exome sequencing (WES) is a powerful, cost-effective, and time-efficient method for molecular diagnosis of genetic syndromes, particularly those with high genetic heterogeneity, such as BBS. It can potentially help identify novel mutations and therefore broaden human knowledge on the genotypic spectrum of genetic diseases. Additionally, for genetic diseases such as BBS in which the underlying genes have not been fully identified, applying WES can lead to the identification of novel genes [7, 8]. Given all these advantages of the method, we used WES for genetic investigation of four Iranian children with clinically suspected BBS.

2. Materials and Methods

Four children with clinically suspected Bardet–Biedl syndrome (cases 1–4), all from consanguineous families, participated in this study approved by the ethics committee of Isfahan University of Medical Science. After obtaining informed consent from their parents, we collected peripheral blood from the probands. Genomic DNA was extracted using the QIAamp DNA Mini Kit (Qiagen, Hilden, Germany) according to the manufacturer's instructions. The DNA samples were then sent to Macrogen (Seoul, South Korea) for library preparation using the SureSelect XT Library Prep Kit (Agilent Technologies, CA, USA), followed by sequencing with the Illumina HiSeq 4000 platform (2x100bp, 100x coverage). The obtained FASTQ raw data files were aligned to the human reference genome GRCh38 using the Burrows–Wheeler Alignment (BWA) tool. Single-nucleotide variants (SNVs) and indels were called and filtered using the Genome Analysis Tool Kit (GATK). We applied GATK hard filtering to remove SNVs with low quality score normalized by depth (QualByDepth < 2), low mapping quality (MQ < 40), strand bias (FisherStrand test > 60), bias in mapping quality (MQRankSum < 12.5), and bias in read position of alternative versus reference allele (ReadPosRankSum < –8). For indels, we removed those with FisherStrand test > 200 and ReadPosRankSum < –20. The variants passing these criteria were annotated using ANNOVAR to obtain gene names, functional consequences (i.e., synonymous/nonsynonymous, frameshift, and stop gain), the potential effects on protein function and conservation scores (SIFT, PolyPhen-2, LRT, MutationTaster, MutationAssessor, GERP++, SiPhy, FATHMM, and CADD), and the frequency in the ExAC database.

For prioritization, first, we excluded nonexonic, noncoding, and synonymous variants. Then, as the pedigrees supported AR inheritance in all cases, we focused on homozygous variants with high depth of coverage (DP > 20). Finally, we further prioritized variants according to overall ExAC and gnomAD frequency, level of deleteriousness, and the association of their genes with BBS or other similar conditions. Using this approach, we detected one previously reported and two novel loss of function (LOF) homozygous variants (stop gain and frameshifting) in known loci for BBS in three out of four children. In the other child, no deleterious variant was found in known genes for BBS. However, we identified a novel variant in the *ALMS1* gene (c.10996delC) indicative of Alström syndrome. All variants were confirmed through Sanger sequencing in the probands. Additionally, for the novel variants, the available first-degree relatives underwent Sanger sequencing for segregation analysis (Figure 1). All variants were categorized as pathogenic according to American College of Medical Genetics and Genomics (ACMG) guidelines [9] (Table 1). The schematic workflow of WES analysis in our study has been presented in Figure 2.

3. Results

The clinical description and genetic testing results of the cases are as follows.

3.1. Case 1. The proband was a 13-year-old boy with obesity, bilateral postaxial polydactyly in the hands, progressive retinitis pigmentosa, mild mental retardation (MR), and renal problems. He had two older brothers—one aged 23 and the other aged 20—who had been suffering from the same symptoms but worse retinopathy that had led to blindness. The proband's WES results revealed a homozygous novel nonsense mutation, c.1196T>G (p.L399X), in exon 5 of the *MKKS* (*BBS6*) gene. Sanger sequencing confirmed the homozygous mutation in the proband and his affected siblings and showed that both parents were carriers.

3.2. Case 2. This case was an 8-year-old boy presented with obesity, postaxial nubbin in both hands, renal impairment, mild MR, and retinitis pigmentosa. His 10-year-old sister had the same symptoms plus poor conditioning. WES analysis showed that the boy was homozygous for a novel nonsense variant, c.1636C>T (p.Q546X), in exon 7 of the *BBS7* gene. Sanger sequencing confirmed the homozygosity of the affected sister and the heterozygosity of the parents for this variant.

3.3. Case 3. This case was a 16-year-old boy with obesity, postaxial polydactyly in the feet, cryptorchidism, distal hypospadias, mild MR, retinitis pigmentosa, and night blindness. He was the only child of a consanguineous marriage. WES analysis revealed that he was homozygous for a previously reported pathogenic variant, c.265-266delTT (p.L89fs), in exon 3 of the *BBS12* gene.

3.4. Case 4. This case was a 2-year-old girl with obesity, mild MR, vision problems, and delayed walking who was clinically diagnosed with BBS. She had a normal sister and a deceased brother who had died at the age of 9. Her brother had been suffering from similar symptoms plus hypogonadism. WES analysis in this case revealed a novel homozygous frameshifting variant, c.10996delC (p.Q3666fs), in exon 16 of the *ALMS1* gene. Exon 16 is a mutational hotspot, accounting for 36% of the total mutations in Alström syndrome [10]. Sanger sequencing confirmed the identified variant in the proband and showed that her parents carry this mutation in a heterozygous state.

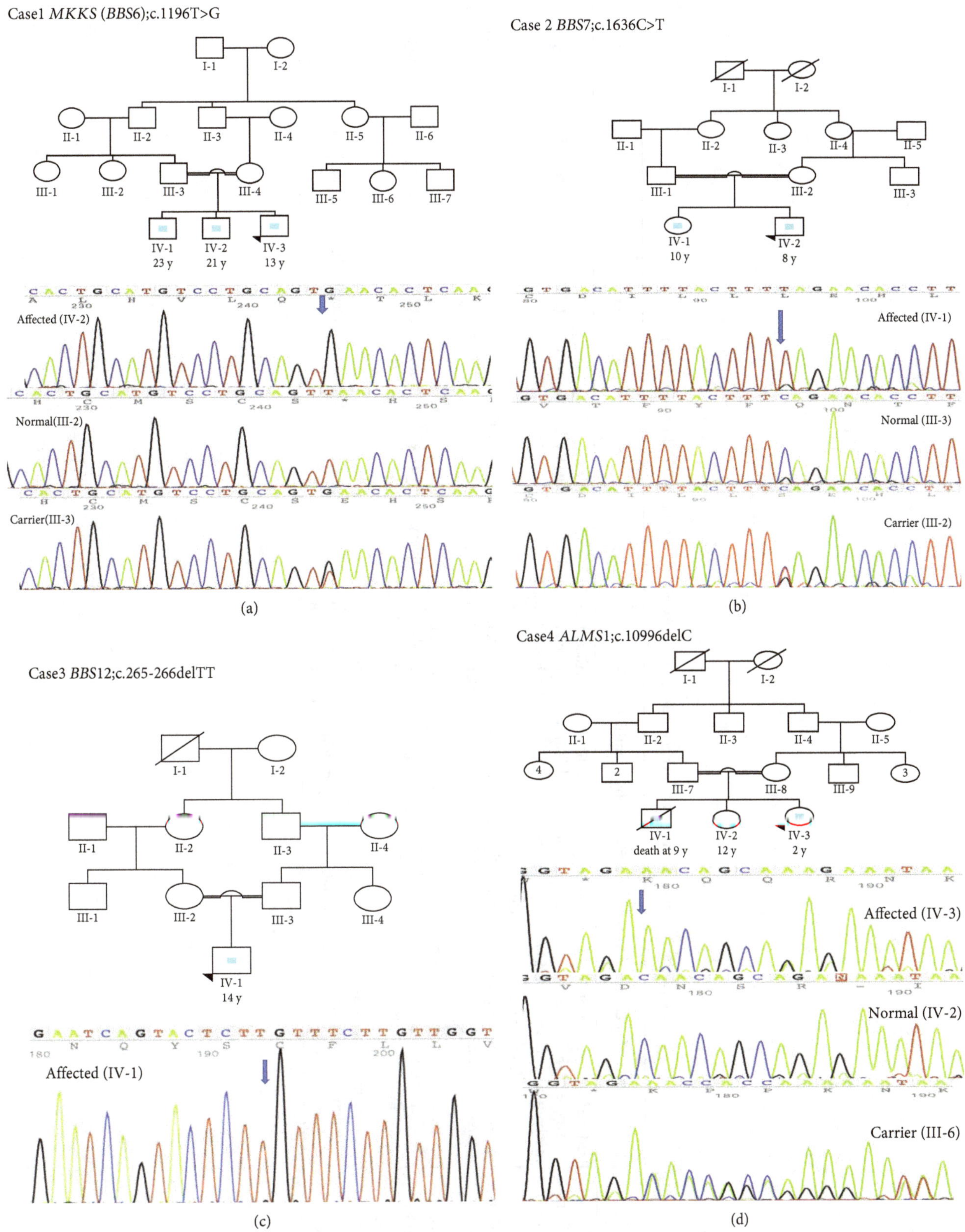

FIGURE 1: Genetic pedigrees supported the autosomal recessive inheritance of syndromic obesity in the cases. (a, b, d) The Sanger sequencing chromatograms of homozygous affected, homozygous normal, and heterozygous carrier individuals for the novel variants in *MKKS* (*BBS6*), *BBS7*, and *ALMS1* genes. (c) The confirmation of the known pathogenic variant in the *BBS12* gene through Sanger sequencing in the proband.

Table 1: The interpretation of variants according to the ACMG guideline. LOF = loss of function.

Case	Candidate variant	The ACMG criteria for pathogenicity met by identified variants			Conclusion
Case 1	c.1196T>G (p.L399X) in *MKKS* (*BBS6*)	Predicted null variant in a gene where LOF is a known mechanism of disease (PVS1)	Cosegregation with disease in multiple affected family members (PP1)	Absent in population databases (PM2)	1 very strong (PVS1) + 1 moderate (PM2) + 1 supporting (PP1) = pathogenic
Case 2	c.1636C>T (p.Q546X) in *BBS7*	Predicted null variant in a gene where LOF is a known mechanism of disease (PVS1)	Cosegregation with disease in multiple affected family members (PP1)	Absent in population databases (PM2)	1 very strong (PVS1) + (moderate (PM2) + 1 supporting (PP1) = pathogenic
Case 3	c.265-266delTT (p.L89fs) in *BBS12*	Predicted null variant in a gene where LOF is a known mechanism of disease (PVS1)	Reported as pathogenic by a reputable source (PP5)	Absent in population databases (PM2)	1 very strong (PVS1) + 1 moderate (PM2) + 1 supporting (PP5) = pathogenic
Case 4	c.10996delC (p.Q3666fs) in *ALMS1*	Predicted null variant in a gene where LOF is a known mechanism of disease (PVS1)	Variant is within a mutational hot spot (PM1)	Absent in population databases (PM2)	1 very strong (PVS1) + 2 moderate (PM1 and PM2) = pathogenic

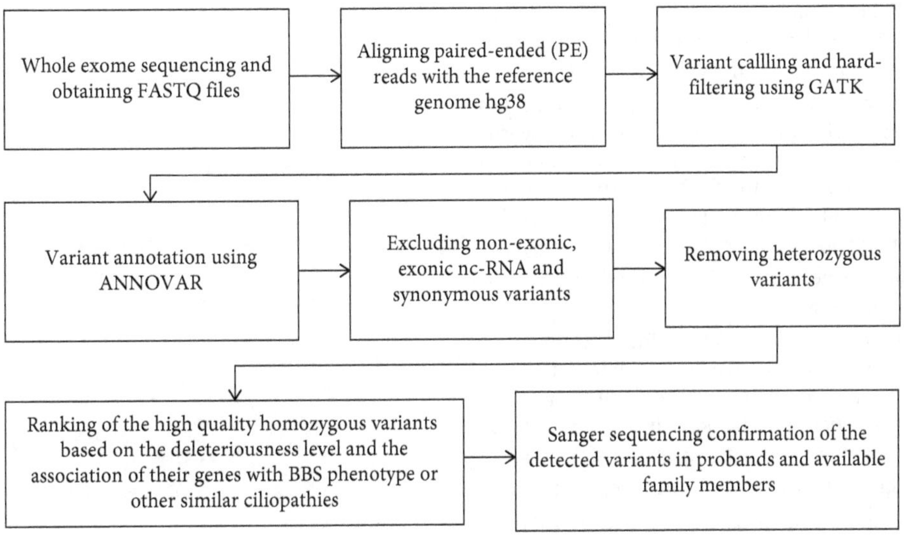

FIGURE 2: The schematic workflow of WES analysis described from obtaining FASTQ files to Sanger sequencing.

4. Discussion

BBS is a genetically heterogeneous disorder with 25 causative genes identified till date [3]. There is some regional variation in the contribution of each gene to the disease. While mutations in *BBS1* and *BBS10* account for most BBS cases (~23% and ~20%, respectively) in Europe and North America, patients originating from Middle Eastern countries are mostly mutated in *BBS4*, *BBS5*, and *BBS8* [11, 12]. So far, there are only limited reports on the mutation profile of BBS genes in Iranian patients. In the largest study including 14 Iranian families with BBS, related mutations were found in *BBS2*, *BBS4*, *BBS12*, and *BBS9* genes in 28.6%, 14%, 21.4%, and ~14% of the patients, respectively [13]. In the present report, we used WES for genetic investigation of four Iranian children suspected to have BBS. After genetic testing, we identified two novel and one reported pathogenic variant in the *MKKS*, *BBS7*, and *BBS12* genes in three out of four children. However, in the other child, a 2-year-old girl clinically diagnosed with BBS, we identified a pathogenic variant in the *ALMS1* gene rather than in the BBS genes; therefore, she was diagnosed with another ciliopathy, Alström syndrome.

Alström syndrome is a rare autosomal recessive single gene disorder that shows a great variability in terms of severity and clinical evolution even among patients within the same family. It has a major clinical overlap with BBS and is characterized by cone-rod dystrophy, hearing impairment, childhood obesity, insulin resistance and hyperinsulinemia, short stature in adulthood, cardiomyopathy, and progressive pulmonary, hepatic, and renal dysfunction [14]. Differential diagnosis of Alström syndrome in children could allow clinicians to provide early follow-up examinations for symptoms such as cardiomyopathy and hearing problems that are late-onset presentations of Alström syndrome but are not frequent in BBS [15].

In conclusion, we report three novel homozygous mutations in the *MKKS*, *BBS7*, and *ALMS1* genes in four Iranian children with clinically suspected Bardet–Biedl syndrome. Furthermore, our study accentuates the importance of genetic testing for differentiating BBS from Alström syndrome. The clinical data in addition to genetic testing results of the four cases presented here have not been previously reported. Our results may contribute to the genetic diagnosis and counselling of families with BBS and Alström syndrome.

Acknowledgments

This research was funded by the Isfahan University of Medical Sciences (grant number 398268).

References

[1] I. H. Koves and C. Roth, "Genetic and syndromic causes of obesity and its management," *Indian Journal of Pediatrics*, vol. 85, no. 6, pp. 478–485, 2018.

[2] E. Forsythe, J. Kenny, C. Bacchelli, and P. L. Beales, "Managing Bardet–Biedl syndrome now and in the future," *Frontiers in Pediatrics*, vol. 6, p. 23, 2018.

[3] M. Dehani, D. Zare-Abdollahi, A. Bushehri et al., "Identification of a novel homozygous mutation in BBS10 gene in an Iranian family with Bardet-Biedl syndrome," *Avicenna Journal of Medical Biotechnology*, vol. 13, no. 4, pp. 230–233, 2021.

[4] "Base Rd," 2022, https://sph.uth.edu/retnet/notes.htm/.

[5] E. Forsythe, K. Sparks, S. Best et al., "Risk factors for severe renal disease in Bardet–Biedl syndrome," *Journal of the American Society of Nephrology*, vol. 28, no. 3, pp. 963–970, 2017.

[6] G. Wheway, J. Lord, and D. Baralle, "Splicing in the pathogenesis, diagnosis and treatment of ciliopathies," *Biochimica et Biophysica Acta (BBA)-Gene Regulatory Mechanisms*, vol. 1862, no. 11-12, p. 194433, 2019.

[7] S. Castro-Sánchez, M. Alvarez-Satta, and D. Valverde, "Performing whole-exome sequencing in Bardet-Bield syndrome," *Cilia*, vol. 4, no. S1, p. 1, 2015.

[8] B. A. Schuler, S. Z. Prisco, and H. J. Jacob, "Using whole exome sequencing to walk from clinical practice to research and back again," *Circulation*, vol. 127, no. 9, pp. 968–970, 2013.

[9] S. Richards, N. Aziz, S. Bale et al., "Standards and guidelines for the interpretation of sequence variants: a joint consensus recommendation of the American College of Medical Genetics and Genomics and the Association for Molecular Pathology," *Genetics in Medicine*, vol. 17, no. 5, pp. 405–424, 2015.

[10] J. D Marshall, P. Maffei, G. B Collin, and J. K Naggert, "Alstrom syndrome: genetics and clinical overview," *Current Genomics*, vol. 12, no. 3, pp. 225–235, 2011.

[11] J. Muller, C. Stoetzel, M. C. Vincent et al., "Identification of 28 novel mutations in the Bardet–Biedl syndrome genes: the burden of private mutations in an extensively heterogeneous disease," *Human Genetics*, vol. 127, no. 5, pp. 583–593, 2010.

[12] E. Forsythe and P. L. Beales, "Bardet-Biedl syndrome," *European journal of Human Genetics*, vol. 21, no. 1, pp. 8–13, 2013.

[13] Z. Fattahi, P. Rostami, A. Najmabadi et al., "Mutation profile of BBS genes in Iranian patients with Bardet-Biedl syndrome: genetic characterization and report of nine novel mutations in five BBS genes," *Journal of Human Genetics*, vol. 59, no. 7, pp. 368–375, 2014.

[14] T. Hearn, "ALMS1 and Alström syndrome: a recessive form of metabolic, neurosensory and cardiac deficits," *Journal of Molecular Medicine*, vol. 97, no. 1, pp. 1–7, 2019.

[15] N. Tahani, P. Maffei, H. Dollfus et al., "Consensus clinical management guidelines for Alström syndrome," *Orphanet Journal of Rare Diseases*, vol. 72, no. 6, pp. 1359–1369, 2003.

31

Polypoidal Choroidal Vasculopathy Complicating Retinal Laser in Quiescent Uveitis

Tomas R. Burke [1] and Susan L. Lightman [1,2]

[1] *Moorfields Eye Hospital, London, UK*
[2] *University College London Institute of Ophthalmology, London, UK*

Correspondence should be addressed to Tomas R. Burke; tomasburke@nhs.net

Academic Editor: Winfried M. Amoaku

A 58-year-old Afro-Caribbean gentleman with a diagnosis of quiescent systemic lupus erythematosus- (SLE-) related occlusive retinal vasculitis was previously treated with sector pan-retinal photocoagulation in his right eye to control temporal retinal neovascularization. At routine review he was found to have a focal area of subretinal fluid in the temporal macula sparing an ischaemic fovea. Fundus fluorescein angiography and indocyanine green angiography confirmed a branching vascular network (BVN) and terminal polys (i.e., polypoidal choroidal vasculopathy (PCV)). Interestingly, the BVN arose within an old laser scar. To our knowledge this is the first report of PCV in uveitis in an Afro-Caribbean patient and of the lesions arising within a laser scar.

1. Introduction

Choroidal neovascularization (CNVM) is a well-recognised complication of inflammatory ocular diseases, particularly those that affect the posterior segment [1]. CNVM are also known to arise secondary to iatrogenic causes such as previous laser therapy [2]. It has been proposed that a discontinuity in the Bruch's membrane-RPE complex is the initiating event in the development of CNVM [3, 4]. Reviewing the literature reveals that there was 1 previous report of of polypoidal choroidal vasculopathy (PCV) in the context of SLE-related uveitis [5], and that patient was of Chinese (i.e. Asian) origin. We present a case of PCV developing in an Afro-Caribbean patient with marked macular ischaemia secondary to SLE-related occlusive retinal vasculitis who has previously been treated with sector pan-retinal photocoagulation (PRP) laser.

2. Case Report

A 58-year-old Afro-Caribbean gentleman attended routine follow-up with a long-standing history of reduced vision (right > left eye), but with no acute visual symptoms. His past ocular history included quiescent bilateral occlusive retinal vasculitis secondary to SLE, with neovascularization in the right temporal retina secondary to a branch retinal vein occlusion that required sector pan-retinal photocoagulation laser 6 years previously. His SLE was also associated with nephritis and was controlled with Mycophenolate Mofetil 1.5g BD.

Best-corrected visual acuity was stable (right eye 6/36, left eye 6/18). No intraocular inflammation was observed. Intraocular pressures were normal. No active neovascularization was observed, though a frond of partially ibrosed neovascularization was present supero-temporally in the right fundus. His maculae were featureless but for a group of faint pinkish lesions in the right temporal macula. Fundus autofluorescence (FAF, Figure 1) and spectral-domain optical coherence tomography (SD-OCT, Figure 2) were carried out using the Heidelberg Spectralis (Heidelberg Engineering, Heidelberg, Germany). FAF revealed laser scars as temporal hypoAF areas and there was a curvilinear group of hyperAF lesions nasal to these. SD-OCT revealed a thinned dry fovea with temporal macular subretinal fluid (SRF) observed over a group of pigment epithelial detachments (PED). As the patient was asymptomatic, observation was initiated and a 4-month follow-up arranged. At review, repeat

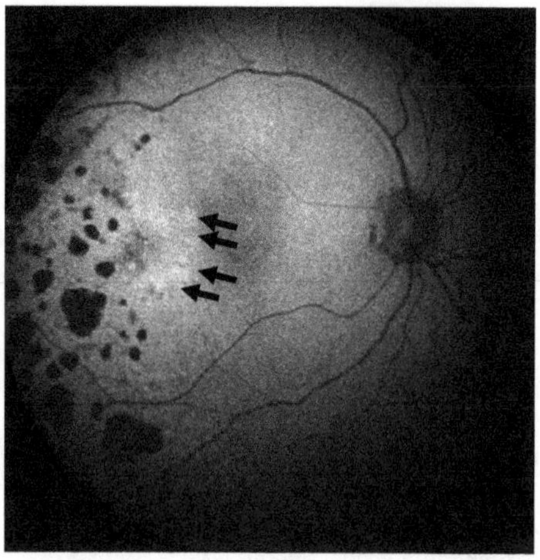

FIGURE 1: Fundus autofluorescence (FAF) right eye at baseline. Note the laser scars appears as heterogeneous hypoAF foci in the temporal fundus of the right eye. Nasal to these, in the temporal macula, note the curvilinear group of faint hyperAF foci (black arrows).

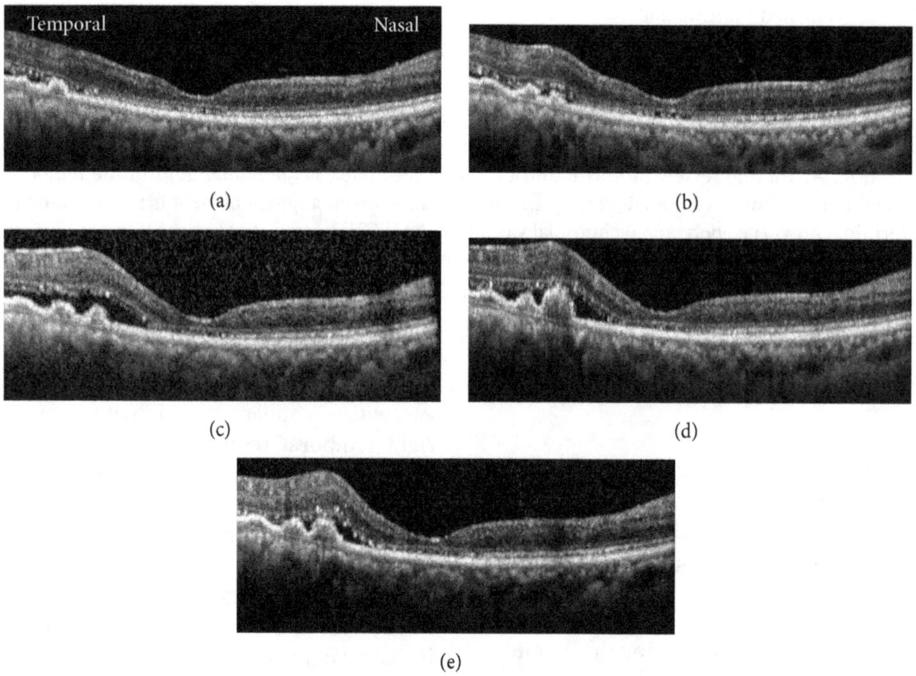

FIGURE 2: Spectral domain-OCT images of right macula from baseline (a) through follow-up at various intervals: +4 months (b), +7 months (c), +8 months (d), and +9 months (e). Note the waxing and waning of subretinal fluid, the variations in the appearance of the temporal pigment epithelial detachments, and the fovea remaining dry throughout follow-up.

imaging revealed progression, though the fovea remained dry (Figure 2). Fundus fluorescein angiography (FFA) and indocyanine green angiography (ICGA) (Heidelberg Spectralis, Heidelberg Engineering, German) revealed a branching vascular network (BVN), arising within a laser scar, with terminal hyperfluorescent polyps (i.e. PCV, Figure 3). Dilated 'pachyvessels' were obvious in the right eye of this patient on ICGA, including areas away from the focus of the BVN. The fellow eye had a normal ICGA without pachyvessels. FFA (Figure 4, Topcon Corp, Tokyo, Japan) performed 4 years previously revealed macular ischemia, active retinal neovascularization and previous laser therapy, however there was no evidence of PCV on that angiogram. Over the course of follow-up (9 months), the subfoveal space and vision were not affected (Figure 2). Enhanced-depth imaging OCT revealed with the 'double-layer' sign and polyps within the temporal macular PEDs (Figure 5). OCT-Angiography images (Zeiss Angioplex) demonstrated widespread macular ischaemia in the right macula, together with the BVN and polyps (Figure 6).

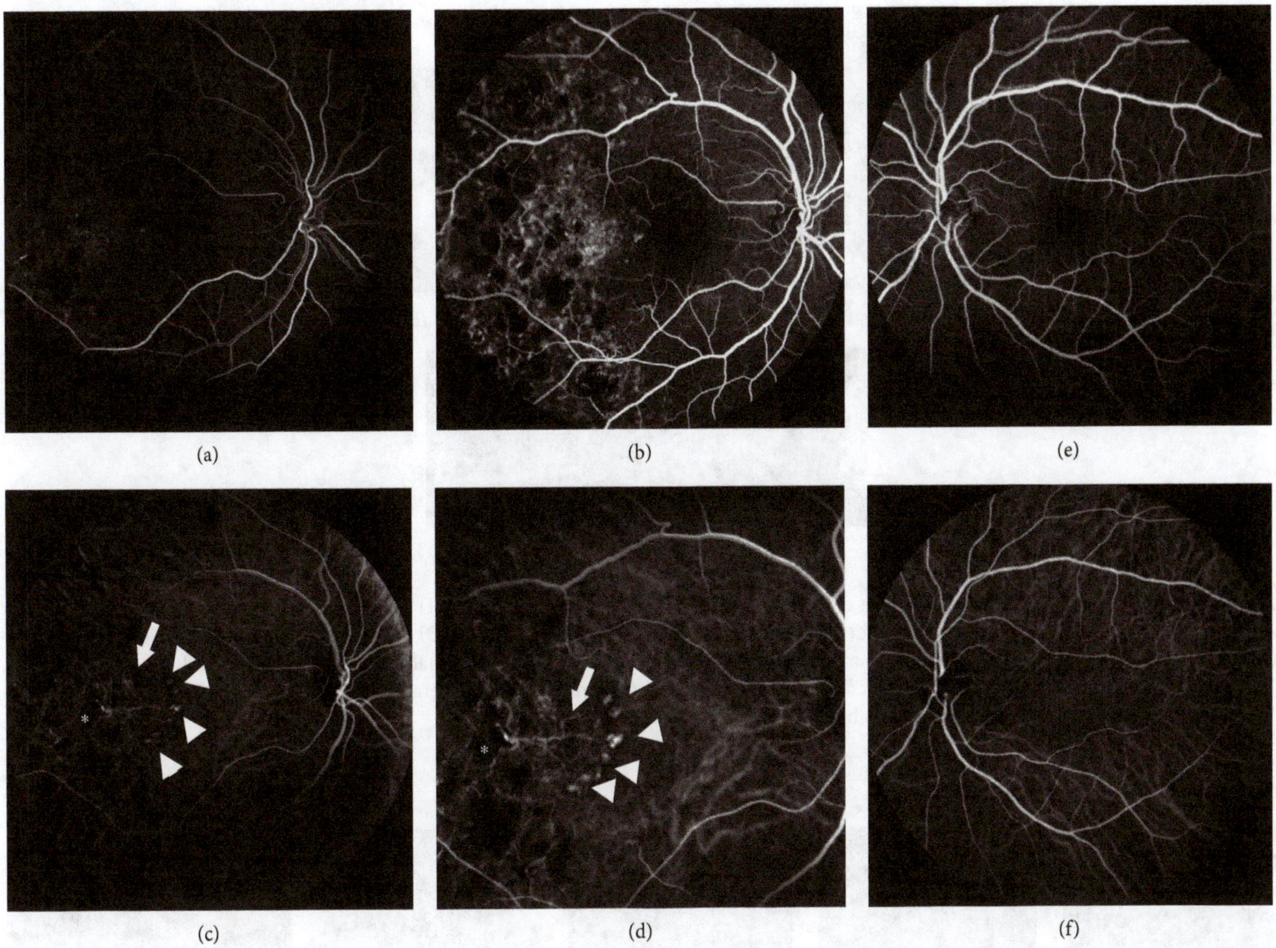

Figure 3: Fundus fluorescein angiogram (55°) of right eye (a, b) and left eye (e). Indocyanine green angiography (ICGA) of right eye (55° c, 30° d) and left eye (f). The branching vascular network (BVN, white arrows) and terminal hyperfluorescent polyps (white arrowheads) were clearly visible on ICGA. These also demonstrated a characteristic hypofluorescent halo. Note that the BVN originates from a hypofluorescent laser scar (∗ in c and d). FFA of the right eye revealed macular ischaemia. FFA and ICGA of the left eye were normal.

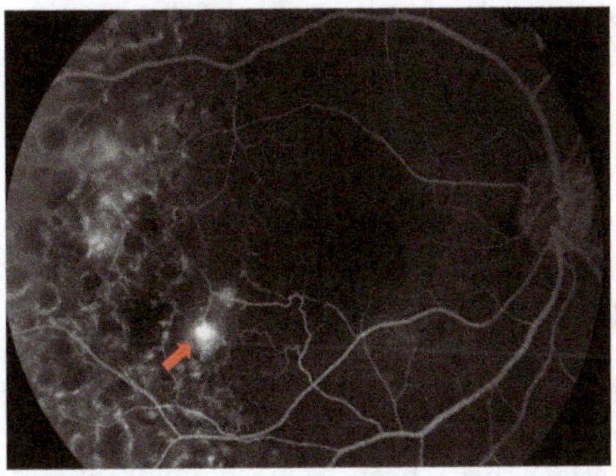

Figure 4: Fundus fluorescein angiogram of the right eye carried out 4 years before development of polypoidal lesions. Macular ischaemia is evident, together with active retinal neovascularization in the infero-temporal macula (red arrow). Previous laser retinal scars are also visible temporally.

3. Discussion

The term PCV was introduced in 1982 (Yannuzzi LA. Idiopathic Polypoidal Choroidal Vasculopathy. Presented at the Macula Society Meeting, Miami, Florida) and published in 1990 to describe a choroidal vasculopathy leading to serous and haemorrhagic pigment epithelial detachments [6]. It is more prevalent in Asian patients, but otherwise there is limited high quality epidemiological data due to the difficulty in confirming the diagnosis [7]. These lesions consist of a

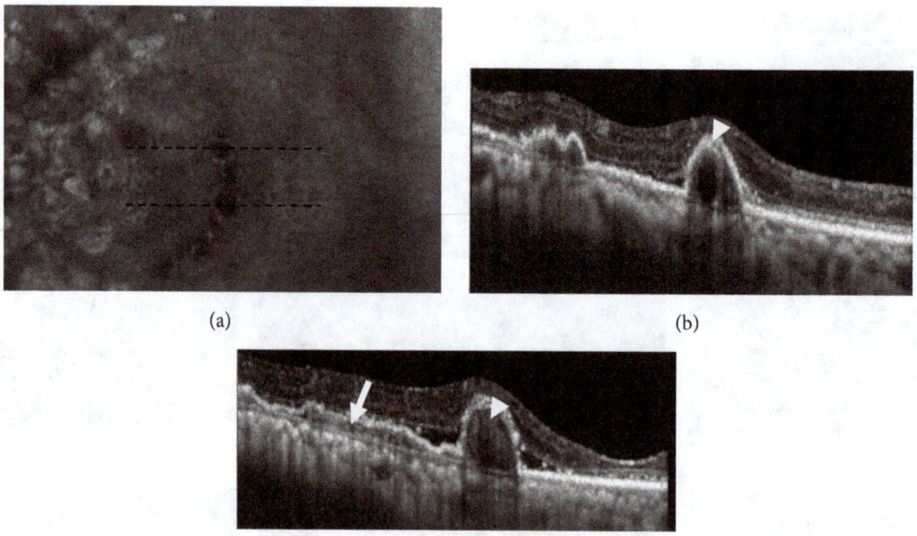

Figure 5: Infra-red image (a) of right eye with corresponding enhanced depth-imaging (EDI) spectral domain-OCT of right macula at the 9 months follow-up time-point. The black dashed line indicates to relevant position of the EDI images (upper b, lower c). Note the "double-layer" sign in image (c) (white arrow) as a hyper-reflective area in the space between the retinal pigment epithelium and Bruch's membrane. This suggests the location of the branching vascular network. Within the pigment epithelial detachments, hyper-reflective lesions can be seen that most likely represent polyps (white arrow-head in b, c).

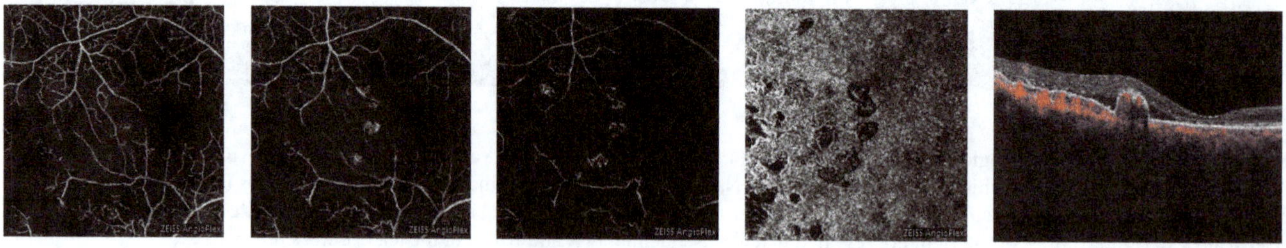

Figure 6: OCT-Angiography (OCT-A) images of the right eye at the 7-month follow-up time-point. The superficial (a) and deep (b) OCT-A slabs revealed macular ischaemia. The polyps were visible in (b), the avascular (c) and choriocapillaris (d) slabs. Flow within the polyps was seen on the cross-sectional OCT-A image (e).

BVN with polypoidal lesion at its edge, and appear under the retinal pigment epithelium. ICGA remains the gold-standard for PCV diagnosis, where the typical finding is that of polypoidal lesions which hyperfluoresce over the run of the angiogram with or without the presence of a BVN. Previously it has been suggested that vascular polyps represent a Type 1 neovascular process [8]. Polypoidal lesions have been reported in a range of conditions [9–13], including those that fall within the pachychoroid spectrum [14–16]. One previous report describes the development of PCV in a Chinese patient with SLE. Choroidal vasculitis was proposed as a mechanism for PCV in SLE incited by common complement pathway activation. Importantly, it has previously been reported that systemic inflammatory markers including C-reactive protein and certain cytokines have been elevated locally and/or systemically in patients with PCV [17, 18]. In our patient, the ICGA highlighted dilated pachyvessels in the right eye away, including regions away from the BVN and laser. This suggests a diffuse pathology of the choroid in the right eye. It is interesting, therefore, that the BVN lesions appeared to arise within a previous laser scar. However, it is not possible to state definitively if the uveitis history+/-laser was relevant for PCV development, particularly as the ocular inflammation had been quiescent for years. Nonetheless this case appears to be the first report of PCV arising within the region of a previous laser scar in the context of uveitis. Debate continues in the literature regarding the exact mechanism of development and even location of the abnormal vessels in PCV [7].

As PCV is more difficult to diagnose than CNVM (often requiring ICGA) and given the divergent management requirements, we must consider that this phenomenon may be under-reported in the iatrogenic- and inflammatory-CNVM literature and maintaining a high index of suspicion for secondary PCV may be justified.

Disclosure

This work was carried out at Moorfields Eye Hospital, London, United Kingdom.

Acknowledgments

The authors do not have any proprietary interest in the materials described in the article. The authors declare that there are no conflicts of interest regarding the publication of this paper.

References

[1] E. D'Ambrosio, P. Tortorella, and L. Iannetti, "Management of uveitis-related choroidal neovascularization: From the pathogenesis to the therapy," *Journal of Ophthalmology*, vol. 2014, Article ID 450428, 6 pages, 2014.

[2] M. P. Varley, E. Frank, and E. W. Purnell, "Subretinal neovascularization after focal argon laser for diabetic macular edema," *Ophthalmology*, vol. 95, no. 5, pp. 567–573, 1988.

[3] J. Pikkel and S. Rumelt, "Intravitreal bevacizumab for choroidal neovascularization secondary to laser photocoagulation for central serous chorioretinopathy," *European Journal of Ophthalmology*, vol. 22, no. 3, pp. 488–491, 2012.

[4] N. Dhingra, S. Kelly, M. A. Majid, C. B. Bailey, and A. D. Dick, "Inflammatory choroidal neovascular membrane in posterior uveitis-pathogenesis and treatment," *Indian Journal of Ophthalmology*, vol. 58, no. 1, pp. 3–10, 2010.

[5] Y. C. Chin, M. Bhargava, C. C. Khor, C. M. G. Cheung, and T. Y. Wong, "Polypoidal choroidal vasculopathy and systemic lupus erythematosus," *Lupus*, vol. 23, no. 3, pp. 319–322, 2014.

[6] L. A. Yannuzzi, J. Sorenson, R. F. Spaide, and B. Lipson, "Idiopathic polypoidal choroidal vasculopathy (IPCV)," *Retina*, vol. 10, no. 1, pp. 1–8, 1990.

[7] C. M. G. Cheung, T. Y. Y. Lai, P. Ruamviboonsuk et al., "polypoidal choroidal vasculopathy," *Ophthalmology*, vol. 125, no. 5, pp. 708–724, 2018.

[8] M. Inoue, C. Balaratnasingam, and K. B. Freund, "Optical coherence tomography angiography of polypoidal choroidal vasculopathy and polypoidal choroidal neovascularization," *Retina*, vol. 35, no. 11, pp. 2265–2274, 2015.

[9] J. G. Wong, X. J. Lai, R. Y. Sarafian, H. S. Wong, and J. B. Smith, "Polypoidal choroidal vasculopathy secondary to a stable choroidal nevus," *Retinal Cases and Brief Reports*, vol. 10, no. 3, pp. 221–224, 2016.

[10] E. Peiretti, M. C. Pozzoni, M. Fossarello, and R. F. Spaide, "Polypoidal choroidal vasculopathy in association with choroidal nevus," *Retinal Cases & Brief Reports*, vol. 3, no. 1, pp. 12–14, 2009.

[11] H. M. Bartlett, B. Willoughby, and N. Mandava, "Polypoidal choroidal vasculopathy in a patient with melanocytoma of the optic nerve," *Retina*, vol. 21, no. 4, pp. 396–399, 2001.

[12] Z. Cebeci, S. Bayraktar, M. Oray, and N. Kir, "Silent polypoidal choroidal vasculopathy in a patient with angioid streaks," *Arquivos Brasileiros de Oftalmologia*, vol. 79, no. 3, pp. 200-201, 2016.

[13] S. Baillif-Gostoli, M. Quaranta-El Maftouhi, and M. Mauget-Faÿsse, "Polypoidal choroidal vasculopathy in a patient with angioid streaks secondary to pseudoxanthoma elasticum," *Graefe's Archive for Clinical and Experimental Ophthalmology*, vol. 248, no. 12, pp. 1845–1848, 2010.

[14] G. J. Manayath, V. S. Shah, V. R. Saravanan, and V. Narendran, "Polypoidal choroidal vasculopathy associated with central serous chorioretinopathy: Pachychoroid spectrum of diseases," *Retina*, vol. 38, no. 6, pp. 1195–1204, 2018.

[15] A. Jean-Charles, H. Merle, I. Audo et al., "Martinique crinkled retinal pigment epitheliopathy: Clinical stages and pathophysiologic insights," *Ophthalmology*, vol. 123, no. 10, pp. 2196–2204, 2016.

[16] C. M. Cheung, W. K. Lee, H. Koizumi, K. Dansingani, T. Y. Y. Lai, and K. B. Freund, "Pachychoroid disease," *Eye*, vol. 33, no. 1, pp. 14–33, 2019.

[17] M. Kikuchi, M. Nakamura, K. Ishikawa et al., "Elevated C-reactive protein levels in patients with polypoidal choroidal vasculopathy and patients with neovascular age-related macular degeneration," *Ophthalmology*, vol. 114, no. 9, pp. 1722–1727, 2007.

[18] Y. Sakurada, Y. Nakamura, S. Yoneyama et al., "Aqueous humor cytokine levels in patients with polypoidal choroidal vasculopathy and neovascular age-related macular degeneration," *Ophthalmic Research*, vol. 53, no. 1, pp. 2–7, 2015.

Physical Incompatibility between Vancomycin and Viscoelastic Mimicking Acute Endophthalmitis: The First Report

Biljana Kuzmanović Elabjer, Dean Šarić, Mladen Bušić, Mirjana Bjeloš, and Andrej Pleše

University Eye Clinic, Faculty of Dental Medicine and Health Care Osijek, Faculty of Medicine Osijek, University Josip Juraj Strossmayer in Osijek, University Hospital "Sveti Duh", Zagreb, Croatia

Correspondence should be addressed to Mladen Bušić; mbusic@kbsd.hr

Academic Editor: Alexander A. Bialasiewicz

This is the first documentation of vancomycin precipitation with viscoelastic in the anterior chamber of the eye. A 34-year-old white male underwent uneventful penetrating keratoplasty. Intracameral instillation of 1 mg/0.1 mL of vancomycin followed no attempts of meticulous viscoelastic irrigation. Six hours later thick white material in the anterior chamber was sedimented. The following criteria excluded the diagnosis of endophthalmitis and TASS: clear and transparent anterior chamber and vitreous body, the absence of ciliary injection and corneal oedema, and unremarkable laboratory tests' results. This iatrogenic complication mimicking endophthalmitis does not require any specific management and should be acknowledged in guidelines for prevention and treatment of endophthalmitis. The objective of this paper is to alert colleagues to this iatrogenic complication of vancomycin mimicking endophthalmitis. Whether this condition should be labelled as positive or negative demands further investigation. As vancomycin is a time-dependent antibiotic, it is possible that this precipitate could serve as a slowly releasing drug depot and viscoelastic as a vehicle for precipitation. This being the case, investigation is needed to analyse its potential to precipitate with another dispersive and cohesive viscoelasticity.

1. Introduction

Vancomycin hydrochloride is a glycopeptide antibiotic used in ophthalmic surgery for postoperative endophthalmitis prophylaxis [1]. It precipitates with gelatine fluid, ciprofloxacin, cloxacillin, and ceftazidime [2–5]. According to medical literature this is the first publication of precipitation of vancomycin with residual viscoelastic (hydroxypropyl methylcellulose IP 2% w/v, Aurovisc®, Madurai, India) in anterior chamber.

2. Case Report

A 34-year-old white healthy male underwent uneventful penetrating keratoplasty for keratoconus of ABCD stage 4 [6]. Preoperatively antisepsis of the periocular skin and eye with 10% povidone-iodine solution was applied for three minutes. The graft was sutured with 10-0 double running nylon (ETHILON® Nylon Suture, Ethicon, USA). For the prophylaxis of endophthalmitis, in this patient vancomycin was indicated due to the allergy to beta-lactam antibiotics and 1 mg/0.1 mL was instilled intracamerally. The vancomycin powder (Vancomycin Kabi 500 mg, Xellia Pharmaceuticals ApS, Denmark) was reconstituted and diluted with 0.9% sodium chloride injection. Six hours after the surgery the patient complained of pain in the operated eye. Photophobia, blepharospasm, and pale lid oedema were present with pinhole visual acuity of logMAR 1.0. No ciliary injection or corneal oedema was present. Graft was secured to the host cornea with equal tension along the suture and negative Seidel test. White, cheese-like material, sedimented and irregularly bordered superiorly to the rest of the clear anterior chamber, was found [Figure 1].

Tyndall was negative, pupil round, and reactive. The lens and the vitreous body were clear. Applanation tonometry was 11 mmHg. Ultrasound documented no pathology of the eye

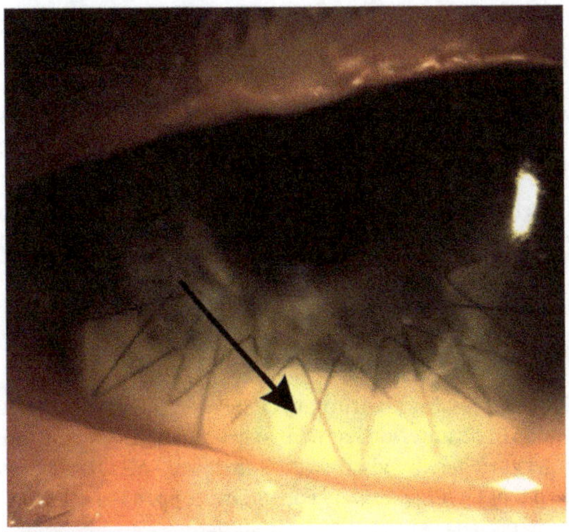

FIGURE 1: The right eye of 34-year-old white male on day zero of the penetrating keratoplasty. Note absence of the corneal oedema. White material at the bottom (black arrow), irregularly bordered superiorly to the rest of the clear anterior chamber.

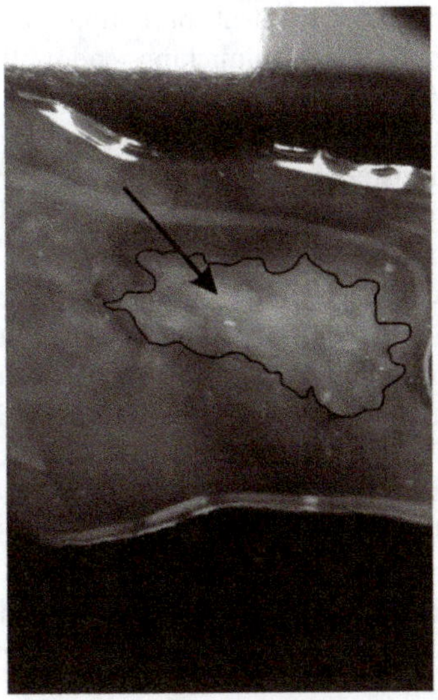

FIGURE 2: In vitro on the glass slide clear vancomycin at the concentration of 1 mg/0.1 mL was instilled in a clear Aurovisc® (black outline). Note opacification (black arrow).

and orbit. The pain decreased on tetracaine drops (Tetrakain® 0.5%, Gradska ljekarna, Zagreb, Croatia). Laboratory tests' results (complete blood count with differential and erythrocyte sedimentation rate) were unremarkable. Under the strong presumption that vancomycin precipitated in the residual viscoelastic no attempts to lavage the anterior chamber were undertaken. Topical dexamethasone with antibiotic (Maxitrol, Alcon Cusi SA, El Masnou, Barcelona, Spain; SA, Alcon-Couvreur NV, Puurs, Belgium) was administered q.i.d. Ophthalmological follow-up was performed hourly for seven hours until the pain resolved. Complete dissolution of precipitates ensued 19 hours following the surgery.

The case report was written with the approval of the institutional research ethics committee, complying with the tenets of the Declaration of Helsinki.

3. Discussion

Patient complaining of pain in the operated eye on the day of surgery with thick white precipitate sedimented in the anterior chamber is an alert for the ophthalmologist to be on standby. Apart from the most obvious infectious endophthalmitis, foreign particles used in surgery and toxic anterior segment syndrome (TASS) must be considered in differential diagnosis [7, 8]. The main distinctions between infectious endophthalmitis and TASS are onset and progression of symptoms as well as the presence of pain and vitritis [7]. However, in both conditions corneal involvement and major inflammatory reaction in the anterior chamber are present [7]. The following criteria excluded the diagnoses of endophthalmitis and TASS: clear and transparent anterior chamber and vitreous body, absence of ciliary injection and corneal oedema, and unremarkable laboratory tests' results as well as the fact that the pain decreased on the tetracaine drops. The material in the anterior chamber, if not of inflammatory origin, had to be iatrogenic. Namely, no meticulous aspiration of viscoelastic was performed due to intraoperative tendency of anterior chamber shallowing. In Aurovisc® instructions for use leaflet acknowledged that the concurrent presence of medication in the chamber or associated ocular structures may interact with Aurovisc® to cause clouding.

It is documented that vancomycin has precipitative properties with different substances, especially those in gelatinous form [2]. Aurovisc® is hydroxyl propyl methyl cellulose viscoelastic solution of 3000–4500 cps at 27°C containing no sodium carbonate. It was advocated that vancomycin and ceftazidime precipitate due to the presence of sodium carbonate in ceftazidime [9]. When vancomycin and ceftazidime were mixed, precipitates formed at a concentration of 10 mg/mL for vancomycin, the same as in this report. However, the precipitation was documented regardless of sodium carbonate presence, favouring alkaline pH as the major element in the precipitation process [5, 10]. The vancomycin–ceftazidime precipitate manifested pH of 6.2, while vancomycin itself, as a salt of hydrochloric acid, is set to pH range 2.5–4.5 [2, 10]. In addition, the study that is more recent evidenced no precipitation of the two drugs, when the drugs were administered in the media one after the complete diffusion of the other [5].

Experimentally, instant precipitation occurred [Figure 2], in vitro on the glass slide when a drop of 1 mg / 0.1 mL vancomycin was added in a clear Aurovisc®.

In our patient, precipitates sedimented in anterior chamber dissolved spontaneously, like the precipitates in vitreous cavity reported earlier [11]. The time required, due to different hemodynamics between vitreous cavity and anterior chamber, was markedly shorter.

In conclusion, this is the first documentation of vancomycin precipitation with viscoelastic in the anterior chamber of the eye. This should be acknowledged in guidelines for prevention and treatment of endophthalmitis as this iatrogenic complication mimicking endophthalmitis does not require any specific management.

The incompatibility developed when the vancomycin drug was administered at the recommended concentration for endophthalmitis prophylaxis, advocating pH and dispersion of vancomycin as two major factors in precipitation process. The objective of this paper is to alert colleagues to this iatrogenic complication of vancomycin mimicking endophthalmitis. Whether this complication should be labelled as positive or negative demands further investigation. As vancomycin is a time-dependent antibiotic, failing to achieve an efficient bactericidal level over at least 11 h, it is possible that this precipitate could serve as a slowly releasing drug depot and viscoelastic as a vehicle for precipitation [10, 12, 13]. This being the case, research is needed to analyse its potential to precipitate with other dispersive and cohesive viscoelastic.

Additional Points

Key Message. This is the first documentation of vancomycin precipitation with viscoelastic in the anterior chamber of the eye. This should be acknowledged in guidelines for prevention and treatment of endophthalmitis as this iatrogenic complication mimicking endophthalmitis does not require any specific management.

Consent

Consent to publish the case report was not obtained. This report does not contain any personal data that could lead to the identification of the patient.

Authors' Contributions

This manuscript has been read and approved by all the authors, and each author believes that the manuscript represents honest work.

References

[1] P. Barry, L. Cordovés, and S. Gardner, *ESCRS Guidelines for Prevention and Treatment of Endophthalmitis Following Cataract Surgery: Data, Dilemmas and Conclusions*, Dublin, Republic of Ireland, 2013.

[2] H.-P. Ng, K.-F. Koh, L.-S. Tham, and M. Harmer, "Vancomycin causes dangerous precipitation when infused with gelatin fluid," *Anaesthesia*, vol. 55, no. 10, pp. 1039-1040, 2000.

[3] M. Hui, A. K. H. Kwok, C. P. Pang et al., "An in vitro study on the compatibility and precipitation of a combination of ciprofloxacin and vancomycin in human vitreous," *British Journal of Ophthalmology*, vol. 88, no. 2, pp. 218–222, 2004.

[4] A. Chan, G. Tawfik, and W. Cheng, "Physical incompatibility between parenteral cloxacillin and vancomycin," *The Canadian Journal of Hospital Pharmacy*, vol. 66, no. 5, pp. 310–312, 2013.

[5] I. Park and S. J. Lee, "Factors affecting precipitation of vancomycin and ceftazidime on intravitreal injection," *Journal of Ocular Pharmacology and Therapeutics*, vol. 29, no. 1, pp. 23–26, 2013.

[6] M. Belin and J. Duncan, "Keratoconus: The ABCD grading system," *Klinische Monatsblätter für Augenheilkunde*, vol. 233, no. 06, pp. 701–707, 2016.

[7] M. H. Lee, D. Cugley, A. Atik, and G. S. Ang, "Endophthalmitis or toxic anterior segment syndrome?" *Clinical and Experimental Optometry*, vol. 100, no. 1, pp. 94-95, 2017.

[8] A. K. Altintas, M. Y. Ciritoglu, Ö. BeyazyildiZ, Ç. Ü. Can, and S. Polat, "Toxic anterior segment synrome outbreak after cataract surgery triggere by viscoelastic substance," *Middle East African Journal of Ophthalmology*, vol. 24, no. 1, pp. 43–47, 2017.

[9] R. G. Fiscella, "Physical incompatibility of vancomycin and ceftazidime for intravitreal injection," *JAMA Ophtalmology*, vol. 111, no. 6, p. 730, 1993.

[10] B. Raju, T. Bali, G. Thiagarajan et al., "Physicochemical properties and antibacterial activity of the precipitate of vancomycin and ceftazidime: implications in the management of endophthalmitis," *Retina*, vol. 28, no. 2, pp. 320–325, 2008.

[11] T. Lifshitz, R. Lapid-Gortzak, Y. Finkelman, and I. Klemperer, "Vancomycin and ceftazidime incompatibility upon intravitreal injection," *British Journal of Ophthalmology*, vol. 84, no. 1, pp. 117-118, 2000.

[12] M. J. Rybak, "The pharmacokinetic and pharmacodynamic properties of vancomycin," *Clinical Infectious Diseases*, vol. 42, no. Supplement_1, pp. S35–S39, 2006.

[13] W. Hachicha, L. Kodjikian, and H. Fessi, "Preparation of vancomycin microparticles: Importance of preparation parameters," *International Journal of Pharmaceutics*, vol. 324, no. 2, pp. 176–184, 2006.

33

Purtscher-Like Retinopathy in a Patient with COVID-19

Alexander R. Bottini, Sean Steinmetz, Kevin J. Blinder, and Gaurav K. Shah

The Retina Institute, St. Louis, MO, USA

Correspondence should be addressed to Kevin J. Blinder; mdblinder.kevinj@rc-stl.com

Academic Editor: Antonio Ferreras

The emerging literature on the novel coronavirus pandemic has reported several cases of varied retinal findings in patients with COVID-19. We report the case of a 59-year-old male who presented with complaint of bilateral blurry vision following hospital discharge after prolonged hospitalization for severe COVID-19 illness. On ocular exam, the patient demonstrated bilateral cotton wool spots localized to the posterior pole of each eye. Multimodal imaging demonstrated findings consistent with retinal nerve fiber layer infarcts in the areas of the cotton wool spots. Exam and imaging of our patient were most consistent with a Purtscher-like retinopathy. We suggest that as ophthalmologists care for increasing numbers of patients recuperating from COVID-19, they monitor for microangiopathic changes similar to those in our patient.

1. Introduction

Purtscher's retinopathy—featuring cotton wool spots, retinal hemorrhages, and inner retinal opacification (Purtscher flecken)—is classically described following significant traumatic injury [1, 2]. Purtscher-like retinopathy describes similar retinal findings associated with a variety of other conditions including pancreatitis, thrombotic thrombocytopenia purpura, and hemolytic uremic syndrome [1, 2]. We present the case of a patient recovering from severe COVID-19 illness requiring prolonged hospitalization who presented with a retinopathy most consistent with Purtscher-like retinopathy.

2. Case Report

A 59-year-old white male presented with complaint of bilateral blurry vision. The patient had noticed a subjective change in visual acuity in the preceding two weeks, which followed his hospital discharge after a prolonged hospitalization for COVID-19.

Past medical history included coronary artery disease, insulin-dependent diabetes mellitus, hypertension, and hyperlipidemia. Six weeks prior to ophthalmic evaluation, the patient presented to the emergency department with fever, cough, and progressive dyspnea. SARS-CoV-2 testing was positive, and chest radiographs demonstrated bilateral infiltrates consistent with COVID-19 pneumonia. The patient's ability to oxygenate quickly deteriorated, and he was admitted to the intensive care unit with acute hypoxemic respiratory failure and intubated shortly thereafter.

The patient's month-long hospital course was complicated by deterioration of his respiratory status, requiring extracorporeal membrane oxygenation for eleven days. His treatment also included convalescent plasma and remdesivir. The patient also developed encephalopathy and coagulopathy requiring full-dose anticoagulation. Blood pressure was labile, and at times, multiple antihypertensive medications were required. His blood glucose levels were well controlled throughout his hospitalization.

At the time of ophthalmic exam, the patient's visual acuity was 20/50 in the right eye and 20/60 in the left eye. Anterior segment examination demonstrated mild nuclear sclerotic cataracts and was notable for the absence of any signs of inflammation. Intraocular pressure by applanation tonometry was 15 in both eyes. Posterior segment examination revealed multiple foci of inner retinal opacification, or cotton wool spots, in the posterior pole of both eyes (Figures 1(a)–1(d)). Apart from these lesions, fundus examination was unremarkable without other signs of retinal

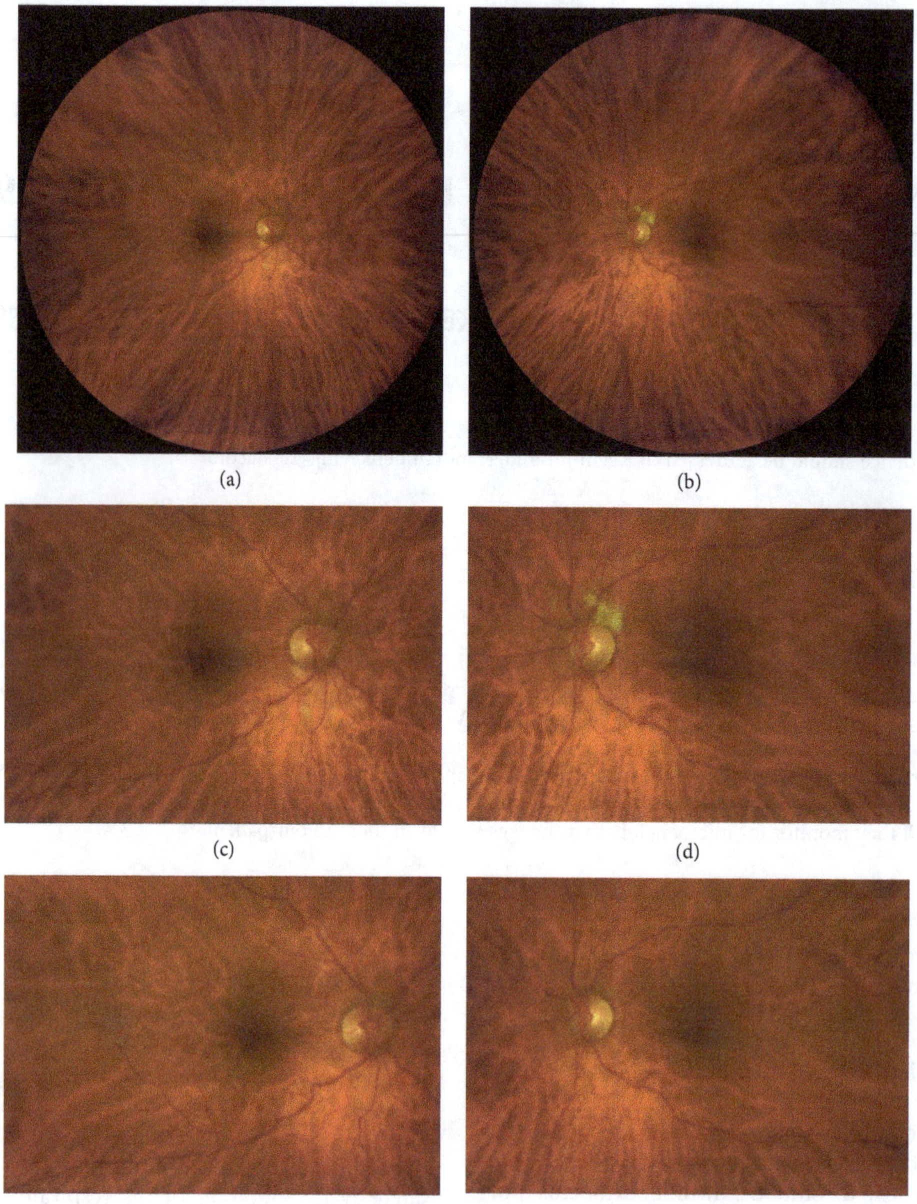

(a) (b) (c) (d) (e) (f)

Figure 1: Fundus photos demonstrating cotton wool spots in the posterior pole of each eye at presentation (a–d) and their interval reduction at two-month follow-up (e, f).

vascular disease or inflammation. Despite the patient's history of hypertension, there was no narrowing of the retinal arterioles or arteriovenous crossing anomalies.

Optical coherence tomography (OCT) revealed no retinal edema (Figures 2(a) and 2(b)). OCT through the lesions revealed thickening and hyperreflectivity of the retinal nerve fiber layer (Figures 2(c) and 2(d)). Fluorescein angiography demonstrated mild obscuration of the retinal vasculature by the peripapillary cotton wool spot in the left eye; otherwise, the study was unremarkable (Figures 2(e)–2(h)). OCT angiography sectioned at the level of the superficial capillary plexus demonstrated flow voids corresponding to the location of the lesions (Figures 2(i)–2(l)).

The patient was counseled on his diagnosis and seen for follow-up two months later. Upon his return, the patient reported improved vision in both eyes. Visual acuity was 20/20 in the right eye and 20/25 in the left eye. On fundus examination (Figures 1(e)–1(f)), there was marked reduction in the size and number of cotton wool spots in both eyes.

3. Discussion

Our patient's clinical course, complicated by multiorgan failure, and ocular findings appear most consistent with a Purtscher-like retinopathy following severe COVID-19

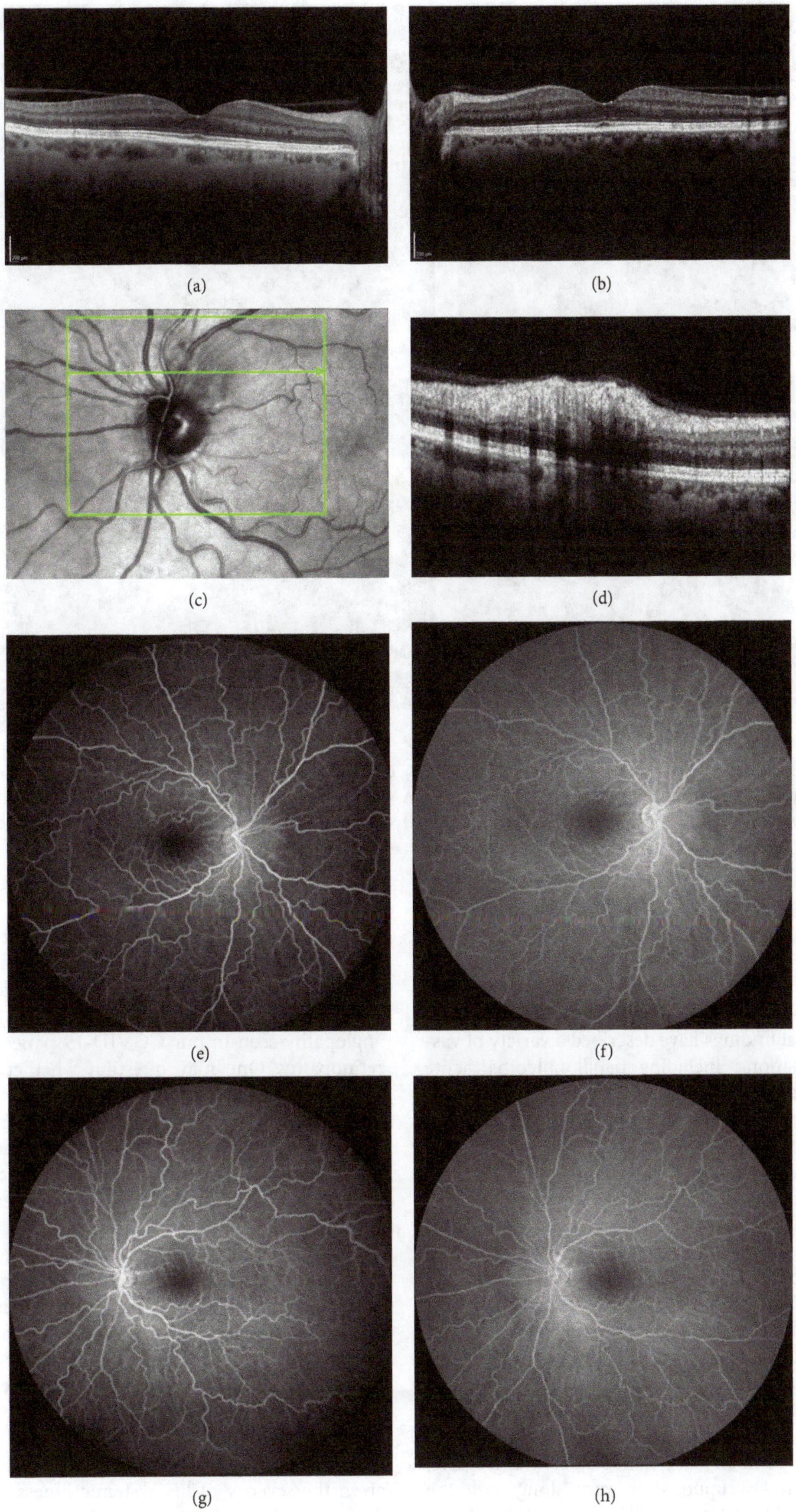

FIGURE 2: Continued.

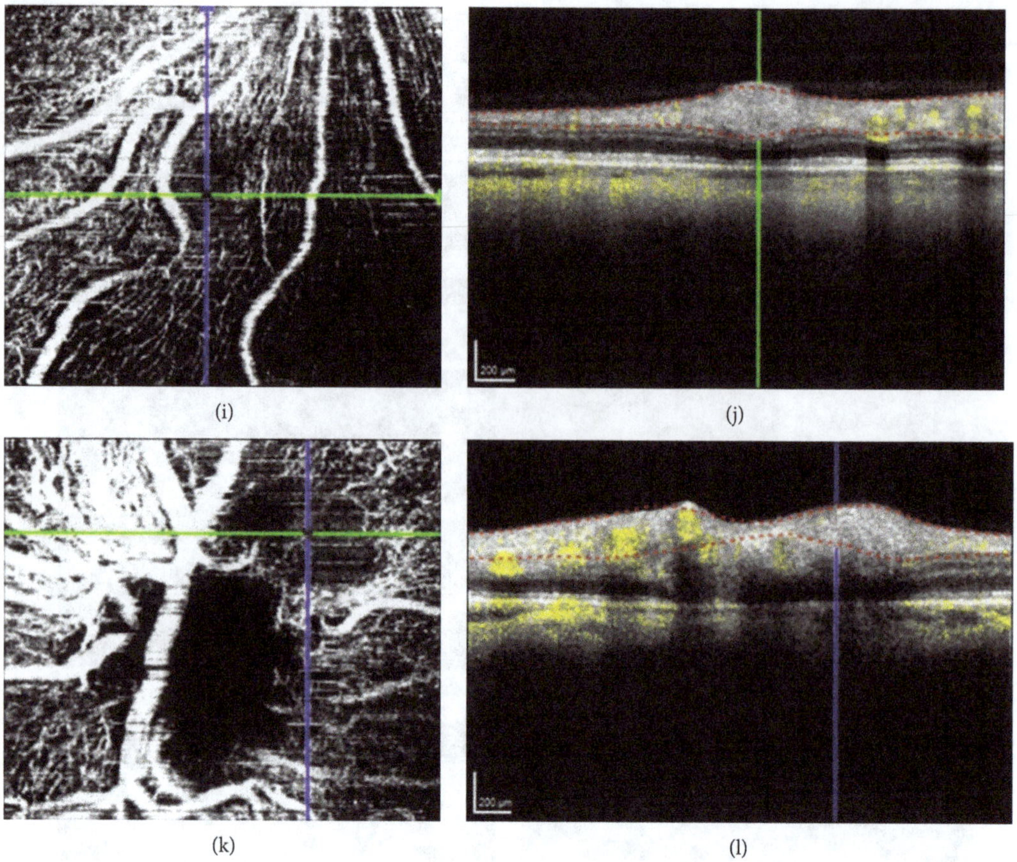

FIGURE 2: OCT demonstrated normal foveal contour in both eyes (a, b). OCT through an area of inner retinal opacification in the left eye (c, d) revealed thickening and hyperreflectivity of the nerve fiber layer. FA was largely unremarkable (e–h) aside from mild obscuration of the retinal vasculature in areas of inner retinal opacification. OCTA (i–l) sectioned at the superficial capillary plexus demonstrated flow voids corresponding to the cotton wool spots.

illness. Retinal anomalies have been among the multitude of reports on the COVID-19 and the novel coronavirus pandemic [3–8]. SARS-CoV-2 has been detected in the retinas of COVID-19 patients on autopsy [4]. Case reports documenting retinal findings have described a variety of vasculopathic presentations, including papillophlebitis, acute ophthalmic artery occlusion, paracentral acute middle maculopathy, acute macular neuroretinopathy, and cotton wool spots [5–8].

In reporting on cotton wool spots in 6 of 27 patients recovered from COVID-19 pneumonia, Landecho et al. suggested that retinal microangiopathic changes may result from the hypercoagulable state seen in cases of COVID-19 or direct viral infection of the vascular endothelium leading to vasculitis [8]. Both of these proposed mechanisms of microangiopathic injury—coagulopathy and vasculitis—are also postulated to be involved in the pathogenesis of Purtscher's and Purtscher-like retinopathy. Microemboli to the retina are suspected to result in the constellation of posterior pole lesions in Purtscher-like retinopathy [1, 2]. The source of the microemboli—air, fat, leukocyte aggregates, platelets, and fibrin—is supposed to vary along with the causes of Purtscher-like retinopathy [2]. Vasculitis, induced by lipase or other inflammatory cytokines, may also lead to thrombosis and vascular occlusion resulting in Purtscher-like retinopathy [2].

Given these similarities in presentation and proposed pathogenesis, it seems appropriate to call the retinal microangiopathy seen in our COVID-19 patient a Purtscher-like retinopathy. One may question whether it is appropriate to ascribe our patient's retinopathy to his COVID-19 infection or to the multiorgan failure and coagulopathy that complicated his clinical course. In considering this question, the report of Landecho et al. is particularly useful, as their patients—whose retinal findings were also consistent with Purtscher-like retinopathy—did not have multiorgan failure or a clinical course as advanced as ours. One may also question if our patient's retinopathy is best described as a Purtscher-like retinopathy or is better attributed to his hypertension or his underlying diabetes. This is a reasonable concern as the diagnosis of Purtscher-like retinopathy is clinical and must consider a wide differential diagnosis. Indeed, our patient lacked the low to moderate number of intraretinal hemorrhages and pathognomonic Purtscher flecken of Purtscher-like retinopathy. However, given the severity of his systemic illness, our patient had a delayed ocular presentation and thus the acute findings of Purtscher-like retinopathy, hemorrhages, and Purtscher flecken may have previously resolved. Furthermore, aside from cotton wool spots, our patient demonstrated none of the characteristic findings of these retinopathies, though the possibility of a delayed presentation of a hypertensive crisis without chronic hypertensive changes remains.

4. Conclusions

In the weeks and months ahead, ophthalmologists will no doubt encounter more and more patients recuperating from COVID-19 infections. We call attention to the findings in our patient and suggest ophthalmologists to be attentive to this Purtscher-like retinopathy. Our observations of micro-angiopathy in these patients may well contribute to a more comprehensive understanding of the burden of COVID-19.

Consent

No written consent has been obtained from the patient as there is no patient identifiable data included in this case report.

References

[1] A. I. M. Miguel, F. Henriques, L. F. R. Azevedo, A. J. R. Loureiro, and D. A. L. Maberley, "Systematic review of Purtscher's and Purtscher-like retinopathies," *Eye (London, England)*, vol. 27, no. 1, pp. 1–13, 2013.

[2] A. Agrawal and M. A. McKibbin, "Purtscher's and Purtscher-like retinopathies: a review," *Survey of Ophthalmology*, vol. 51, no. 2, pp. 129–136, 2006.

[3] P. M. Marinho, A. A. Marcos, A. C. Romano, H. Nascimento, and R. Belfort, "Retinal findings in patients with COVID-19," *Lancet*, vol. 395, no. 10237, p. 1610, 2020.

[4] M. Casagrande, A. Fitzek, K. Püschel et al., "Detection of SARS-CoV-2 in human retinal biopsies of deceased COVID-19 patients," *Ocular Immunology and Inflammation*, vol. 28, no. 5, pp. 721–725, 2020.

[5] A. Insausti-Garcia, J. A. Reche-Sainz, C. Ruiz-Arranz, A. L. Vazquez, and M. Ferro-Osuna, "Papillophlebitis in a COVID-19 patient: inflammation and hypercoagulable state," *European Journal of Ophthalmology*, p. 112067212094759, 2020.

[6] O. M. Dumitrascu, O. Volod, S. Bose, Y. Wang, V. Biousse, and P. D. Lyden, "Acute ophthalmic artery occlusion in a COVID-19 patient on apixaban," *Journal of Stroke and Cerebrovascular* ... 2, 2020.

... acentral acute middle maculo- ... oretinopathy following SARS- ... vol. 34, no. 12, pp. 2352-2353, ...

... Gándara et al., "COVID-19 ret- ... ivo biomarker of systemic vas- ... *rnal Medicine*, vol. 289, no. 1,

34

Visual Snow-Like Symptoms and Posterior Uveitis following COVID-19 Infection

Kathryn Kelani Braceros, Masumi G. Asahi, and Ron P. Gallemore

Retina Macula Institute, Torrance, California, USA

Correspondence should be addressed to Ron P. Gallemore; rongallemoremd@gmail.com

Academic Editor: Huban Atilla

Visual snow (VS) is a neurologic condition consisting of a constant positive visual disturbance described as "static" with diagnosis requiring exclusion of competing neurologic and ophthalmologic disorders. The authors describe the first case of visual snow-like symptoms in a patient following coronavirus disease 2019 (COVID-19) infection. He was found to have a transient subtle mild inflammatory reaction in the vitreous and optic nerve edema which resolved, but the VS persisted. Our findings suggest that COVID-19 may precipitate a transient autoimmune response in some patients with resultant ocular inflammation as well as long-term symptoms of VS. This has potential implications for the understanding and treatment of complications related to COVID-19 and in VS.

1. Introduction

Visual snow (VS) is a neurologic condition consisting of a constant positive visual disturbance described as "static" or innumerable small dots throughout the visual field [1]. There are often associated visual symptoms such as palinopsia, entoptic phenomena, photophobia, and nyctalopia [1, 2]. The current diagnosis of visual snow requires exclusion of competing neurologic and ophthalmological disorders [2]. Here, we report the first case of visual snow-like symptoms with associated posterior uveitis shortly after coronavirus disease 2019 (COVID-19) infection with persistent VS after resolution of ocular inflammation.

2. Case Presentation

The case is a 28-year-old Chinese male with no past medical or psychiatric history presenting with complaints of constant "static" in his entire field of vision which he subsequently described as "a subtle overlay of an out-of-signal TV screen over my entire vision." Symptoms began shortly following diagnosis with COVID-19 infection. The patient developed symptoms of COVID-19 (fever, cough, loss of sense of taste, and smell) on March 12, 2020, and was confirmed positive for COVID-19 via nasopharyngeal swab on March 20, 2020, by way of a nasopharyngeal swab tested for the coronavirus with reverse transcription-polymerase chain reaction RNA testing. He was subsequently hospitalized for 2 days and treated with IV azithromycin and hydroxychloroquine. The patient was discharged home and eventually tested negative for COVID-19 on April 11, 2020, also via nasopharyngeal swab and RNA, RT PCR. He then reported associated photophobia and palinopsia (after images). He denied prior visual symptoms prior to COVID-19 infection. He was also found to have decreased vision in the left eye by his optometrist and was referred for further evaluation.

The patient presented with best-corrected visual acuity (BCVA) of 20/20 in both eyes (OU). Intraocular pressure (IOP) was 17 mmHg in the right eye (OD) and 16 mmHg in the left eye (OS). Confrontation visual field was full, extraocular motility intact, and pupils equal reactive a reactive to light. Slit lamp exam (SLE) was with clea OU and with rare to trace white blood cells (WBC vitreous OU, but otherwise unremarkable. The only noted with complete darkness and the patient inspection of the vitreous over

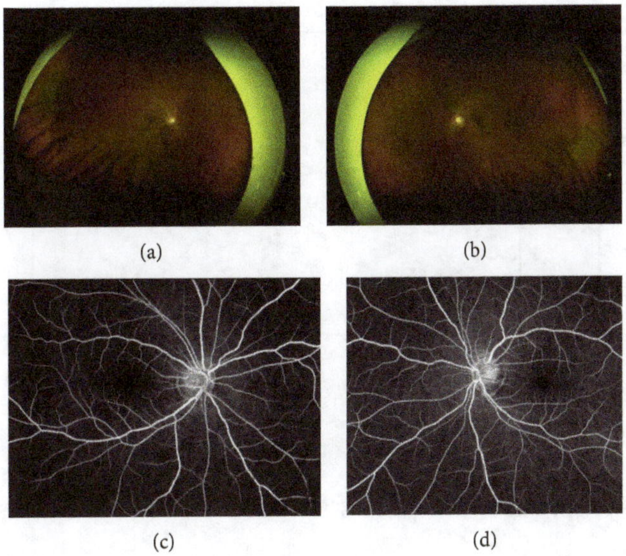

FIGURE 1: Fundus photo of the (a) right and (b) left eyes at presentation. Late recirculation phase fluorescein angiogram taken at 3 minutes showing subtle staining of the nerve of the (c) right and (d) left eyes.

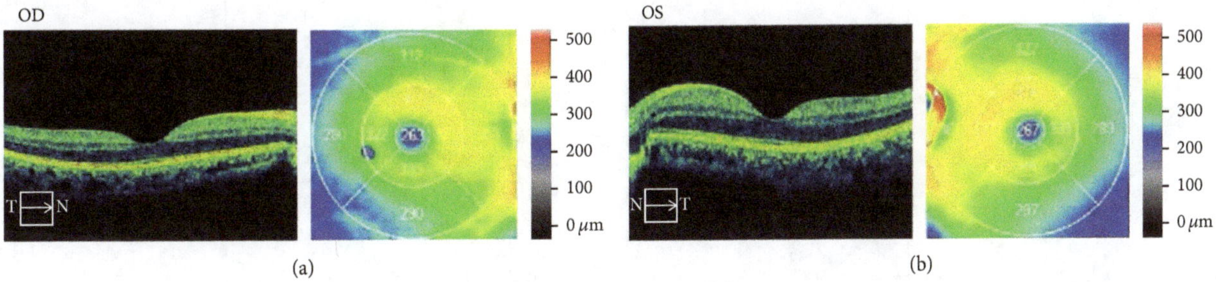

FIGURE 2: Optical coherence tomography with associated topographical map at presentation showing normal foveal contour with mild macular thickening of the (a) right eye and (b) left eye.

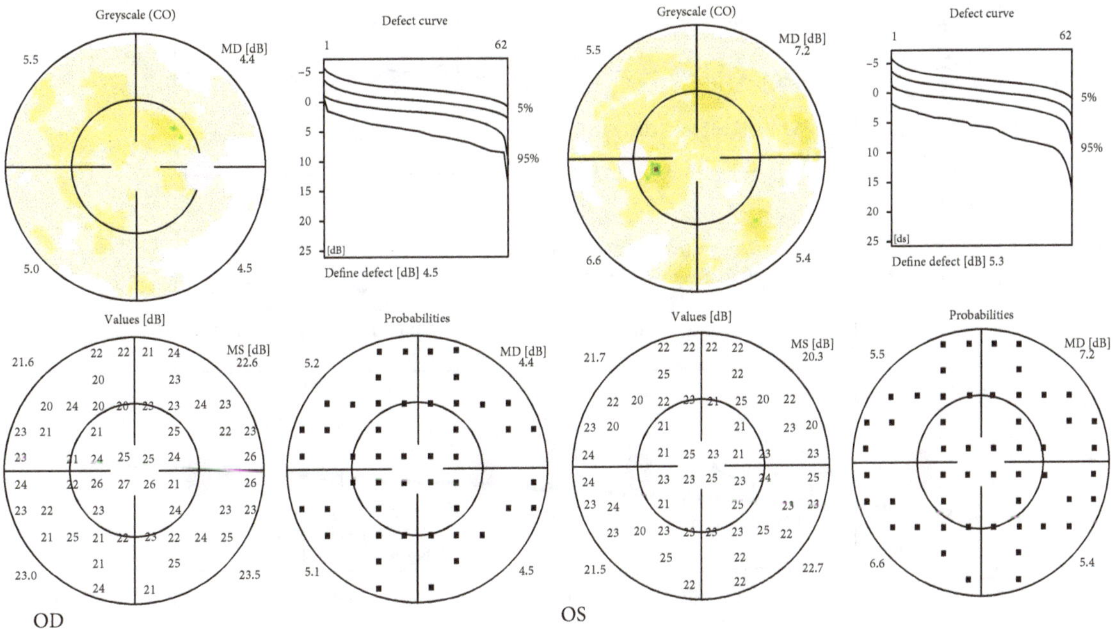

FIGURE 3: Octopus 30-2 visual field at presentation showing diffuse nonspecific suppression in the right eye (OD) and left eye (OS).

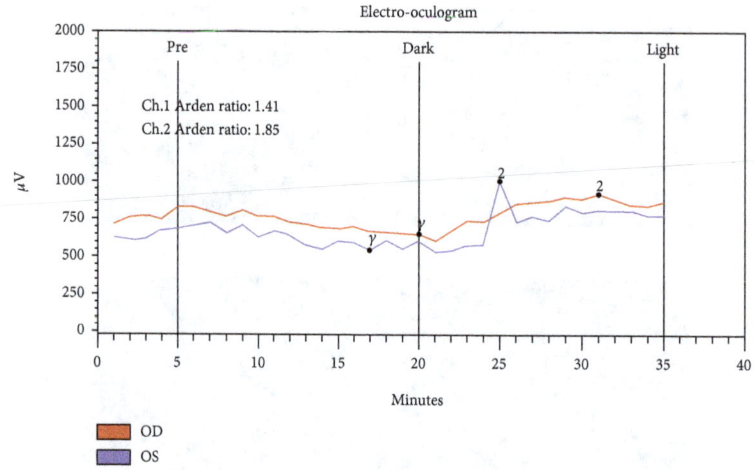

FIGURE 4: Electrooculogram (EOG) showing suppression in the right eye (OD) and borderline suppression in the left eye (OS) with Arden ratio of 1.41 (OD) and 1.85 (OS).

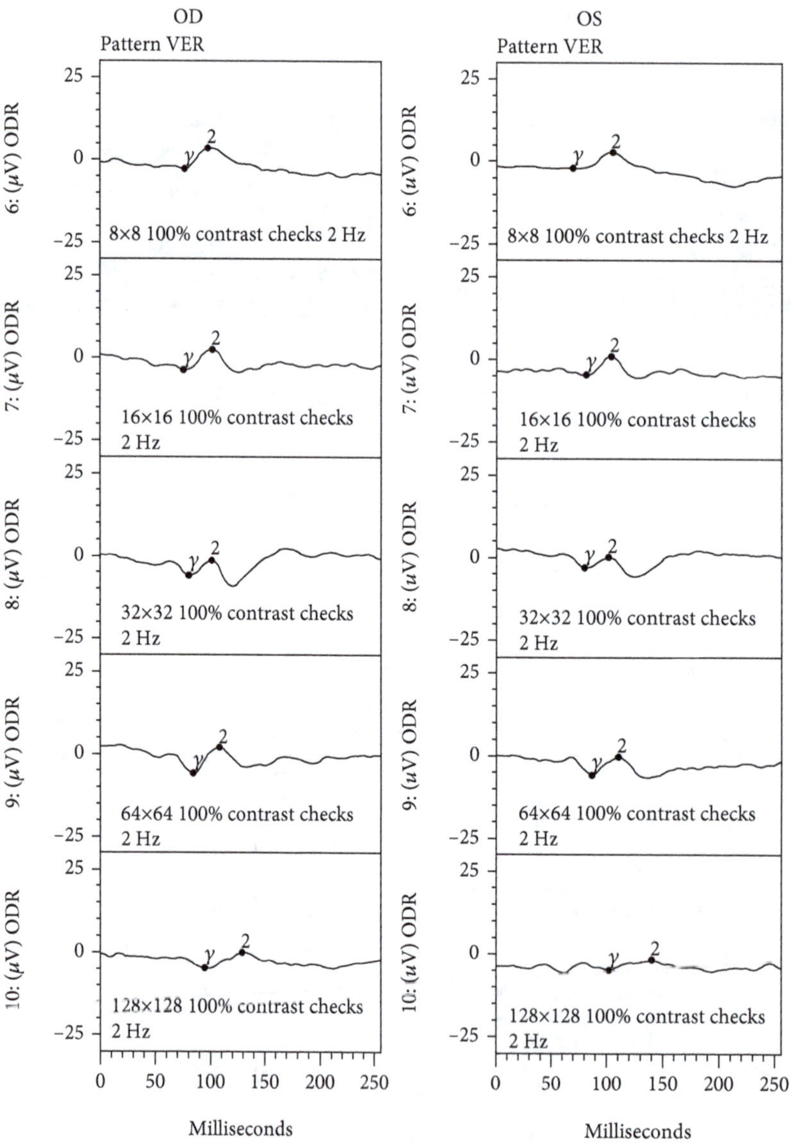

FIGURE 5: Visual evoked potential/response (VEP/VER) demonstrated mild suppression in the right and left eyes (OD and OS, respectively).

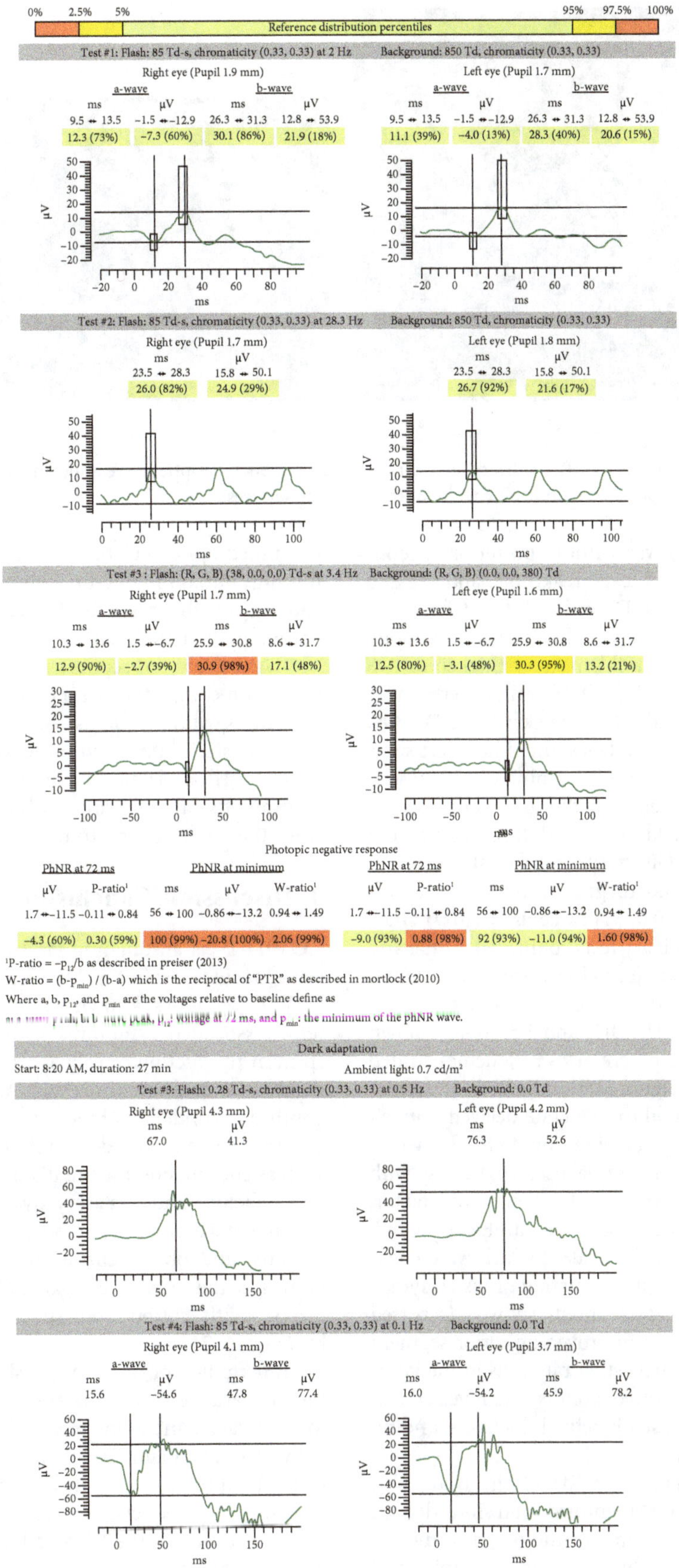

FIGURE 6: Handheld flash full field electroretinogram (ERG) showing mild to moderate delayed implicit time with reduced photopic negative response OU.

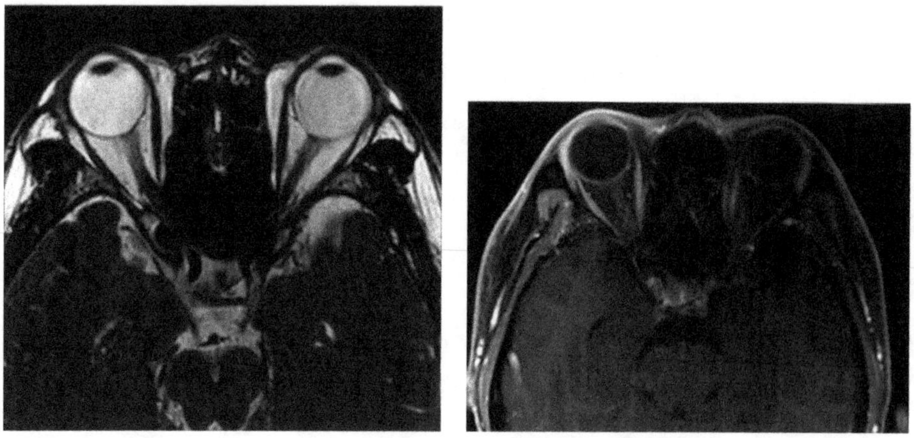

Figure 7: Magnetic resonance imaging (MRI) of head and orbits without evidence of optic nerve abnormality on (a) T2 image and without perineural enhancement of the optic nerve on (b) T1 with contrast and fat suppression.

Dilated fundus exam (DFE) was without posterior vitreous detachment (PVD) and retinal tear/break/hole, and the cup to disc (c/d) ratio was 0.6 OD and 0.7 OS (shown in Figures 1(a) and 1(b)). Optical coherence tomography (OCT) of the macula showed mild macular thickening OS (shown in Figures 2(a) and 2(b)). OCT retinal nerve fiber layer (RNFL) analysis showed RNFL thickening OD > OS. Fluorescein angiography (FA) studies showed no overt signs of retinal vascular leakage, but subtle staining of retinal vessels and subtle hyperfluorescence of the disc were present. The Octopus 30-2 visual field showed diffuse suppression OU (shown in Figure 3). Given the subtle inflammatory changes on clinical exam and diagnostic imaging, he was trialed on topical bromfenac 0.075% twice daily (BID) OU.

At a subsequent visit, ancillary tests confirmed retinal and optic nerve dysfunction including an electrooculogram (EOG) which showed suppression OD and borderline suppression OS with an Arden ratio of 1.41 (OD) and 1.85 (OS) (shown in Figure 4). Visual evoked potential (VEP) demonstrated mild suppression (shown in Figure 5). Handheld flash electroretinogram (ERG) showed mild to moderate delayed implicit time with reduced photopic negative response OU (shown in Figure 6). The patient underwent laboratory testing with ACE, HLA-B27, ANA, lysozyme, CRP, rheumatoid factor, HIV 1 and 2, ESR, syphilis Ab IgG, QuantiFERON Gold, mitogen, TB1 Ag, TB2 Ag, and CBC, all of which were negative for another cause of ocular inflammation or visual symptoms. Follow-up examination at one month showed decreased retinal thickness consistent with improved posterior segment inflammation but some mild persistent rare cells in the vitreous, and a final follow-up visit three months later revealed resolution of inflammatory cells, stable retinal thickness, and no change in the visual symptoms.

Magnetic resonance imaging (MRI) of the brain and orbits with and without contrast identified mild sinus disease and an incidental 1.6 cm by 1.7 cm arachnoid cyst in the left anterior temporal region. Orbits were unremarkable, and optic nerve was negative for perineural contrast enhancement (shown in Figure 7). The patient was also seen by a neuroophthalmologist who initially diagnosed the patient with presumed optic neuritis in the left eye despite negative MRI findings but, on follow-up, confirmed the diagnosis of visual snow given the absence of ocular inflammation and other pathology that could account for his symptoms.

The patient did report subjective improvement in symptoms with compliance with topical bromfenac and subjective worsening without the use of the topical bromfenac. Symptoms of "static" persisted on follow-up despite resolution of vitreous cells and a normal ophthalmologic exam. Symptoms continue to date of writing, which is more than ten months since the onset of symptoms.

3. Discussion/Conclusion

COVID-19 is an ongoing viral pandemic that is caused by severe acute respiratory syndrome coronavirus 2 (SARS-CoV-2) that is best known for its effect on the respiratory system. Associated symptoms include fever, cough, dyspnea, sputum production, myalgia, arthralgia, headache, diarrhea, rhinorrhea, and sore throat [1]. As clinicians and researchers continue to understand the virus, new clinical manifestations continue to be reported, including neurologic manifestations such as encephalitis, meningitis, acute cerebrovascular disease, and olfactory and gustatory dysfunction [1–5]. Ophthalmic findings have also been reported including anterior uveitis, retinitis, and optic neuritis in animals and hyperreflective lesions at the level of the ganglion cell and inner plexiform layers, subtle cotton wool spots, and microhemorrhages in humans [6, 7].

Emerging reports have also shown COVID-19 preceding the appearance of various autoimmune and autoinflammatory diseases, including pediatric inflammatory syndrome (PIMS) and Guillain-Barre syndrome [8, 9]. This raises questions about the nature of its link with autoimmune and autoinflammatory sequelae. Infectious diseases have long been considered one of the triggers for autoimmune and autoinflammatory diseases, mainly via molecular mimicry, and we hypothesize that an autoimmune response to the recent COVID-19 infection played a primary role in the development of the ocular inflammatory changes noted in our patient [10], specifically the mild vitritis, optic nerve leakage, and mild disc edema as manifested by an increase in the relative nerve fiber layer thickness as well as mild macular edema which manifested as an increase in macular thickness that reduced with treatment with the anti-inflammatory (NSAID) drop, bromfenac.

Posterior uveitis has been reported in patients following COVID-19 infection, and there are reports suggesting retinal inflammation as well. Bakhoum et al. stated that patients have subclinical inflammation in the vitreous detected with SD-OCT, and this is consistent with our findings [11]. There is also a report of intraretinal changes the authors associated with COVID-19 infection, specifically hyperreflective lesions at the level of ganglion cell and inner plexiform layers though subsequent correspondence by others related to the publication questions their origin and significance, raising the possibility of artifact or association with other systemic diseases like diabetes or hypertension [7]. Nonetheless, the report of retinal findings is consistent with our case suggesting posterior segment inflammation associated with prior infection with COVID-19. Of note, animal studies have shown evidence for retinitis and optic neuritis associated with COVID-19, also suggesting retinal involvement with systemic COVID-19 infection [6].

The ocular inflammation in our patient was subtle and difficult to detect—on first glance, the examination appeared normal, but careful inspection of the vitreous under dark-adapted conditions did reveal some cells. Additional data indicated posterior segment dysfunction including the abnormal ERG implicit times for both a- and b-waves, suppressed EOG amplitude, reduced VEP amplitude, generalized suppression of static visual field perimetry, and mild subtle leakage from the optic nerve and retinal vessels on fluorescein angiography. The patient did have a reduction of macular thickness on OCT studies after initiation of treatment with the topical nonsteroidal anti-inflammatory drop, bromfenac, but the visual snow symptoms persisted arguing that the posterior segment inflammation was not the cause of the visual snow symptoms. There is a case of posterior segment inflammation initially diagnosed as visual snow that ultimately was diagnosed as a case of uveitis, birdshot choroidopathy, with resolution of symptoms after treatment [12].

Visual snow has been reported to have a prevalence of 2.2% with symptoms commonly appearing during the late teenage years and early adulthood [13, 14]. The exact etiology has yet to be elucidated. There are strong associations with migraine and tinnitus, suggesting that they may share some common pathophysiologic mechanism with VS [1]. Others have suggested hypermetabolism of the right lingual gyrus, a thalamocortical dysrhythmia, or a feature of hallucinogenic persisting perception disorder [13, 15, 16]. It is a seemingly benign condition, but this condition can be debilitating for patients and may even be the first manifestation of a serious brain disease given a case report confirming Creutzfeldt-Jakob disease on postmortem examination in a patient who developed VS four years after the symptom onset [17]. Given our findings and the others reported above, underlying conditions must be tested before visual snow is made as the diagnosis.

It should be noted that the patient was treated with azithromycin and hydroxychloroquine for COVID-19 prior to presentation to ophthalmology. These medications are not benign and are known to have neurocognitive effects which, however, are less likely contributors to the patient's development of VS. Although clinical trials for azithromycin revealed no neurologic, audiometric, or ophthalmologic side effects [18] [Hopkins], azithromycin has been rarely shown to have cognitive side effects including delirium, disorientation, and impaired concentration typically present within a week of drug ingestion and resolution within three days [19] [Warstler]. Hydroxychloroquine is known to cause retinal toxicity with well-established characteristics and screening guidelines [20] [Marmor]. A recent literature review on hydroxychloroquine found neuropsychiatric effects to be very uncommon with reports of psychosis limited to several case reports [21] [Hamm].

In summary, we present a case of subtle posterior segment inflammation following COVID-19 infections with symptoms suggesting visual snow. Careful examination and ancillary testing confirmed the presence of retinal and optic nerve dysfunction. We propose that an autoimmune response was the culprit. Treatment with anti-inflammatory drops reduced symptoms. This has potential implications for the understanding and treatment of complications related to COVID-19.

Consent

The authors confirm that the patient has given his written informed consent to publish his case report (including publication of images).

Authors' Contributions

All authors attest that they meet the current ICMJE criteria for Authorship.

References

[1] J. R. Lechien, C. M. Chiesa-Estomba, D. R. De Siati et al., "Olfactory and gustatory dysfunctions as a clinical presentation of mild-to-moderate forms of the coronavirus disease (COVID-19): a multicenter European study," *European Archives of Oto-Rhino-Laryngology*, vol. 277, no. 8, pp. 2251–2261, 2020.

[2] I. H. Solomon, E. Normandin, S. Bhattacharyya et al., "Neuropathological features of COVID-19," *New England Journal of Medicine*, vol. 383, no. 10, pp. 989–992, 2020.

[3] A. Giacomelli, L. Pezzati, F. Conti et al., "Self-reported olfactory and taste disorders in Patients With Severe Acute Respiratory Coronavirus 2 Infection: a cross-sectional study," *Clinical Infectious Diseases*, vol. 71, no. 15, pp. 889-890, 2020.

[4] M. U. Ahmed, M. Hanif, M. J. Ali et al., "Neurological manifestations of COVID-19 (SARS-CoV-2): a review," *Frontiers in Neurology*, vol. 11, 2020.

[5] L. Wang, Y. Shen, M. Li et al., "Clinical manifestations and evidence of neurological involvement in 2019 novel coronavirus SARS-CoV-2: a systematic review and meta-analysis," *Journal of Neurology*, vol. 267, no. 10, pp. 2777–2789, 2020.

[6] P. M. Marinho, A. A. A. Marcos, A. C. Romano, and H. Nascimento, *Belfort R. Retinal findings in patients with COVID-19*, Elsevier Ltd., Lancet (London, England), 2020.

[7] I. Seah and R. Agrawal, "Can the coronavirus disease 2019 (COVID-19) affect the eyes? A review of coronaviruses and ocular implications in humans and animals," *Ocular immunology and inflammation*, vol. 28, no. 3, pp. 391–395, 2020.

[8] C. Galeotti and J. Bayry, "Autoimmune and inflammatory diseases following COVID-19," *Nature Reviews Rheumatology*, vol. 16, no. 8, pp. 413-414, 2020.

[9] G. Toscano, F. Palmerini, S. Ravaglia et al., "Guillain-Barré syndrome associated with SARS-CoV-2," *New England Journal of Medicine*, vol. 382, no. 26, pp. 2574–2576, 2020.

[10] R. S. Fujinami, M. G. von Herrath, U. Christen, and J. L. Whitton, "Molecular mimicry, bystander activation, or viral persistence: infections and autoimmune disease," *Clinical Microbiology Reviews*, vol. 19, no. 1, pp. 80–94, 2006.

[11] M. F. Bakhoum, M. Ritter, A. Garg, A. X. Chan, C. Y. Bakhoum, and D. Smith, *Subclinical ocular inflammation in persons recovered from ambulatory COVID-19*, MedRxiv, 2020, https://www.medrxiv.org/content/10.1101/2020.09.22.20128140v2.

[12] R. C. Patel, A. T. Vitale, D. J. Creel, and K. B. Digre, "Not all that flickers is snow," *Journal of Neuro-Ophthalmology*, vol. 41, no. 1, 2021.

[13] F. Puledda, C. Schankin, and P. J. Goadsby, *Visual snow syndrome: a clinical and phenotypical description of 1,100 cases*, Neurology, Lippincott Williams & Wilkins, 2020.

[14] D. Kondziella, M. H. Olsen, and J. P. Dreier, "Prevalence of visual snow syndrome in the UK," *European Journal of Neurology*, vol. 27, no. 5, pp. 764–772, 2020.

[15] C. J. Schankin, F. H. Maniyar, K. B. Digre, and P. J. Goadsby, *Visual snow–a disorder distinct from persistent migraine aura*, OUP Academic, Oxford University Press, 2014.

[16] A. I. Metzler and C. E. Robertson, "Visual Snow Syndrome: Proposed Criteria, Clinical Implications, and Pathophysiology," *Current Neurology and Neuroscience Reports*, vol. 18, no. 8, 2018.

[17] B. S. Chen, S. Lance, B. Lallu, and N. E. Anderson, "Visual snow: Not so benign," *Journal of Clinical Neuroscience*, vol. 64, pp. 37–39, 2019.

[18] S. Hopkins, "Clinical toleration and safety of azithromycin," *The American Journal of Medicine*, vol. 91, no. 3, pp. S40–S45, 1991.

[19] A. Warstler and J. Bean, "Antimicrobial-induced cognitive side effects," *Mental Health Clinician*, vol. 6, no. 4, pp. 207–214, 2016.

[20] M. F. Marmor, U. Kellner, T. Y. Lai, and R. B. Melles, "Recommendations on screening for chloroquine and hydroxychloroquine retinopathy (2016 revision)," *Ophthalmology*, vol. 123, no. 6, pp. 1386–1394, 2016.

[21] B. S. Hamm and L. J. Rosenthal, "Psychiatric aspects of chloroquine and hydroxychloroquine treatment in the wake of coronavirus disease-2019: psychopharmacological interactions and neuropsychiatric sequelae," *Psychosomatics*, vol. 61, no. 6, pp. 597–606, 2020.

Choroidal Vascular Changes in Acute Idiopathic Maculopathy as Demonstrated by Multimodal Imaging including Optical Coherence Tomography Angiography

Tahsin Khundkar,[1] **Syed R. Hasan**,[2] **Mark P. Breazzano**,[3] **Constance Mei**,[4] **and Brandon B. Johnson**[5]

[1]*Department of Ophthalmology, University of Minnesota, 516 Delaware Street SE, Minneapolis, MN 55455, USA*
[2]*AdvantageCare Physicians, 180-05 Hillside Avenue, Queens, NY 11432, USA*
[3]*Department of Ophthalmology, Johns Hopkins University School of Medicine, 87 Thomas Johnson Drive, Frederick, MD 21702, USA*
[4]*Department of Ophthalmology, New York Medical College-Jamaica Hospital Medical Center, 134-20 Jamaica Avenue, Richmond Hills, NY 11418, USA*
[5]*New York Retina Center, 161 E 32nd St, New York, NY 10016, USA*

Correspondence should be addressed to Tahsin Khundkar; tkhundkar9@gmail.com

Academic Editor: Maurizio Battaglia Parodi

Purpose. To present a case of acute idiopathic maculopathy (AIM) and illustrate primary choroidal perfusion defect using multimodal imaging. *Case Description.* We report a case of a 24-year-old man with a paracentral scotoma of the right eye and recent flu-like illness. The patient was found to have a unilateral ovoid-shaped, placoid lesion just inferior to the fovea. Multimodal imaging confirmed findings most consistent with a diagnosis of acute idiopathic maculopathy (AIM). Serologic studies confirmed a strongly positive immunoglobulin G (IgG) titer for coxsackievirus A. Spectral domain optical coherence tomography angiography (SD-OCTA) showed bilateral areas of vascular reduction at the level of the choriocapillaris and choroid, sparing the retinal circulation. *Conclusions and Importance.* The changes in outer retina and retinal pigment epithelium, classically described in AIM, are likely secondary to choroidal hypoperfusion.

1. Introduction

Acute idiopathic maculopathy (AIM) is a rare, inflammatory disorder classically thought to involve the retinal pigment epithelium (RPE) and outer retina [1]. AIM was initially described by Yannuzzi et al. [1] in a group of healthy, young adults who experienced sudden, unilateral loss of central vision following a flu-like illness with neurosensory retinal detachment and focal, yellow-white thickening at the level of the RPE. The clinical spectrum of the condition was later expanded to include bilateral disease [2]. Coxsackievirus seropositivity on laboratory testing has been described in association with AIM [2, 3]. Most patients experience spontaneous recovery over several weeks to months; however, the use of systemic steroids may hasten recovery [1, 4]. We describe a case of AIM with bilateral, asymmetric findings using multimodal imaging.

2. Case Presentation

A 24-year-old, healthy, Caucasian man presented with a "blurred spot" in the vision of his right eye for two days. There were no other ocular complaints. The patient endorsed a recent flu-like episode 12 weeks prior to presentation.

On examination, best-corrected visual acuity was 20/20 in each eye. No relative afferent pupillary defect was observed. Amsler grid testing revealed a superior wedge-shaped paracentral scotoma in the right eye. The anterior segment examination and intraocular pressure were normal in both eyes. No cells in the vitreous were observed. Fundus

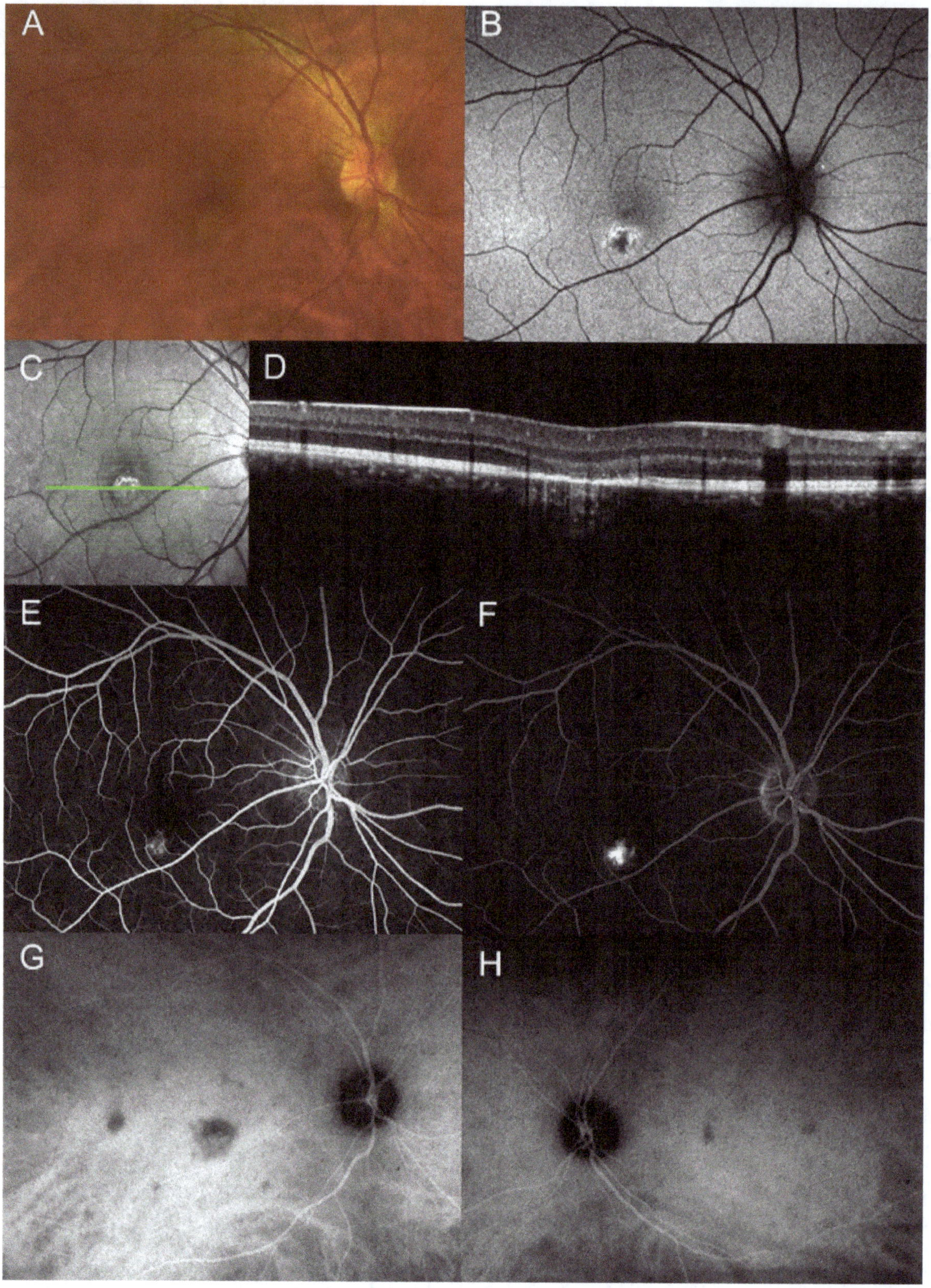

(a)

FIGURE 1: Continued.

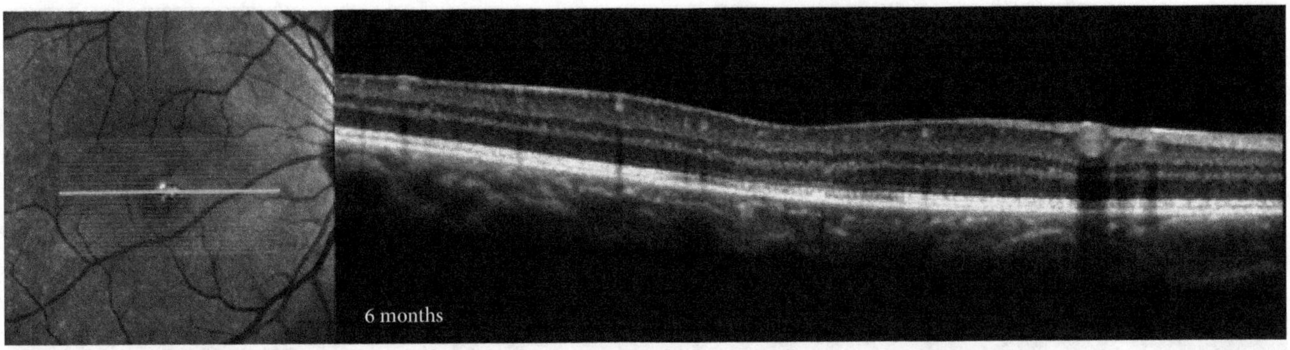

(b)

Figure 1: Wide-field fundus photography of the right eye (A) shows an ovoid, hypopigmented placoid lesion adjacent to the fovea. FAF (B) reveals corresponding hypoautofluorescence and surrounding areas of hyperautofluorescence with irregular borders. Near-infrared reflectance (C) and spectral-domain optical coherence tomography (D) reveal speckled hyperreflectivity within the lesion and significant disruption of the outer retina, including the outer nuclear layer, ellipsoid zone, and retinal pigmented epithelium with choroidal hypertransmission. Early hyperfluorescence with FA (E) precedes increased hyperfluorescence of the macular lesion with discrete borders upon recirculation phase (F). Late-phase indocyanine green angiography shows multiple areas of hypocianescence in the right (G) greater than the left eye (H), including the area corresponding to the lesion. (b) Spectral-domain optical coherence tomography at 6 months after initial presentation shows improved attenuation in the outer plexiform layer.

examination revealed an ovoid-shaped, tan, hypopigmented lesion just inferior to the fovea in the right eye (Figure 1).

Fundus autofluorescence (FAF) showed a corresponding wedge-shaped area of hypoautofluorescence surrounded by a margin of hyperautofluorescence. Near-infrared reflectance (NIR) showed a stippled hyperreflective lesion with a hyporeflective border. Corresponding cross-sectional imaging with spectral-domain optical coherence tomography (SD-OCT) revealed choroidal hypertransmission and outer retinal attenuation from the outer plexiform layer to the retinal pigment epithelium. Fluorescein angiography (FA) of the right eye demonstrated a hyperfluorescent macular lesion and increasing hyperfluorescence mostly within the margins upon recirculation. Late-phase indocyanine green angiography (ICG) showed multiple areas of hypocianescence corresponding to choroidal nonperfusion—worse on the right, but present in both eyes (Figure 1).

SD-OCTA of the right eye was obtained one month after the initial presentation and demonstrated normal-appearing retinal circulation, including deep capillary plexus (DCP). Notably, there was a vascular perfusion defect at the level of the choriocapillaris and choroid in the area corresponding to the lesion (Figure 2). Similar involvement of the choriocapillaris with sparing of the DCP was also seen on SD-OCTA slabs of the left eye, corresponding to areas of hypocianescence seen on late-phase ICG.

The patient was found to have strongly positive IgG titers for coxsackievirus A7 (1:800), A9 (1:1600), A64 (1:1600), and A24 (1:1600). Respective IgM titers were negative. An extensive laboratory workup was otherwise normal. An oral prednisone (1 mg/kg) taper was initiated, and the patient was monitored closely. Six months after initial presentation, patient's subjective complaints of a scotoma had resolved and SD-OCTA revealed improved perfusion of the choriocapillaris and choroid and OCT showed improvement in the attenuation of the ellipsoid zone (Figures 1(b) and 2).

3. Discussion

Acute idiopathic maculopathy is a rare, self-limited, macular disease disproportionately affecting young men [1]. It has been postulated that AIM exists on a spectrum of acute multifocal placoid pigment epitheliopathy (APMPPE) [5] and our case illustrates this point. The lesions in APMPPE clinically appear yellow-white and may have a complex outer boundary due to confluence of smaller lesions. In contrast, the lesion in our case is solitary with an ovoid shape and smooth border. Despite the lack of classically described subretinal fluid or neurosensory detachment, the angiographic and autofluorescence findings were consistent with previously reported cases of AIM [2, 3]. In this report, early arteriovenous phase FA showed hyperfluorescence of the lesion and a staining pattern in the late recirculation phase. This is in contrast to APMPPE in the acute stage, which reveals an intense, homogeneous hypofluorescence at the site of the placoid lesions. The FAF in this case was similar to findings in APMPPE and demonstrated a mixed pattern of hyperautofluorescence corresponding to deposition of lipofuscin from RPE cell thickening or duplication and hypoautofluorescence from RPE cell loss [6].

This case further supports the growing speculation that the pathogenesis of AIM is primarily a choroiditis with the changes to overlying RPE and outer retina occurring secondarily to choroidal ischemia [7–9]. The multiple, bilateral areas of choroidal hypoperfusion, as demonstrated by moth-eaten areas of hypocianescence on ICG, also point to a primary choroidal insult. More impressively, SD-OCTA shows hypoperfusion in the choroid and choriocapillaris of both eyes, without involvement of the DCP in the subacute phase—similar to findings in APMPPE [10, 11]. Lee et al. also concluded a primarily choroidal insult in acute macular neuroretinopathy by studying OCTA findings but noted that choriocapillaris flow loss persisted [12]. After 6 months of follow-up, we observed a partial return of choroidal perfusion voids, with

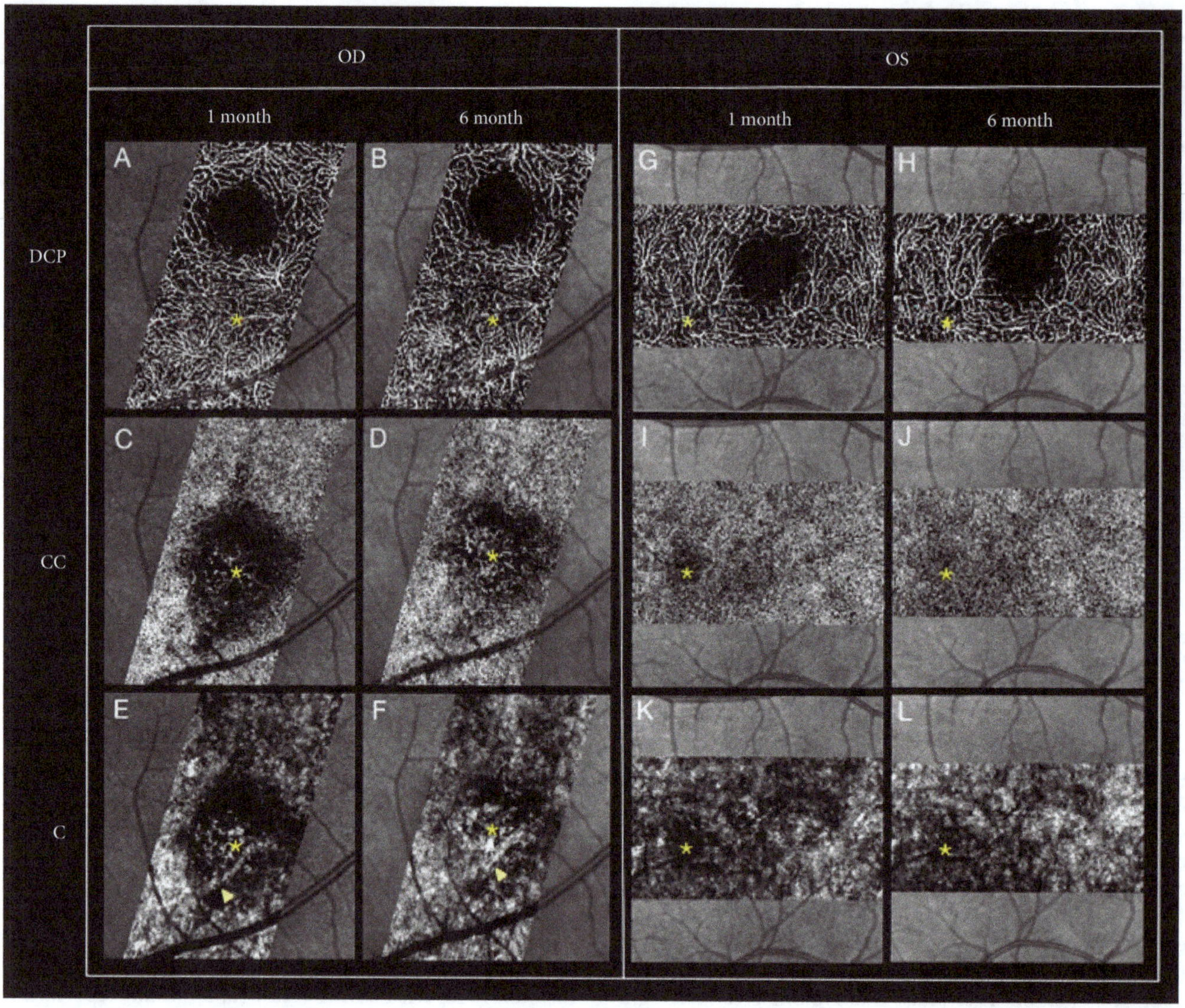

FIGURE 2: Spectral domain-optical coherence tomography angiography findings at various levels during the 1-month and 6-month follow-up. An asterisk marks the center of the lesion. Normal perfusion is seen in the deep capillary plexus (DCP) of the right eye at 1 month (A) and at 6-month (B) follow-up, as well as in the left eye at 1 month (G) and 6 months (H). Perfusion deficit of the right eye is noted at the area of the lesion in the choriocapillaris (C) and choroid (E), with choroidal vascular dilatation (arrowhead). Similar areas of choriocapillaris (I) and choroidal (K) hypoperfusion is seen in the fellow eye. Improved perfusion is noted at 6-month follow-up in both eyes (D, F, J, L), with persistent choroidal vascular dilatation in the right eye (F, arrowhead).

concomitant resolution of visual symptoms. Hashimoto et al. demonstrated a similar change in choroidal perfusion with recovery in cases of AIM [8] as well as APMPPE [11], further suggesting an overlap between these diseases.

The relatively good visual recovery and reconstruction of the outer retinal layers in this case suggest that the disease process is reversible in AIM. Jung and colleagues hold that the preservation of the external limiting membrane may indicate that the inner retina, cell nuclei, and cellular structures necessary for outer segment regeneration remain intact [13]. Furthermore, restoration of the RPE pump function likely occurs following resolution of the acute inner choroidal inflammatory process.

Multiple reports have documented positive coxsackievirus serologies in association with AIM [2, 3]. In our case, the patient endorsed a viral prodrome prior to visual symptoms and was found to have strongly positive IgG titers for coxsackievirus A7, A9, A64, and A24. Whether due to direct viremia or by an aberrant response due to molecular mimicry in the setting of viral infection, the exact mechanism by which coxsackievirus causes tissue insult remains unclear.

Limitations of any case report include overinterpretation and an inability to imply a cause-effect relationship. In this report, the interval from viral illness and onset of eye symptoms was 12 weeks—a longer lag time than is usually seen. The positive coxsackie IgG titers are only suggestive of an association but not definitive. Lastly, the OCTA images were obtained one month after the onset of symptoms, allowing time for vascular reorganization.

4. Conclusion

We present a case of AIM and use multimodal imaging including OCTA as well as serologic testing to make the challenging diagnosis. Our findings suggest that the pathogenesis of AIM involves a primary insult to the inner choroid with secondary RPE and outer retinal damage, similar to the mechanism suggested in APMPPE [7–9, 11].

Consent

Consent was given by patient to use anonymized clinical details and photographs.

Disclosure

All authors attest that they meet the current ICMJE criteria for authorship.

References

[1] L. A. Yannuzzi, L. M. Jampol, M. F. Rabb, J. A. Sorenson, C. Beyrer, and L. M. Wilcox Jr., "Unilateral acute idiopathic maculopathy," *Archives of Ophthalmology*, vol. 109, no. 10, pp. 1411–1416, 1991.

[2] K. B. Freund, L. A. Yannuzzi, G. R. Barile, R. F. Spaide, S. A. Milewski, and D. R. Guyer, "The expanding clinical spectrum of unilateral acute idiopathic maculopathy," *Archives of Ophthalmology*, vol. 114, no. 5, pp. 555–559, 1996.

[3] A. P. Beck, L. M. Jampol, D. A. Glasser, and J. S. Pollack, "Is coxsackievirus the cause of unilateral acute idiopathic maculopathy?," *Archives of Ophthalmology*, vol. 122, no. 1, pp. 121–123, 2004.

[4] M. A. Fuente and R. Cuadrado, "Unilateral acute idiopathic maculopathy: angiography, optical coherence tomography and microperimetry findings," *Journal of Ophthalmic Inflammation and Infection*, vol. 1, no. 3, pp. 125–127, 2011.

[5] A. L. Li, N. V. Palejwala, J. G. Shantha et al., "Long-term multimodal imaging in acute posterior multifocal placoid pigment epitheliopathy and association with coxsackievirus exposure," *PLoS One*, vol. 15, no. 8, article e0238080, 2020.

[6] R. Spaide, "Autofluorescence imaging of acute posterior multifocal placoid pigment epitheliopathy," *Retina*, vol. 26, no. 4, pp. 479–482, 2006.

[7] H. Haruta, M. Sawa, Y. Saishin, N. Ohguro, and Y. Tano, "Clinical findings in unilateral acute idiopathic maculopathy," *International Ophthalmology*, vol. 30, no. 2, pp. 199–202, 2010.

[8] Y. Hashimoto, W. Salito, M. Salito et al., "Increased choroidal blood flow velocity with regression of unilateral acute idiopathic maculopathy," *Japanese Journal of Ophthalmology*, vol. 59, no. 4, pp. 252–260, 2015.

[9] M. Srour, G. Querques, O. Rostaqui, and E. Souied, "Early spectral-domain optical coherence tomography findings in unilateral acute idiopathic maculopathy," *Retina*, vol. 33, no. 10, pp. 2182–2184, 2013.

[10] T. R. Burke, C. J. Chu, S. Salvatore et al., "Application of OCT-angiography to characterise the evolution of chorioretinal lesions in acute posterior multifocal placoid pigment epitheliopathy," *Eye*, vol. 31, no. 10, pp. 1399–1408, 2017.

[11] K. Hirooka, W. Saito, M. Saito et al., "Increased choroidal blood flow velocity with regression of acute posterior multifocal placoid pigment epitheliopathy," *Japanese Journal of Ophthalmology*, vol. 60, no. 3, pp. 172–178, 2016.

[12] S. Y. Lee, J. L. Cheng, K. M. Gehrs et al., "Choroidal features of acute macular neuroretinopathy via optical coherence tomography angiography and correlation with serial multimodal imaging," *JAMA Ophthalmology*, vol. 135, no. 11, pp. 1177–1183, 2017.

[13] C. S. Jung, J. F. Payne, C. S. Bergstrom et al., "Multimodality diagnostic imaging in unilateral acute idiopathic maculopathy," *Archives of Ophthalmology*, vol. 130, no. 1, pp. 50–56, 2012.

36

Multimodal Imaging of Waldenstrom Macroglobulinemia-Associated Hyperviscosity-Related Retinopathy Treated with Plasmapheresis

Michael J. Schatz, Carl S. Wilkins, Oscar Otero-Marquez, Toco Y. P. Chui, Richard B. Rosen, and Meenakashi Gupta

The New York Eye and Ear Infirmary, 310 East 14th Street, New York, NY 10003, USA

Correspondence should be addressed to Michael J. Schatz; mschatz@nyee.edu

Academic Editor: Stephen G. Schwartz

While plasmapheresis is well known to significantly improve both retinal findings and systemic manifestations associated with Waldenstrom macroglobulinemia, few reports exist documenting changes in optical coherence tomography angiography (OCT-A). The authors present a case of a patient with Waldenstrom macroglobulinemia who had resolution of white-centered peripheral retinal lesions and parafoveal outer nuclear layer hyperreflective material following plasmapheresis. Applying image analysis software to before and after OCT-A images, the authors were able to show an objective decrease in retinal capillary and large vessel density following plasmapheresis. This technique can be used to guide treatment and surveillance for patients with hyperviscosity-related retinopathy.

1. Introduction

Waldenstrom macroglobulinemia is a lymphoplasmacytic lymphoma, with an incidence of 2-5 cases per million person years [1], median age of diagnosis of approximately 69 years old, and a male-to-female ratio of approximately 2 : 1 [2]. It results in unregulated production of IgM which increases the viscosity of the blood. Hyperviscosity is thought to cause autoregulatory venous dilation, subsequent venous stasis, and a rise in intravascular pressure [3]. The resultant retinal hypoxia of the vascular endothelial cells leads to vascular tortuosity, retinal hemorrhage, exudates, and retinal vein occlusion. Previous studies have shown that as serum viscosity and serum IgM levels rise, both peripheral hemorrhages and venous dilation increases [3]. Though treating hyperviscosity improves the clinical appearance of the retina, some patients ultimately suffer from decreased vision due to ischemic maculopathy. OCT-A can aid in the noninvasive evaluation of retinal perfusion deficits and potentially guide treatment courses by monitoring microvascular integrity.

2. Case Report

A 55-year-old man with an ocular history of posterior vitreous detachment, lattice degeneration with atrophic hole, and glaucoma suspect was referred for evaluation of retinal vascular tortuosity. Several months later, the patient was diagnosed by his oncologist with Waldenstrom macroglobulinemia. Upon reexamination, new vitreous hemorrhage, white-centered peripheral lesions, and increasing vascular tortuosity were noticed (Figures 1(a) and 1(b)). Fluorescein angiography from this time is shown in Figure 2. The patient also started to notice "waviness," episodic dizziness, and headaches. His oncologist started one round of intravenous immunoglobulin, followed by three rounds of plasmapheresis.

Pre- and one week posttreatment OCT-A scans nasal to the fovea were obtained with a commercial spectral domain OCT system (Avanti RTVue-XR; Optovue, Fremont, CA). The full retinal vascular layer OCT-A located between the inner limiting membrane and 9 μm below the posterior

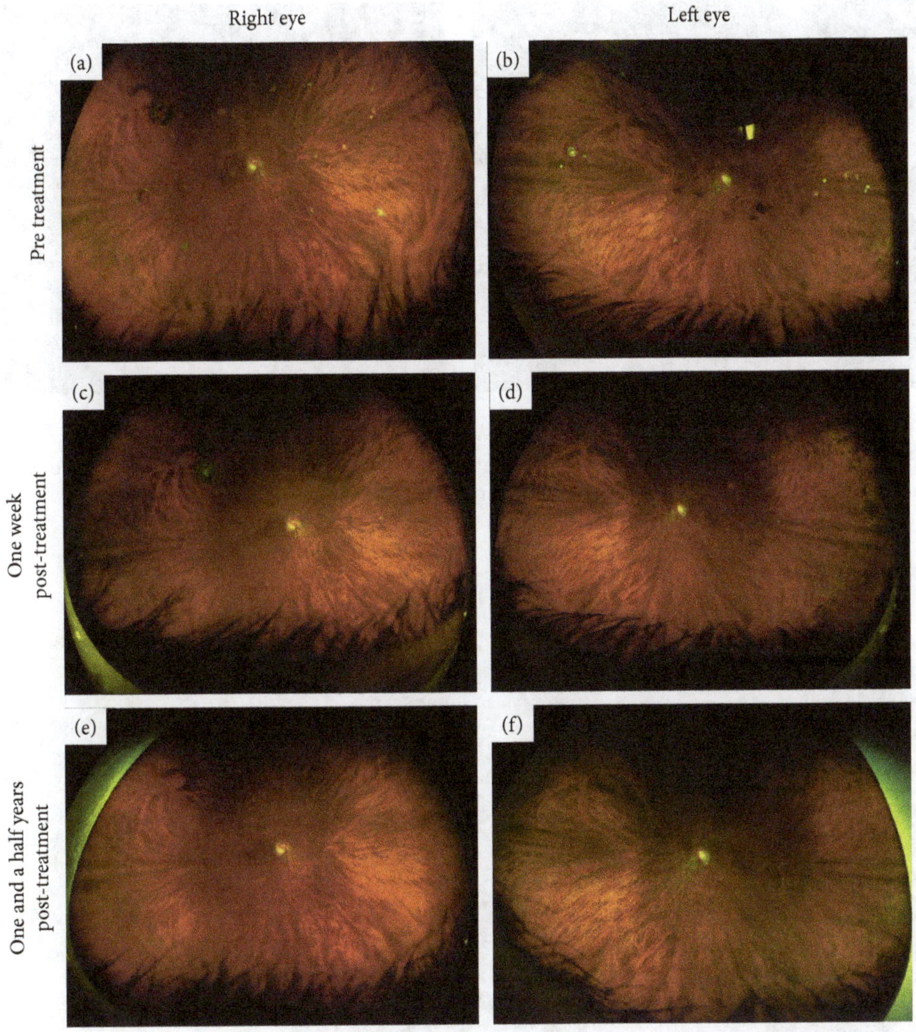

FIGURE 1: Fundus photos of right and left eyes. (a, b) Three days before beginning plasmapheresis. Prominent vascular tortuosity and white centered peripheral lesions. Faint sclerotic vessels with box-carring-like changes apparent in the far nasal and temporal periphery of both eyes, possibly the result of pseudovasoocclusive events in the setting of venous stasis. (c, d) One week after finishing the third round of plasmapheresis. Dramatic improvement in the white-centered peripheral lesions is apparent. There is also a reduction in the box-carring-like changes in the periphery. (e, f) One and a half years later, there is sustained resolution of the white-centered peripheral lesions, but still some vascular tortuosity.

boundary of the outer plexiform layer (Figures 3(b) and 3(e)) was used to measure the capillary and large vessel density. First, image registration was performed using ImageJ [4].

Segmentation of capillaries was performed after removal of the large blood vessels using local thresholding (MATLAB 2018b; MathWorks, Natick, MA) [5]. Next, computation of capillary and large vessel densities was performed. A color-coded density map was created for a rapid qualitative assessment (Figures 3(c) and 3(f)). After treatment, capillary density decreased from 47.62% to 45.35%, and large vessel density decreased from 18.87% to 10.16%. Pre- and post-treatment en face OCT (Figures 3(a) and 3(d)) and spectral domain OCT (Figures 4(a) and 4(b)) over the white-centered peripheral lesions showed significant resolution of the parafoveal outer nuclear layer hyperreflective material.

Following plasmapheresis, the patient noticed improvements in metamorphopsia, headaches, and dizzy spells. Visual acuity improved from 20/25 OU to 20/20 OU. The patient was started on five months of rituximab and bendamustine. The resolution of his white-centered peripheral lesions was sustained nearly one and a half years later (Figures 1(e) and 1(f)).

3. Discussion

We present a case of a patient with hyperviscosity-related retinopathy secondary to Waldenstrom macroglobulinemia that had dramatic improvement in both ocular and systemic symptoms following plasmapheresis. Plasmapheresis has been known for more than a decade to significantly reduce serum viscosity and hyperviscosity-related retinopathy. A

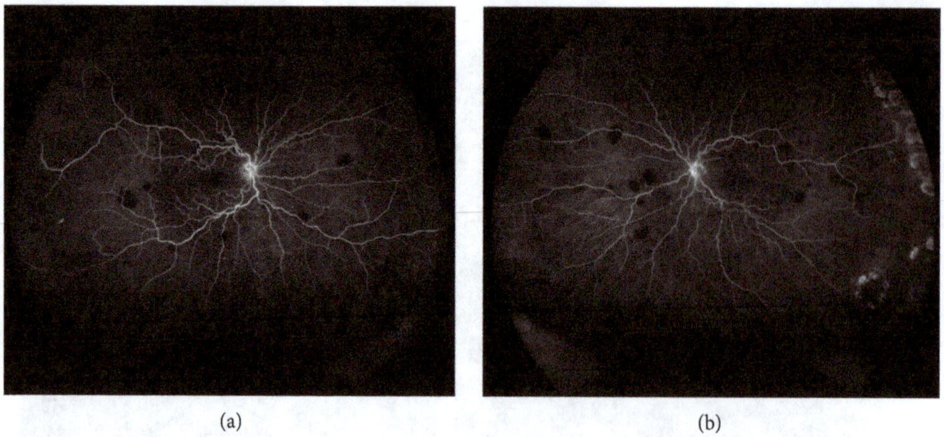

FIGURE 2: Fluorescein angiography of right (a) and left (b) eyes, three days before beginning plasmapheresis. Blockage is noted in areas of peripheral white-centered lesions. Capillary drop-out as well as peripheral staining are also apparent.

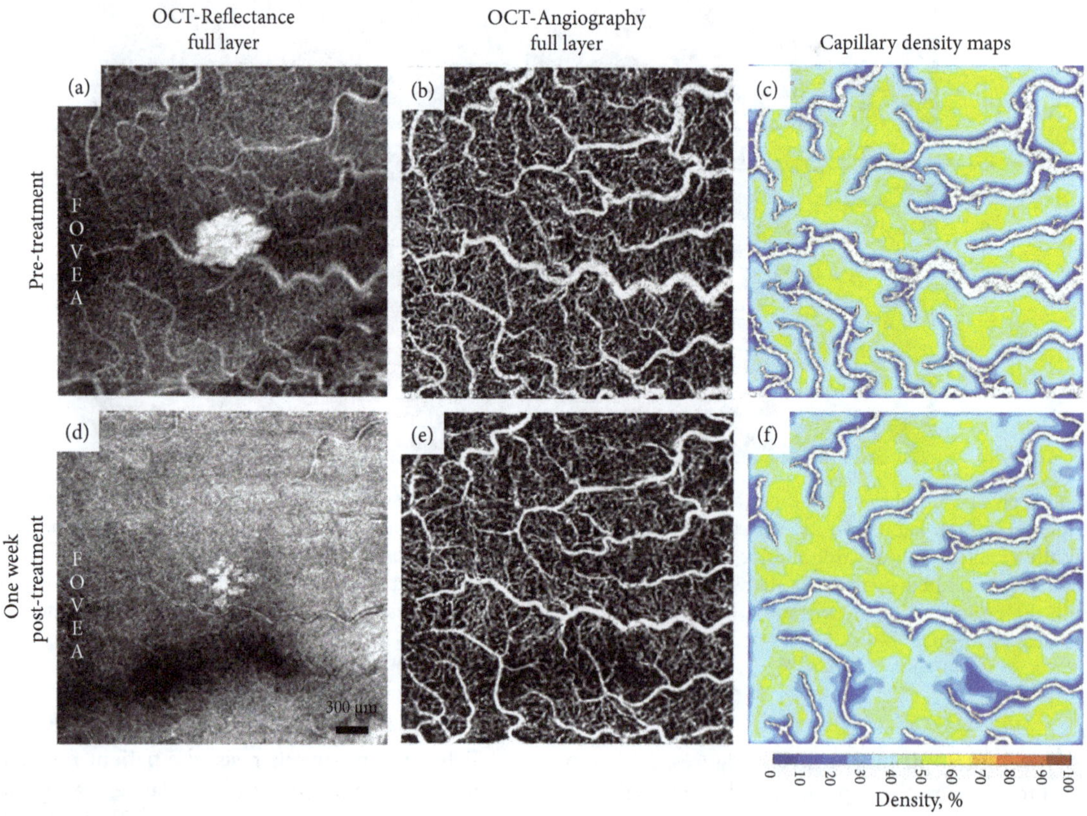

FIGURE 3: OCT angiography of the right retina, nasal to the fovea, before and one week after finishing plasmapheresis. (a, d) OCT reflectance full layer before (a) and after (d) plasmapheresis. One week after treatment, there was a significant decrease in the hyperreflective lesion nasal to the fovea. (b, e) Full vascular OCT-A layer before (b) and after (e) plasmapheresis. Qualitatively, there is a noticeable decrease in vessel diameter. (c, f) Capillary density maps before (c) and after (f) plasmapheresis. Capillaries are color-coded; large vessels are excluded and shown in white. After treatment, capillary density decreased from 47.62% to 45.35% and large vessel density decreased from 18.87% to 10.16%.

2008 case series of nine patients showed that plasmapheresis decreases the retinal venous diameter by an average of 15.3%, with those having the greatest reduction in serum viscosity showing the greatest reduction in retinal venous diameter [6]. One prior report of multimodal imaging in Waldenstrom macroglobulinemia-associated retinopathy demonstrated thickened choroid and shed retinal photoreceptors within serous retinal detachments and also showed a reduction in subretinal fluid and remaining outer retinal atrophy following local treatment with intravitreal bevacizumab [7].

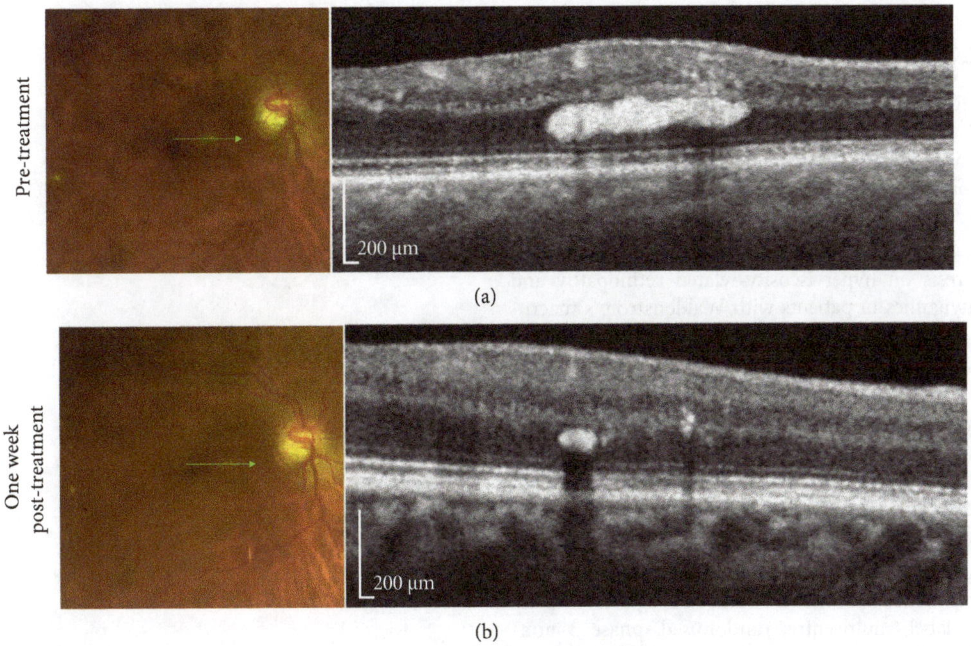

FIGURE 4: Color fundus photos and spectral domain OCT over white-centered peripheral lesions over the right nasal fovea three days before (a) and one week after (b) plasmapheresis show significant resolution of the outer nuclear layer hyperreflective material.

Our patient did not have any associated serous detachment; however, serial imaging demonstrated a reduction in the average capillary diameter within the superficial plexus as well as a decrease in capillary and large vessel density following plasmapheresis. The decrease in vessel diameter is explained by the reduction in serum viscosity and hence a reduction in the venous stasis. A cause for the decrease in capillary and large vessel density, however, is less obvious. One possible explanation is that the hypoxia and pseudoocclusive events induced by the hyperviscosity led to the permanent destruction of capillary and large retinal vessels. Another explanation is that the reduction in capillary and large vessel density is artifactual, reflecting the decrease in vessel diameter more than a true decrease in the number of vessels. Even in the latter instance, the algorithm used in this report is still significant as it serves as an objective, proxy measurement for vessel diameter, which normally has only been compared qualitatively.

Long-term therapy traditionally consisted of R-CHOP (rituximab, cyclophosphamide, doxorubicin, vincristine, and prednisone) therapy, though recent studies show increased progression-free survival with bendamustine plus rituximab [8], which is what our patient received. The exact length of sustained improvement of hyperviscosity-related retinopathy following plasmapheresis, with or without adjuvant chemotherapy, as well as the frequency of intermittent therapy remains unknown. There is no standard of care established regarding how to monitor patients with hyperviscosity-related retinopathy undergoing treatment. OCT-A is a more sensitive modality to detect vascular integrity which may otherwise be missed with conventional imaging. We propose applying algorithms to OCT-A images to objectively measure the retinal vessel diameter and density to guide treatment duration and monitor for recurrence in patients with hyperviscosity-related retinopathy.

Disclosure

The content is solely the responsibility of the authors and does not necessarily represent the official views of the National Institutes of Health.

Acknowledgments

This study was supported by the National Eye Institute of the National Institutes of Health (award number R01EY027301). Additional funding for this research was provided by the New York Eye and Ear Infirmary Foundation Grant, the Marrus Family Foundation, the Challenge Grant award from Research to Prevent Blindness, and the Jorge N. Buxton Microsurgical Foundation.

References

[1] L. J. Herrinton and N. S. Weiss, "Incidence of Waldenstrom's macroglobulinemia," *Blood*, vol. 82, no. 10, pp. 3148–3150, 1993.

[2] R. García-Sanz, S. Montoto, A. Torrequebrada et al., "Waldenström macroglobulinaemia: presenting features and outcome in a series with 217 cases," *British Journal of Haematology*, vol. 115, no. 3, pp. 575–582, 2001.

[3] M. N. Menke, "Hyperviscosity-related retinopathy in Waldenström macroglobulinemia," *Archives of Ophthalmology*, vol. 124, no. 11, p. 1601, 2006.

[4] C. T. Rueden, J. Schindelin, M. C. Hiner et al., "ImageJ2: ImageJ for the next generation of scientific image data," *BMC Bioinformatics*, vol. 18, no. 1, 2017.

[5] J. S. Andrade Romo, R. E. Linderman, A. Pinhas, J. Carroll, R. B. Rosen, and T. Y. P. Chui, "Novel development of parafoveal capillary density deviation mapping using an age-group and eccentricity matched normative OCT angiography database," *Science and Technology*, vol. 8, no. 3, p. 1, 2019.

[6] M. N. Menke, G. T. Feke, J. W. McMeel, and S. P. Treon, "Effect of plasmapheresis on hyperviscosity-related retinopathy and retinal hemodynamics in patients with Waldenström's macroglobulinemia," *Investigative Ophthalmology & Visual Science*, vol. 49, no. 3, p. 1157, 2008.

[7] L. T. Xu, R. J. Courtney, and J. P. Ehlers, "Bevacizumab therapy and multimodal ultrawide-field imaging in immunogammopathy maculopathy secondary to Waldenström's macroglobulinemia," *Ophthalmic Surgery, Lasers & Imaging Retina*, vol. 46, no. 2, pp. 262–265, 2015.

[8] M. J. Rummel, N. Niederle, G. Maschmeyer et al., "Bendamustine plus rituximab versus CHOP plus rituximab as first-line treatment for patients with indolent and mantle-cell lymphomas: an open-label, multicentre, randomised, phase 3 non-inferiority trial," *The Lancet*, vol. 381, no. 9873, pp. 1203–1210, 2013.

37

Vitreous Hemorrhage following High-Altitude Retinopathy

Arjun Shrestha,[1] **Rinkal Suwal**,[1] **and Biju Shrestha**[2]

[1]*BP Eye Foundation, Hospital for Children, Eye, ENT & Rehabilitation Services, Bhaktapur, Nepal*
[2]*Department of Physiology, Kathmandu Medical College, Kathmandu, Nepal*

Correspondence should be addressed to Arjun Shrestha; arjundr@gmail.com

Academic Editor: Kevin J. Blinder

Purpose. To report a case of high-altitude retinopathy with vitreous hemorrhage. *Methods.* An apparently healthy 29-year-old boy presented with a history of floater and slight diminution of vision in the left eye after climbing the mountain 4760 meters high. *Results.* The visual acuity at presentation was 20/20 in the right eye and 20/30 in the left eye. Anterior segment findings of both eyes were unremarkable. Fundus evaluation revealed bilaterally dilated major retinal veins. The right eye revealed clear, quiet vitreous, healthy macula, and pink and smooth optic disc. There was fresh vitreous hemorrhage confined just one disc diameter away at the superior and inferior part of the optic nerve in the left eye. The macula and optic nerve head of this eye grossly looked normal. Complete blood count, haemoglobin, ESR, CRP, sugar, renal function test, lipid panel, and serology for HIV, HCV, VDRL, and HBsAg were normal. The Mantoux test and chest X-ray also revealed normal findings. Physician consultation did not reveal other abnormalities. On the 3rd week of follow-up, his vision was 20/20 in both eyes. Fundus examination revealed clear vitreous in both eyes though some venous dilation and tortuosities were still evident in the left eye. A macular OCT scan showed almost normal-appearing fundus. *Conclusions.* Vitreous hemorrhage following climbing high altitude can be one of the manifestations of high-altitude retinopathy.

1. Introduction

High-altitude retinopathy (HAR) is a manifestation of high-altitude sickness, with other presentations like high-altitude pulmonary edema, high-altitude cerebral edema, and acute mountain sickness. HAR constitutes numerous retinal vascular decompensations related to hypoxia, with developing sudden onset symptoms like headache, nausea, anorexia, insomnia, and fatigue. The acute ocular manifestations are mainly retinal hemorrhages, peripapillary hyperemia, and dilated vessels, which mostly occur in individuals with mountain climbers who are exposed to high altitude above 3,000 meters (m) [1].

Intra- and preretinal hemorrhages are generally seen at the peripheral retina. Macular and vitreous hemorrhage, papilledema, and cotton wool spots can also occur in severe cases. According to severity, Weidman and Tabin [2] have classified HAR in four different grades: grade one—dilated retinal veins with hemorrhages within one disc area, grade two—moderate dilated retinal veins with hemorrhages in 2 disc areas, grade three—advanced dilated retinal veins with hemorrhages in 3 disc areas and paramacular and vitreous hemorrhage, and grade four—engorged retinal veins with hemorrhages greater than three-disc areas, macular and vitreous hemorrhage, or papilledema.

At high altitudes, due to inadequate oxygen levels, the body's metabolic state demands a sequence of physiological changes, which consequently increases cardiac output and then pulmonary ventilation. HAR was first described by Singh et al. [3] in 1969, where they outlined the ocular deformities in 24 soldiers, accounted with high-altitude illness. They reported three cases with vitreous hemorrhage and four cases with papilledema. The etiopathogenesis of HAR is unknown. However, it is suggested that, like in other oxygen-dependent retinal diseases (e.g., von Hippel-Lindau disease, retinopathy of prematurity, proliferative diabetic retinopathy, and glaucoma), factors like heterodimeric transcription and hypoxia-inducible factor could be the mediator for the changes in HAR [4]. Here, we have reported a case of bilateral HAR in a mountain climber.

2. Case Report

We report a case of bilateral-altitude retinopathy with vitreous hemorrhage in the left eye in a 29-year-old boy. He presented to us with a history of floaters in the left eye after five days of climbing the Himalaya of 4760 meters in Nepal. He also complained of slight diminution of vision in the same eye. He disclosed that climbing mountain was his hobby and he was not using supplemental oxygen either. He denied a history of similar complaints in the past and did not give systemic symptoms like headache, giddiness, vomiting, or any discomfort.

On examination, the best-corrected visual acuity (BCVA) was 20/20 in the right eye and 20/30 in the left eye. Intraocular pressure was 12 mmHg in both eyes. Slit-lamp biomicroscopic examination of the anterior segment of both eyes revealed the normal finding. Dilated fundus examination revealed bilaterally dilated major retinal veins, and the retinal vein and artery ratio showed 3 : 1 in both eyes. The right eye revealed clear, quiet vitreous, healthy macula, and pink and smooth optic disc. There was fresh vitreous hemorrhage confined just one disc diameter away at the superior and inferior part of the optic nerve in the left eye. The macula and optic nerve head of this eye grossly looked normal. The peripheral retinal finding also revealed no tears or other abnormalities.

Color fundus photographs were taken and are shown in Figure 1. Macular optical coherence tomography (OCT) was not taken in this visit due to vitreous hemorrhage. Full blood count, haemoglobin, sugar, creatinine, urea, lipids, CRP, and serology for HIV, HCV, VDRL, and HBsAg were normal. The tuberculin test and chest X-ray also appeared normal. Consultation of an internal medicine specialist did not give any abnormalities.

The patient was counselled for a wait and watch schedule and asked to be followed up in 3 weeks or as soon as possible if flashes, curtain-like visual block, or poor vision was noticed.

On the 3rd week, his BCVA was 20/20 in both eyes. Vitreous was clear in both eyes; however, retinal venous tortuosities and dilation were still present in the left eye. The macular OCT scan showed normal-appearing fundus. The retinal vein and artery ratio changed to 3:2. Color photos and OCT are shown in Figure 2.

3. Discussion

HAR represents numerous retinal vascular deformities associated with hypoxia. HAR is familiar findings among travelers at high altitudes, who exceed higher than 5000 m and are prone to developing severe high-altitude sickness like pulmonary edema, which could be life-threatening. Symptoms of individuals with HAR are mainly headache, insomnia, lassitude, and gastrointestinal upset. These symptoms generally begin from 8 to 24 hours and clear over four to eight days after exposure to high altitude [5].

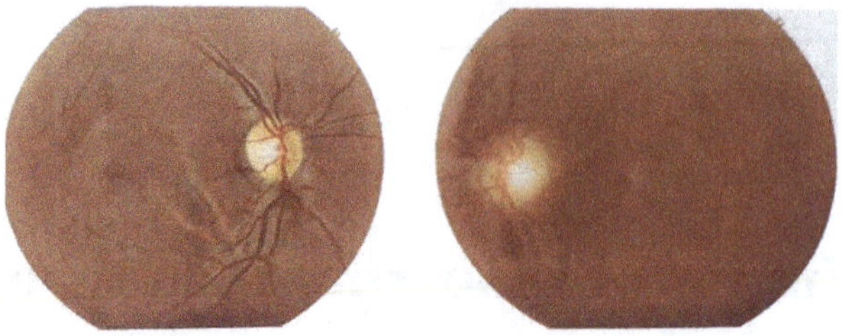

Figure 1: Fundus color photograph.

Patients with HAR are generally presented with sudden diminution of vision after exposure to high altitude and then regress after travelling to a lower altitude. Nonetheless, HAR can be misdiagnosed. So, other causes should be ruled out before establishing a diagnosis of HAR because of similar presentations in other ocular pathology.

The retina has a higher metabolic activity than other human tissues. Furthermore, there is a vascular regulatory mechanism and close anatomical correlation on supplying vascular blood to both the brain and retina. Retinal changes in HAR are associated with possible ocular dysregulation, described in mountaineers with the increase in all hemodynamic parameters. However, in hypoxic conditions like in high altitudes, autoregulation of choroidal and retinal flow was stable in oxygen delivery. In addition, an increase in the level of hematocrit, which leads to an increase in blood viscosity, could also be one of the factors for causing HAR [6].

Available incidence has suggested that retinal hemorrhages are due to arteriole side leakage of the vascular bed or capillary rupture. Due to an increase in the volume and rate of blood flow, these capillaries might become more vulnerable. Increased intraocular pressure could also be a common cause of HAR for individuals after ascent to high altitude. Changes and deformities in retinal hemodynamics and hypoxia create several adjustments in circulatory and respiratory physiology, leading to increased cerebral blood flow and increased cerebral venous pressure [7]. These effects then decrease the cerebrospinal absorption, and then, hypoxia induces capillary permeability increasing cerebrospinal fluid resulting in papilledema. Hemorrhagic retinopathy is set because of an increase in retinal venous pressure. Yet the definite pathological changes are not still explained and remain an area for requiring further research.

HAR can be both mild and transient. Still, it could lead to permanent damage. A study done by Ho et al. [5] found that the BCVA was nearly restored in individuals with HAR to the baseline after three weeks. Yet there was the presence of vascular tortuosity and engorgement of the blood vessels in the retina. They also found defects in the retinal nerve fiber layer and optic nerve while examining through scanning laser polarimeter (GDx). Retinal vein occlusions have also been delineated in HAR [8]. In 1989, Butler et al. had done a prospective study on all fourteen individuals after six weeks of climbing Mount Everest. They reported intraretinal hemorrhages in five eyes in four climbers, and central retinal vein occlusion was found in one of these climbers. They suggested

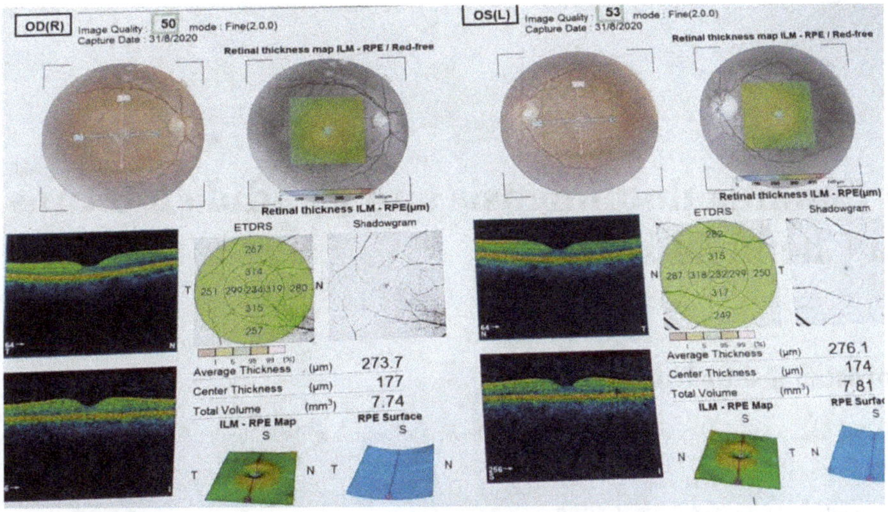

FIGURE 2: Macular OCT and color photograph showing normal findings.

that increased intraocular pressure and usage of nonsteroidal anti-inflammatory drugs could be the significant risk factors for the occurrence of HAR [2]. Frayser et al. [9] also delineated retinal hemorrhages in nine out of twenty-five climbers ascending 5,335 meters on Mt. Logan. However, there was no relation between retinal hemorrhage and speed of ascent. In another study, retinal hemorrhages accounted for 36% of 39 individuals climbing above 4,329 m on Mt. McKinley [10]. Here, they found a positive correlation between the occurrence of retinal hemorrhage and the severity of headache. They also discovered that individuals with a history of migraine, increased physical exertion, and rapid ascent are more prone to developing retinal hemorrhages.

4. Conclusion

Individuals having ascents to high altitudes have a high risk of developing HAR. Therefore, a detailed ocular examination with proper history is needed for all of them.

References

[1] R. K. Seth and R. A. Adelman, "High-altitude retinopathy and optical coherence tomography findings," *Seminars in Ophthalmology*, vol. 25, no. 1-2, pp. 13–15, 2010.

[2] M. Wiedman and G. C. Tabin, "High-altitude retinopathy and altitude illness," *Ophthalmology*, vol. 106, no. 10, pp. 1924–1927, 1999.

[3] I. Singh, P. Khanna, M. Srivastava, M. Lal, S. B. Roy, and C. Subramanyam, "Acute mountain sickness," *New England Journal of Medicine*, vol. 280, no. 4, pp. 175–184, 1969.

[4] O. Arjamaa and M. Nikinmaa, "Oxygen-dependent diseases in the retina: role of hypoxia-inducible factors," *Experimental eye research*, vol. 83, no. 3, pp. 473–483, 2006.

[5] T.-Y. Ho, W.-F. Kao, S.-M. Lee, P.-K. Lin, J.-J. Chen, and J.-H. Liu, "High-altitude retinopathy after climbing Mount Aconcagua in a group of experienced climbers," *Retina*, vol. 31, no. 8, pp. 1650–1655, 2011.

[6] G. E. Lang and G. B. Kuba, "High-altitude retinopathy," *American journal of ophthalmology*, vol. 123, no. 3, pp. 418–420, 1997.

[7] L. G. C. E. Pugh, "Physiological and medical aspects of the Himalayan Scientific and Mountaineering Expedition," *British medical journal*, vol. 2, no. 5305, pp. 621–627, 1962.

[8] R. Arora, K. Jha, and B. Sathian, "Retinal changes in various altitude illnesses," *Singapore Medical Journal*, vol. 52, no. 9, pp. 685–688, 2011.

[9] R. Frayser, C. S. Houston, A. C. Bryan, I. D. Rennie, and G. Gray, "Retinal hemorrhage at high altitude," *New England Journal of Medicine*, vol. 282, no. 21, pp. 1183-1184, 1970.

[10] G. A. Schumacher and J. H. Petajan, "High altitude stress and retinal Hemorrhage," *Archives of Environmental Health: An International Journal*, vol. 30, no. 5, pp. 217–221, 1975.

38

Combined Candida dubliniensis and Candida albicans Keratitis following a Chemical Injury

Justin Torosian and Thomas Mauger

West Virginia University Eye Institute, 1 Medical Center Drive, Morgantown, WV 26506, USA

Correspondence should be addressed to Justin Torosian; justin.torosian@wvumedicine.org

Academic Editor: Alexander A. Bialasiewicz

Candida dubliniensis is an uncommon source of ocular infections and has only been reported in a single previous case of keratitis. This report documents the course of a combined *Candida dubliniensis* and *Candida albicans* keratitis following a chemical injury. Antifungal sensitivities of the two different *Candida* species are also demonstrated.

1. Introduction

Fungal keratitis is a challenging clinical condition. The diagnosis and initiation of appropriate treatment may be delayed due to the insidious nature of the disease. Once identification of the organism is obtained and specific treatment is initiated, the course of therapy is often prolonged and clinical outcome may be poor. Fungal keratitis may be caused by either filamentous or yeast species. Filamentous fungi are more commonly associated with refractive contact lens wear and ocular trauma while yeasts are more commonly encountered in cases of chronic ocular surface disease [1, 2].

2. Case Presentation

A 43-year-old female presented to the emergency department with a history of a liquid chemical exposure to the right eye with a household liquid cleaner containing 6% sodium hypochlorite. Examination demonstrated a central 5 mm corneal epithelial defect and diffuse conjunctival injection. The corneal stroma was edematous. The eye was treated with topical atropine 1% BID, prednisolone acetate 1% QID, tobramycin-dexamethasone ointment QHS, ofloxacin QID, doxycycline 100 mg by mouth BID, vitamin C 1 tab by mouth daily, and preservative-free artificial tears QID. The patient was seen two days later and a 3 mm central stromal infiltrate was noted. Fortified vancomycin 50 mg/ml and tobramycin 15 mg/ml were added topically every hour while awake. The patient was referred to our clinic two days later and found to have a 3 mm anterior stromal infiltrate with fluffy borders with an overlying 5 mm epithelial defect consistent with infectious keratitis. A one millimeter hypopyon was present (Figure 1). The cornea was cultured for bacteria and fungus. All steroid containing medications were stopped. Cultures were negative. The cornea remained unchanged over the next week. The patient was taken to surgery for a corneal biopsy, repeat corneal cultures, cryotherapy, and a conjunctival flap. These cultures grew *Candida dubliniensis* and *Candida albicans*. Sensitivities to antifungal agents were obtained (Table 1).

The eye was treated with hourly topical natamycin 5% and the infection resolved over the next three weeks (Figure 2). She is awaiting a corneal transplant due to resultant corneal opacity.

3. Discussion

To our knowledge, *C. dubliniensis* has been described only once previously in the literature as a cause of fungal keratitis and never in combination with *C. albicans*. In this previous case, the patient's condition worsened despite topical antifungal therapy and required cryotherapy, penetrating keratoplasty, and instillation of intracameral antimicrobial

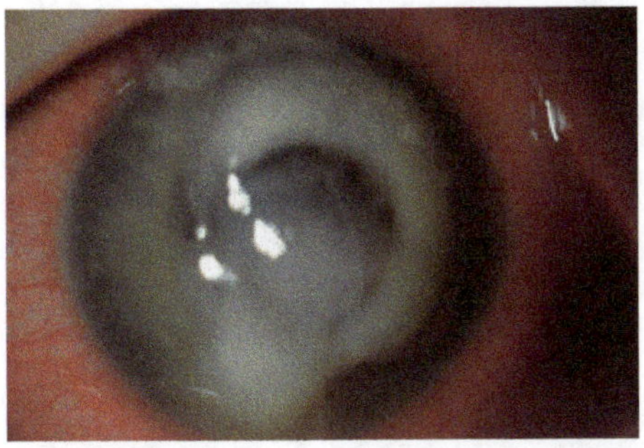

FIGURE 1: Central corneal epithelial defect with stromal infiltrate and hypopyon.

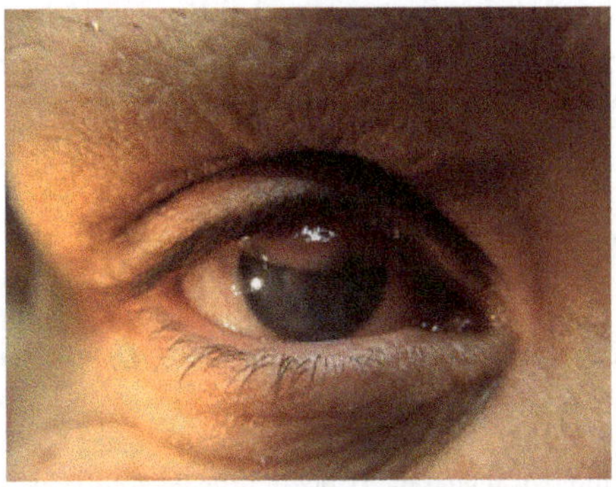

FIGURE 2: Corneal ulcer after Cryo treatment and conjunctival flap.

TABLE 1: Anti-Fungal Susceptibilities.

Anti-Fungal	Candida albicans MIC SUSCEPTIBILITY (mcg/mL)	Candida dubliniensis MIC SUSCEPTIBILITY (mcg/mL)
5 Flucytosine	0.5	0.06
Amphotericin B	0.5	0.225
Caspofungin	0.06	0.12
Fluconazole	0.25	0.12
Itraconazole	0.12	0.03
Voriconizole	0.008	0.008

and antifungal agents, as well as partial conjunctival flap placement [3].

C. dubliniensis was first designated as a unique organism in the United Kingdom in 1995, where it was identified as a causative agent of oral candidosis [4]. More recently, it has been identified as an uncommon cause of fungemia in cancer patients undergoing treatment, though it remains far rarer than various other candida species [5].

Regarding ocular involvement, *C. dubliniensis* has been known to be a potential causative organism of endophthalmitis, described multiple times in the ophthalmology literature in North America since 2012 [6–8]. In this case presentation, multiple aspects of the clinical presentation as well as the innate properties of *C. dubliniensis* become of interest. *C. dubliniensis* is a novel cause of fungal keratitis that can be difficult to identify and treat but is felt to be less virulent than *C. albicans* and generally susceptible to available antifungal therapies.

C. dubliniensis has been shown to produce germ tubes and chlamydospores, which has typically been thought of as a property of *C. albicans*. However, this novel species has been shown to be less robust on warmer temperature cultures [4]. It is interesting that both *C. albicans* and *C. dubliniensis* were shown to have grown in this patient. Furthermore, the particular culture of *C. dubliniensis* isolated was found to be less susceptible to caspofungin, but more susceptible to 5 flucytosine, amphotericin B, fluconazole, and itraconazole, and equally susceptible to voriconazole compared to the *C. albicans* isolate.

In vitro, *C. dubliniensis* has been shown to develop resistance to fluconazole in a multifactorial fashion similar to *C. albicans*, including both upregulation of efflux transporters and mutations in the gene encoding for lanosterol demethylase [9]. Furthermore, *C. dubliniensis* has been shown to be less virulent than *C. albicans*, which has been postulated maybe in part due to lower efficiency in hyphae formation [10]. Interestingly, recent literature has illuminated that *C. dubliniensis* hyphae formation is limited in nutrient-rich media due to changes in expression of transcriptional regulatory protein UME6 [11].

Of interest, as opposed to the first reported case of *C. dubliniensis* keratitis, our patient had both *C. dubliniensis* and *C. albicans* isolated in the corneal biopsy culture. The previously reported case in the literature was referred to the authors for nonhealing corneal ulcer, but the initial mechanism of injury is unclear. In this case, the initial injury to the eye was a severe chemical burn from an alkaline solution, sodium hypochlorite. It is reasonable to consider that the severe disruption of corneal architecture allowed for the growth of multiple infectious organisms. Furthermore, it begs the question of how many cases of fungal keratitis first begin as multiorganism infections. It is unclear how commonly multiple candidal species coexist in other modes of infection; however, *C. dubliniensis* and *C. albicans* have been shown to do so in oral samples taken from children with dental caries [12]. Previously, murine models have shown an inability for *C. dubliniensis* to cause keratitis as a single organism in immunocompetent mice. However, there was an ability to cause keratitis in immunocompromised models [13]. Perhaps the severe chemical injury in our patient provided a relative lack of blood flow and therefore created isolation from the body's typical immune response.

Of note, there are several limitations to this case study. First is that the organisms were detected and isolated by corneal culture. Perhaps in the future, additional collateral information including histology or sampling of other sites, including the mouth, nares, and any eye medications the patient may have used, would be of interest. Finally, given the ubiquitous nature of various candida species, the possibility of a culture contaminant must be considered.

Fortunately, the previous reported case of *C. dubliniensis* keratitis had a positive outcome following instillation of intracameral antifungals and antibiotics as well as penetrating keratoplasty. Indeed, although *C. dubliniensis* keratitis is an uncommon cause of fungal keratitis, it tends to be less virulent of a species and remains largely sensitive to common antifungal agents.

References

[1] E. W. Gower, L. J. Keay, R. A. Oechsler et al., "Trends in Fungal keratitis in the United States, 2001 to 2007," *Ophthalmology*, vol. 117, no. 12, pp. 2263–2267, 2010.

[2] L. J. Keay, E. W. Gower, A. Iovieno et al., "Clinical and microbiological characteristics of fungal keratitis in the United States, 2001-2007: A multicenter study," *Ophthalmology*, vol. 118, no. 5, pp. 920–926, 2011.

[3] T. D. Oostra, L. R. Schoenfield, and T. F. Mauger, "Candida dubliniensis: A novel cause of fungal keratitis," *IDCases*, vol. 14, Article ID e00440, 2018.

[4] D. J. Sullivan, T. J. Westerneng, K. A. Haynes, D. E. Bennett, and D. C. Coleman, "Candida dubliniensis sp. nov.: phenotypic and molecular characterization of a novel species associated with oral candidosis in HIV-infected individuals," *Microbiology*, vol. 141, no. 7, pp. 1507–1521, 1995.

[5] D. S. Jung, D. Farmakiotis, Y. Jiang, J. J. Tarrand, and D. P. Kontoyiannis, "Uncommon Candida species fungemia among cancer patients, Houston, Texas, USA," *Emerging Infectious Diseases*, vol. 21, no. 11, pp. 1942–1950, 2015.

[6] B. D. McMillan, G. J. Miller, and J. Nguyen, "Rare case of exogenous Candida dubliniensis endophthalmitis: a case report and brief review of the literature," *Journal of Ophthalmic Inflammation and Infection*, vol. 4, no. 1, pp. 1–4, 2014.

[7] T. P. Moloney and J. Park, "Candida dubliniensis endophthalmitis: Five cases over 15 years," *Journal of Ophthalmic Inflammation and Infection*, vol. 3, no. 1, pp. 1–6, 2013.

[8] E. Rosenberger, D. A. Youssef, S. Safdar, C. R. Larzo, and J. Myers, "Third case of Candida dubliniensis endogenous endophthalmitis in North America: Case report and review of the literature," *International Ophthalmology*, vol. 34, no. 4, pp. 945–950, 2014.

[9] S. Perea, J. L. López-Ribot, B. L. Wickes et al., "Molecular mechanisms of fluconazole resistance in *Candida dubliniensis* isolates from human immunodeficiency virus-infected patients with oropharyngeal candidiasis," *Antimicrobial Agents and Chemotherapy*, vol. 46, no. 6, pp. 1695–1703, 2002.

[10] C. Stokes, G. P. Moran, M. J. Spiering, G. T. Cole, D. C. Coleman, and D. J. Sullivan, "Lower filamentation rates of Candida dubliniensis contribute to its lower virulence in comparison with Candida albicans," *Fungal Genetics and Biology*, vol. 44, no. 9, pp. 920–931, 2007.

[11] L. O'Connor, N. Caplice, D. C. Coleman, D. J. Sullivan, and G. P. Moran, "Differential filamentation of Candida albicans and Candida dubliniensis is governed by nutrient regulation of UME6 expression," *Eukaryotic Cell*, vol. 9, no. 9, pp. 1383–1397, 2010.

[12] A. Al-Ahmad, T. M. Auschill, R. Dakhel et al., "Prevalence of Candida albicans and Candida dubliniensis in caries-free and caries-active children in relation to the oral microbiota—a clinical study," *Clinical Oral Investigations*, vol. 20, no. 8, pp. 1963–1971, 2016.

[13] Y.-L. Chen, A. Brand, E. L. Morrison et al., "Calcineurin controls drug tolerance, hyphal growth, and virulence in *Candida dubliniensis*," *Eukaryotic Cell*, vol. 10, no. 6, pp. 803–819, 2011.

Pseudomonas aeruginosa Scleritis following Pterygium Surgery with Mitomycin C or Beta Irradiation: Three-Case Report

Winai Chaidaroon, Somsanguan Ausayakhun, Napaporn Tananuvat, Phit Upaphong, and Kittipong Thabsuwan

Department of Ophthalmology, Faculty of Medicine, Chiang Mai University, Chiang Mai 50200, Thailand

Correspondence should be addressed to Winai Chaidaroon; hanumanthai777@gmail.com

Academic Editor: Maurizio Battaglia Parodi

Purpose. To report three cases of culture-positive *Pseudomonas aeruginosa* scleritis following pterygium surgery. *Patients and Methods.* A retrospective study of all patients of *Pseudomonas aeruginosa* scleritis after pterygium surgery presented from May 2017 to May 2020 was performed. Patient demographics and clinical characteristics included age, gender, time between prior surgery and onset, adjunctive therapy, risk factors, initial visual acuity, final visual acuity, clinical features, medical treatment, and surgical intervention were analyzed. *Results.* Three eyes of three patients with clinical characteristics and laboratory-confirmed *Pseudomonas aeruginosa* scleritis were identified. Two patients were related with mitomycin C application after pterygium surgery, and only one had beta irradiation. Antibiotic administration and scleral debridement were required in 3 patients. One eye was enucleated. Final visual outcomes of two patients were improved. *Conclusions. Pseudomonas aeruginosa* scleritis after pterygium surgery is a crucial ophthalmic disease. An early diagnosis with a prompt intensive antibiotic treatment in combination with surgical interventions may improve visual outcome.

1. Introduction

Scleritis, an inflammatory ocular disease of the sclera, is a devastating disorder that can cause permanent visual loss [1]. It has a diversity of clinical manifestations and causative factors. The major etiology is the immunological origin. However, scleritis caused by infections accounts for 5-10%. Infectious scleritis may occur after accidental or surgical injuries, severe endophthalmitis, or primary corneal infection, which can cause several vision-threatening complications such as cataract, glaucoma, and loss of the eye [2, 3]. Among a variety of organisms that have been isolated from infectious scleritis, *Pseudomonas aeruginosa* remains the most common infectious pathogen [4].

Pterygium is an ocular surface condition manifested by a triangular-shaped fibrovascular formation arising from the conjunctiva onto the cornea [5, 6]. A widely accepted risk factor for this disease is prolonged exposure to ultraviolet or sunlight, which damages the limbal stem cell barrier [7]. Thus, pterygium excision is one of the most common ophthalmic operations in patients who live in tropics and subtropics [2]. The bare sclera technique is the first surgical intervention associated with high rates of pterygium recurrence and postoperative infection [8]. *Pseudomonas aeruginosa* scleritis is commonly associated with the excision of pterygium and may occur years after surgery.

The main objective of this study is to report three cases of *Pseudomonas aeruginosa* scleritis following pterygium excision. The clinical characteristics, previous surgery with adjunctive treatments, treatments (medical and surgical therapy), and visual outcomes are described.

2. Patients and Methods

A retrospective descriptive study was conducted on the computer-encoded medical records of patients who had culture-proven *Pseudomonas aeruginosa* scleritis at the Ophthalmology Clinic, Chiang Mai University Hospital. The study protocol was conducted in accordance with the tenets of the Declaration of Helsinki, and the protocol was approved by the Ethics Committee of the Faculty of Medicine, Chiang Mai University (Study code: OPT-2564-08608). Written informed consents were obtained from all patients before the publication. In order to find recent cases of this rare disease, the database of medical records of clinical case summaries between May 2017 and May 2020 was cross-referenced against computer-coded cases with a diagnosis of *Pseudomonas* scleritis. Three patients (3 infected eyes) were identified. The computer records containing patient demographics and clinical characteristics were downloaded and analyzed. These data included age, gender, the time between prior surgery and onset, adjunctive therapy, initial visual acuity, final visual acuity, clinical features, medical treatment, and surgical intervention. Clinical notes for cases 1–3 were demonstrated. The summaries of all cases have been included in this report.

3. Case Presentation

3.1. Case 1. A 67-year-old male was referred to the tertiary hospital with severe pain, redness, and blurred vision in his right eye. He had a 12-year history of pterygium excision with the mitomycin C eye drops. At a secondary hospital, the doctor treated him as necrotizing scleritis with 0.5% moxifloxacin eye drops hourly in the right eye and ciprofloxacin (500 mg) one tablet twice daily for seven days without improvement before referral.

On his initial examination, the best-corrected visual acuity (BCVA) was 6/36, OD and 6/12, OS and marked injection of the conjunctiva with severe mucopurulent discharge. Slit-lamp biomicroscopy revealed necrotic scleral thinning surrounded by edematous necrotic tissue at the temporal sclera near the limbus in the right eye without anterior chamber reaction (Figure 1). The cornea was normal. Fundoscopic examination showed normal fundus. The left eye had a mild cataract, and the fundoscopy was also normal. The intraocular pressures were normal in both eyes. Scraping was obtained from the necrotic sclera and the base of the active lesion for microscopic examination and culture. The result of bacterial culture revealed *Pseudomonas aeruginosa* which was sensitive to amikacin, colistin, ceftazidime, imipenem, meropenem, ciprofloxacin, and levofloxacin. The patient was admitted to the hospital, and initial treatment was initiated with fortified amikacin (20 mg/mL) eye drops hourly and intravenous ceftazidime 1 g every eight hours. After four days of unresponsive medical treatment, superficial necrotic scleral tissue debridement was performed. The BCVA improved from 6/36 to 6/12 in the right eye, with an improvement in scleral thinning three weeks after admission. Fortified amikacin (20 mg/mL) eye drops were tapered within one month and replaced with levofloxacin eye drops four times daily. The BCVA of the right eye was 6/12, and the scleral lesion was healed completely without further thinning two months after treatment.

3.2. Case 2. A 68-year-old female, with a history of previous pterygium excision with mitomycin C application in the right eye five years ago, was referred to the ophthalmology clinic with right eye pain, redness, and decreased vision for three days. She was treated by a general ophthalmologist with 0.3% gentamicin eye drops hourly for a few days, but increased pain and redness and decreased vision occurred. She denied a history of systemic diseases.

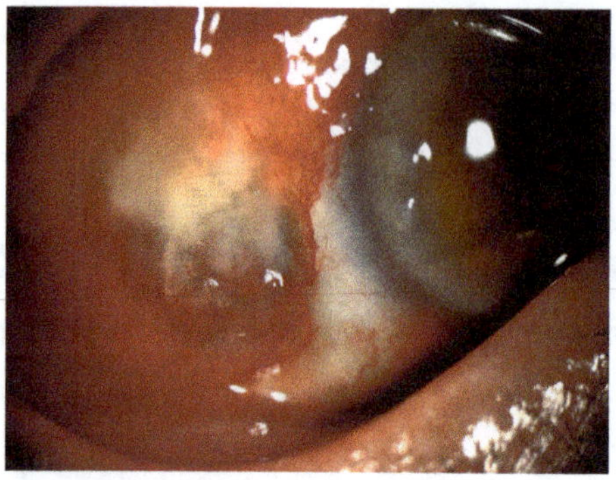

FIGURE 1: Slit-lamp photograph of the right eye of case 1, necrotic scleral thinning surrounded by edematous necrotic tissue was found at the temporal sclera near the limbus.

On eye examination, the BCVA was 6/18, OD and 6/9, OS. Slit-lamp biomicroscopy of the right eye showed a necrotic scleral ulcer in the area of previous pterygium excision and marked congestion of temporal conjunctival vessels with severe mucopurulent discharge. No hypopyon was found (Figure 2). The intraocular pressure and fundoscopy were normal. The fellow eye was normal.

Scleral specimens collected from the scleral ulcer disclosed many Gram negative bacilli and culture yielded *Pseudomonas aeruginosa*, which was sensitive to amikacin, gentamicin, ceftazidime, imipenem, meropenem, ciprofloxacin, and levofloxacin. As *Pseudomonas aeruginosa* scleritis was a definite diagnosis, the empirical treatment was initiated with topical fortified gentamicin (14 mg/mL) and cefazolin (33 mg/mL) eye drops hourly. Superficial necrotic scleral tissue debridement was performed. After four days, the frequency of eye drops was gradually decreased to every two hours with clinical improvement. Intravenous amikacin and ceftazidime were administered for three days. After four weeks of admission, the scleral ulcer turned to dark discoloration with less inflammation. The patient was discharged with BCVA of 6/6 in the right eye.

3.3. Case 3. A 70-year-old male had a history of right nasal pterygium excision with bare sclera technique and beta irradiation application 25 years ago. He also had a history of complicated cataract surgery in his right eye for five years prior to this admission. He presented at our hospital with severe right eye pain, blurred vision, redness, and swelling of the eyelids for seven days. With uncontrolled diabetes mellitus, the fasting blood sugar was 200 mg/dL and hemoglobin A1c was 7.1%. At presentation, the BCVA was hand movement, OD and 6/12, OS. Slit-lamp biomicroscopy of the right eye revealed conjunctival hyperemia, severe eyelid swelling, marked chemosis, and necrotic scleral ulcer size of 3 × 4 mm with calcified plaques at the nasal side of the previous pterygium excision (Figure 3). Mild corneal opacity was found without hypopyon. The fundoscopy showed severe vitritis that obscured fundus findings. Examination

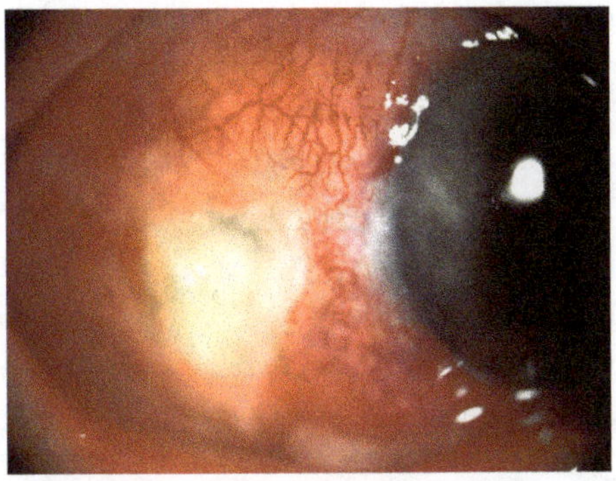

Figure 2: Slit-lamp photograph of the right eye of case 2 showed severe congestion of temporal conjunctival vessels, mucopurulent discharge, and necrotic scleral ulcer in the area of previous pterygium excision.

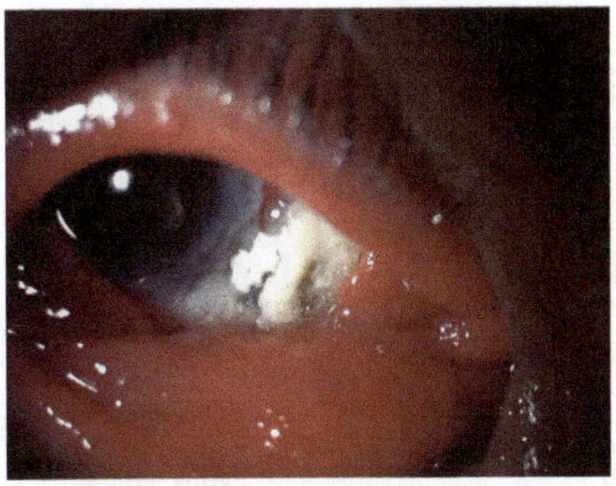

Figure 3: Slit-lamp photograph of the right eye of case 3 demonstrated severe eyelid swelling, marked chemosis, and scleral necrotic scleral ulcer size of 3 × 4 mm with calcified plaques at the nasal side of the previous pterygium excision.

of the left eye was normal. He was admitted for diabetic monitoring and proper eye treatment. He was brought to the operating room for microbial work up on the scleral site and the vitreous after a well glycemic control. The necrotic scleral tissues were debrided with ceftazidime irrigation. Vitreous tapping and a combination of intravitreal ceftazidime and vancomycin injection were performed. The specimens from vitreous, and sclera exhibited heavy Gram negative rod organisms. The culture findings illustrated *Pseudomonas aeruginosa*. The initial topical therapy was started with fortified amikacin (20 mg/mL) eye drops hourly and intravenous ceftazidime 1 g every eight hours. Four days later, the patient suffered severe eye pain with no light perception. He preferred to have his right eye removed by an enucleation procedure after a lengthy discussion.

Patient demographics and clinical characteristics are summarized in Table 1. Table 2 illustrates the antimicrobial susceptibility of *Pseudomonas aeruginosa* obtained from scleral tissues determined by using microdilution with microblot assay.

4. Discussion

Pseudomonas aeruginosa scleritis is a rare disorder that may cause marked thinning and melting of the sclera, leading to endophthalmitis, and the resulting loss of vision. Many studies revealed that advanced age may be a contributing factor to *Pseudomonas* scleritis [9–11]. Additionally, in a large retrospective study of infectious scleritis, Hodson et al. found that the median age of the patients who suffered from infectious scleritis was 70 years [12]. All cases in our study were over 60 years old. These findings may reflect that age could be one of the risk factors for *Pseudomonas aeruginosa* scleritis or the nature of a certain latency period after pterygium excision. *Pseudomonas aeruginosa* was detected in diabetic subjects more predominantly than nondiabetic subjects, demonstrated by the study of Noche et al. [13]. One patient in our study also had diabetes that may be a risk factor for *Pseudomonas aeruginosa* scleritis. Nuzzi and Tridico showed that there was a high recurrent rate of pterygium after simple pterygium excision [14]. Consequently, adjunctive therapy such as mitomycin C and beta irradiation had been used to prevent the recurrence. In this study, two patients had clear histories of mitomycin C and only one had beta irradiation application as the adjuvant therapy for at least 20 years. *Pseudomonas aeruginosa* scleritis following pterygium surgery with mitomycin C and beta irradiation had been proposed [15–17]. Several reasons suggested by Meallet indicated that the application of either mitomycin C or beta irradiation was inclined to compromise conjunctival blood vessels and subconjunctival connective tissues, thus restraining normal conjunctival wounding healing and leaving bare sclera for facile infection [18]. Bare sclera without intact conjunctival epithelium may be susceptible to infection. *Pseudomonas aeruginosa* employs neutrophil-activated collagenases to damage ocular tissues, in particular, compromised sclera [19]. Moreover, *Pseudomonas* bacteria could produce extracellular proteases. These destructive enzymes may contribute to the extension of subconjunctival *Pseudomonas* scleritis [2]. An animal experiment study by Kessler et al. indicated that the destruction of ocular tissue by *Pseudomonas* involved the protease produced by *Pseudomonas* and host response of both collagenolytic and proteoglycanolytic enzymes [20]. The duration between the previous surgical procedure and the onset in our study varied from 5 to 25 years. Alsagoff et al. and O'Donoghue et al. reported that the longest latent period was 40 years [21, 22]. The explanation for such a long latent period was undetermined; however, systemic autoimmune diseases or the surgery itself could stimulate or modify the hypersensitivity reaction associated with pathogens [23].

The clinical characteristics of *Pseudomonas aeruginosa* scleritis usually exhibit localized scleral inflammation and necrosis. In this study, two patients had severe pain and necrotic scleral melting consistent with typical *Pseudomonas* scleritis. Another was a diabetic patient with a severe scleral infection and endophthalmitis at presentation.

Initial management of *Pseudomonas aeruginosa* scleritis in our study included topical fortified antibiotics in all cases. Huang et al. reported that early surgical debridement and antibiotic irrigation should be highly encouraged in patients with severe scleritis which was poorly responded to aggressive medical treatment [2]. Regarding surgical intervention, three eyes in our study had undergone debridement of

TABLE 1: Demographics, clinical characteristics, treatments, and outcomes of three cases with *Pseudomonas aeruginosa* scleritis.

Case	Sex/ age (yr)/ eye	Adjunctive therapy	Latent period (yr)	Associated risk factors	BCVA initial-final	Clinical features	Treatments	Additional procedures
1	M/ 67/ OD	Mitomycin C	12	None	6/36-6/ 12	Scleral thinning surrounded by edematous necrotic tissue	Fortified amikacin eye drops and intravenous ceftazidime	Superficial necrotic scleral debridement
2	F/ 68/ OD	Mitomycin C	5	None	6/18-6/ 6	Necrotic scleral ulcer with severe mucopurulent discharge	Fortified gentamicin and cefazolin and intravenous amikacin and ceftazidime	Superficial necrotic scleral debridement
3	M/ 70/ OD	Beta irradiation	25	Diabetes mellitus	Hm	Severe lids swelling, marked chemosis, scleral ulcer with calcium plaques	Fortified gentamicin and cefazolin and intravenous amikacin and ceftazidime	Vitreous tapping with intravitreal antibiotics injection and scleral debridement with ceftazidime irrigation Enucleation

BCVA: best-corrected visual acuity; F: female; Hm: hand movement; M: male; OD: right eye; yr: year.

TABLE 2: Drug sensitivity patterns of *Pseudomonas* isolates of three cases by microdilution with microblot assay.

Drug	Case 1	Case 2	Case 3
Gentamicin	S	S	R
Cefepime	S	S	R
Amikacin	S	S	S
Ciprofloxacin	S	S	R
Colistin	S	R	R
Doripenem	S	S	R
Ceftazidime	S	R	R
Imipenem	S	S	I
Levofloxacin	S	S	R
Piperacillin-tazobactam	S	R	I
Meropenem	S	S	R

I: intermediate; R: resistant; S: sensitive.

necrotic scleral tissue. Surgical debridement not only had a good expedition of antibiotic penetration but also removed the volume of infected necrotic tissues. A unique collagen fiber arrangement of the sclera and a less vascular layer of an outer coat of the eye causes poor penetration of antibiotics for *Pseudomonas* scleritis treatment. A previous study confirmed the persistence of *Pseudomonas* pathogen despite laborious antibiotic treatment [17]. However, one eye in our study did not respond to both intensive antibiotic therapy and surgical interventions, which may be related to a strong virulence of *Pseudomonas aeruginosa* and/or host immune response to the microorganisms. The literature reviewed by Reynolds and Alfonso showed that nearly 60% of intensively treated eyes had undergone evisceration or enucleation [24]. Interestingly, all cases in this study had clinical improvement without corticosteroid treatment, except one case that had diabetes with severe endophthalmitis. The role of treatment with antibiotics and corticosteroids in ocular *Pseudomonas aeruginosa* infection remains uncertain [25, 26]; thus, we agreed not to use corticosteroids in three cases, especially in case 3 who had diabetes.

5. Conclusion

We highlighted three cases of *Pseudomonas aeruginosa* scleritis following pterygium surgery with the history of the application of either mitomycin C or beta irradiation. Early diagnosis with rapid intensive antibiotic treatment in conjunction with surgical interventions may improve visual outcomes.

Consent

We obtained written and informed consent from the patient for the publication of case details and images.

Acknowledgments

The authors thank Dr. Robert P Batzinger, PhD. for English manuscript revision and Mrs. Sunthari Upaphong, R.N. for kind assistance in photograph preparation.

References

[1] S. Ahmad, M. Lopez, M. Attala et al., "Interventions and outcomes in patients with infectious *Pseudomonas* scleritis: a 10-year perspective," *Ocular Immunology and Inflammation*, vol. 27, no. 3, pp. 499–506, 2019.

[2] F. C. Huang, S. P. Huang, and S. H. Tseng, "Management of infectious scleritis after pterygium excision," *Cornea*, vol. 19, no. 1, pp. 34–39, 2000.

[3] Z. A. Syed and C. J. Rapuano, "Umbilical amnion and amniotic membrane transplantation for infectious scleritis and scleral melt: a case series," *American Journal of Ophthalmology Case Reports*, vol. 21, article 101013, 2021.

[4] V. Jain, P. Garg, and S. Sharma, "Microbial scleritis-experience

from a developing country," *Eye (London, England)*, vol. 23, no. 2, pp. 255–261, 2009.

[5] J. C. Sánchez-Thorin, G. Rocha, and J. B. Yelin, "Meta-analysis on the recurrence rates after bare sclera resection with and without mitomycin C use and conjunctival autograft placement in surgery for primary pterygium," *The British Journal of Ophthalmology*, vol. 82, no. 6, pp. 661–665, 1998.

[6] T. Y. Wong, P. J. Foster, G. J. Johnson, S. K. Seah, and D. T. Tan, "The prevalence and risk factors for pterygium in an adult Chinese population in Singapore: the Tanjong Pagar survey," *American Journal of Ophthalmology*, vol. 131, no. 2, pp. 176–183, 2001.

[7] N. Dushku and T. W. Reid, "Immunohistochemical evidence that human pterygia originate from an invasion of vimentin-expressing altered limbal epithelial basal cells," *Current Eye Research*, vol. 13, no. 7, pp. 473–481, 1994.

[8] T. Shahraki, A. Arabi, and S. Feizi, "Pterygium: an update on pathophysiology, clinical features, and management," *Therapeutic Advances in Ophthalmology,*, vol. 13, 2021.

[9] S. C. Huang, H. C. Lai, and I. C. Lai, "The treatment of Pseudomonas keratoscleritis after pterygium excision," *Cornea*, vol. 18, no. 5, pp. 608–611, 1999.

[10] H. Siatiri, N. Mirzaee-Rad, S. Aggarwal, and A. Kheirkhah, "Combined tenonplasty and scleral graft for refractory *Pseudomonas* scleritis following pterygium removal with mitomycin C application," *Journal of Ophthalmic & Vision Research*, vol. 13, no. 2, pp. 200–202, 2018.

[11] P. L. Farrell and R. E. Smith, "Bacterial corneoscleritis complicating pterygium excision," *American Journal of Ophthalmology*, vol. 107, no. 5, pp. 515–517, 1989.

[12] K. L. Hodson, A. Galor, C. L. Karp et al., "Epidemiology and visual outcomes in patients with infectious scleritis," *Cornea*, vol. 32, no. 4, pp. 466–472, 2013.

[13] C. Domngang Noche, B. Tchatchouang, P. R. Fotsing Kwetche, G. Kagmeni, and A. L. Bella, "Ocular bacterial flora and antimicrobial susceptibility profile of a diabetic population in Cameroon: an analytical study," *International Journal of Biological and Chemical Sciences*, vol. 13, no. 4, pp. 2082–2091, 2019.

[14] R. Nuzzi and F. Tridico, "How to minimize pterygium recurrence rates: clinical perspectives," *Clinical Ophthalmology (Auckland, NZ)*, vol. 12, pp. 2347–2362, 2018.

[15] A. P. Moriarty, G. J. Crawford, I. L. McAllister, and I. J. Constable, "Severe corneoscleral infection. A complication of beta irradiation scleral necrosis following pterygium excision," *Archives of Ophthalmology*, vol. 111, no. 7, pp. 947–951, 1993.

[16] K. H. Tarr and I. J. Constable, "Pseudomonas endophthalmitis associated with scleral necrosis," *The British Journal of Ophthalmology*, vol. 64, no. 9, pp. 676–679, 1980.

[17] C. H. Hsiao, J. J. Chen, S. C. Huang, H. K. Ma, P. Y. Chen, and R. J. Tsai, "Intrascleral dissemination of infectious scleritis following pterygium excision," *The British Journal of Ophthalmology*, vol. 82, no. 1, pp. 29–34, 1998.

[18] M. A. Meallet, "Subpalpebral lavage antibiotic treatment for severe infectious scleritis and keratitis," *Cornea*, vol. 25, no. 2, pp. 159–163, 2006.

[19] E. R. Ramenaden and V. R. Raiji, "Clinical characteristics and visual outcomes in infectious scleritis: a review," *Clinical Ophthalmology*, vol. 7, pp. 2113–2122, 2013.

[20] E. Kessler, B. J. Mondino, and S. I. Brown, "The corneal response to Pseudomonas aeruginosa: histopathological and enzymatic characterization," *Investigative Ophthalmology & Visual Science*, vol. 16, no. 2, pp. 116–125, 1977.

[21] Z. Alsagoff, D. T. Tan, and S. P. Chee, "Necrotising scleritis after bare sclera excision of pterygium," *The British Journal of Ophthalmology*, vol. 84, no. 9, pp. 1050–1052, 2000.

[22] E. O'Donoghue, S. Lightman, S. Tuft, and P. Watson, "Surgically induced necrotising sclerokeratitis (SINS)–precipitating factors and response to treatment," *The British Journal of Ophthalmology*, vol. 76, no. 1, pp. 17–21, 1992.

[23] C. Y. Su, J. J. Tsai, Y. C. Chang, and C. P. Lin, "Immunologic and clinical manifestations of infectious scleritis after pterygium excision," *Cornea*, vol. 25, no. 6, pp. 663–666, 2006.

[24] M. G. Reynolds and E. Alfonso, "Treatment of infectious scleritis and keratoscleritis," *American Journal of Ophthalmology*, vol. 112, no. 5, pp. 543–547, 1991.

[25] E. J. Cohen, "The case against the use of steroids in the treatment of bacterial keratitis," *Archives of Ophthalmology*, vol. 127, no. 1, pp. 103-104, 2009.

[26] N. Ni, M. Srinivasan, S. D. McLeod, N. R. Acharya, T. M. Lietman, and J. Rose-Nussbaumer, "Use of adjunctive topical corticosteroids in bacterial keratitis," *Current Opinion in Ophthalmology*, vol. 27, no. 4, pp. 353–357, 2016.

40

Paramacular Acute Middle Maculopathy Associated with Glyceryl Trinitrate

Tryfon Rotsos,[1] Ioannis Giachos,[1] Konstantinos Tyrlis,[1] Chrysanthos Symeonidis,[2] Ekaterini Mani,[1] and Ilias Georgalas[1]

[1]1st Department of Ophthalmology, National and Kapodistrian University of Athens, Athens, Greece
[2]2nd Department of Ophthalmology, Aristotle University of Thessaloniki, Thessaloniki, Greece

Correspondence should be addressed to Chrysanthos Symeonidis; chrys2209@gmail.com

Academic Editor: Cristiano Giusti

An unusual case of nitroglycerin-induced Paracentral Acute Middle Maculopathy (PAMM) is presented. A 50-year-old patient with sudden vision loss and scotoma was followed up with swept-source optical coherence tomography (SS-OCT), optical coherence tomography-angiography (OCT-A), and fluorescein angiography (FA). An anal fissure treated with glyceryl trinitrate (GTN) 0.2% ointment with headache and dizziness after application was reported. Fundoscopy OS revealed mild retinal venous dilatation and tortuosity with scattered blot hemorrhages and subtle, parafoveal, whitish lesions in the outer retina. SS-OCT revealed diffuse, hyperreflective lesions in the inner plexiform (IPL), inner nuclear (INL), and outer plexiform layers (OPL). OCT-A revealed focal dropout in the deep capillary plexus. FA showed masking due to blot hemorrhages and early punctuate leakage in the inner retina. This entity was identified as nitroglycerin-induced PAMM. Over the following 8 months, after discontinuation of the ointment application, the patient was symptom-free with stable visual acuity. OCT revealed INL/OPL thinning and confirmed complete lesion resolution. This first report of retinal vascular abnormalities due to nitrite ointment provides an insight into an unknown side effect of nitroglycerin ointment use. A dose-dependent correlation between GTN application and retinal vascular abnormalities remains to be confirmed.

1. Introduction

Glyceryl trinitrate (GTN) is a nitric oxide-releasing drug which is mainly used in the management of angina pectoris, acute myocardial infarction, severe hypertension, and acute coronary artery spasms by dilating the venous system and decreasing ventricular preload. GTN is a prodrug which after denitration produces the active metabolite nitric oxide (NO). Organic nitrates that undergo these two steps within the body are called nitrovasodilators. GTN has also applications in the treatment of benign anal diseases such as anal ulcer and hemorrhoids [1]. An abnormal pressure response of the internal anal sphincter (IAS) plays a role in the pain sensation that characterizes these lesions. In the setting of anal fissure, chemical sphincterotomy leads to reduced anal canal pressure, relieves pain, and promotes localized healing. The IAS is innervated by nitric oxide-releasing nerves, and the release of NO triggers IAS to relaxation [2]. Administration of exogenous NO, via glyceryl trinitrate, has a similar effect [3].

The most common side effect of topical GTN is headache [1]. This is indicative of systemic absorption of the drug and its potential for clinical manifestations in other organs. Specifically, in the eye, nitroglycerin has the ability to cross the blood-ocular barrier and have a vasodilatory effect to the retinal vessels [4]. In contrast to retinal arteries, retinal veins and capillaries lack any elastic or smooth muscle tissue [5]. They are, however, covered with pericytes that express a contractile filamentous component called alpha-smooth muscle actin (αSMA). This component acts as a major indicator of vascular smooth muscle cells and is the reason why retinal capillaries are affected by vasoregulators like GTN [6].

The case of a patient with possible nitroglycerin-induced Paracentral Acute Middle Maculopathy (PAMM) after treatment with nitroglycerin ointment is presented [7]. To our best knowledge, this is the first report of a patient presenting with retinal and vascular abnormalities due to nitrite ointment.

2. Case Report

A 50-year-old Caucasian male presented to the emergency department, complaining of sudden vision loss and the presence of scotoma in his left eye (OS) with no ocular pain or discomfort. His past ophthalmic history was unremarkable. The patient had a history of painful anal fissure under treatment with GTN 0.2% ointment three times daily for the previous 2 months. After almost every application of the ointment, he was symptomatic with headache and dizziness that were partially relieved by common analgesics. He also reported that during the previous 15 days, pain from the fissure was significantly stronger, especially after bowel movement, which caused him to apply the ointment more often (up to 6 times daily). During the last 3 days, he reported episodes of transient postural hypotension. He was under no other medications and reported only occasional consumption of caffeine. He had no history of smoking, excessive drinking, or substance abuse.

Best-corrected visual acuity (BCVA) was 85 ETDRS letters OD and 75 ETDRS letters OS. Intraocular pressure was within normal limits. RAPD was negative in both eyes, and Ishihara plates showed no apparent dyschromatopsia. Anterior chamber examination of both eyes was unremarkable. There were no significant fundoscopic findings OD. Fundoscopy OS revealed mild retinal venous dilatation and tortuosity with scattered blot hemorrhages (Figures 1(a) and 1(b)). In the outer retina, subtle, parafoveal, whitish lesions were noted. Extensive multimodal imaging which included OCT, fundus autofluorescence (FAF), optical coherence tomography-angiography (OCT-A), and fluorescein angiography (FA) was performed (Figures 1(c)–1(h)).

Swept-source-optical coherence tomography (DRI OCT Triton, SS-OCT) demonstrated diffuse, hyperreflective lesions at the level of the inner plexiform layer (IPL), inner nuclear layer (INL), and outer plexiform layer (OPL) compatible with Paracentral Acute Middle Maculopathy (PAMM, Figures 2(a) and 2(b)). Fundus autofluorescence did not reveal any hyper- or hypofluorescent lesions of the Retinal Pigment Epithelium (RPE). Optical coherence tomography-angiography (DRI OCT Triton, SS-OCT) revealed a focal, small area of capillary dropout in the deep capillary plexus. Superficial capillary plexus, outer retina, and choriocapillaris appeared normal. No other vascular abnormalities were apparent. Fluorescein angiography revealed normal arteriovenous transit time, masking effect due to blot hemorrhages, and early punctuate leakage in the inner retina (Figure 3).

An extensive haematological workup which included complete blood count, fasting blood sugar and hemoglobin A1c, ESR, CRP, LDL, HDL, plasma homocysteine level, rheumatoid factor, ANA, ANCA, SACE, FTA-ABS, VDRL, antiphospholipid antibodies, protein C and S levels, factor V Leiden, cryoglobulins and a thrombophilia screen was performed. Moreover, plasma protein electrophoresis, chest X-ray (for the exclusion of sarcoidosis, tuberculosis, and left ventricular hypertrophy), and a magnetic resonance angiography (for any vascular stenosis) with contrast dye were also performed. The patient was also referred to cardiology for a full assessment with electrocardiogram, carotid Doppler imaging, cardiac echocardiogram, and rhythm and blood pressure Holter monitoring. There was no cardiological or vascular disease diagnosed. Haematological workup, X-ray, and MRA revealed no pathological findings.

The patient was advised to immediately discontinue any application of the drug. During the following month, the patient did not experience any of his previous symptoms and his visual acuity OS was 80 ETDRS letters with no RAPD. Fundoscopy revealed partial resolution of blot hemorrhages. The macula appeared normal. OCT revealed retinal disruption and thinning at the level of INL and OPL and partial resolution of the hyperreflective lesions (Figure 2(c)). OCT-A remained unaltered (Figure 1(i)).

Six months later, the patient was free of symptoms. Visual acuity OS was 80 ETDRS letters. Fundoscopy revealed complete resolution of the hemorrhages and the whitish lesions (Figure 1(j)). OCT showed INL and OPL thinning and complete resolution of the hyperreflective lesions (Figure 2(d)).

The patient mentioned that 8 months after the initial diagnosis, he had an exacerbation of symptoms regarding his anal fissure. He applied the ointment twice during a day for 4 days, which led to the remission of headaches and transient reduction of his visual acuity. He discontinued the drug application.

3. Discussion

Based on the clinical findings, multimodal imaging approach, laboratory results, and medical history of the patient, this disorder was identified as nitroglycerin-induced PAMM. Differential diagnosis included central retinal vein occlusion, branch retinal vein occlusion, ocular ischemic syndrome, retinal angiitis, diabetic retinopathy, and hypertensive retinopathy. Diabetic retinopathy and hypertensive retinopathy were excluded on the basis that the patient did not suffer from diabetes mellitus or hypertension and on the fact that the right eye remained asymptomatic and with no clinical signs. Central or branch retinal vein occlusion was excluded because of the atypical fundoscopic and fluorescein angiography findings, the presence of PAMM on presentation, the correlation of visual symptoms with the application of the ointment and improvement of symptoms, and findings after discontinuation of the drug. Ocular ischemic syndrome was excluded since the carotid Doppler ultrasound imaging and MRA were normal. A wide array of imaging and laboratory examinations were performed which failed to identify any obvious ocular disease. Valsalva retinopathy was excluded on the basis that the patient reported no episodes of constipation, only pain during defecation.

To our knowledge, this is the first reported case of nitroglycerin-related PAMM. It is conceivable that the

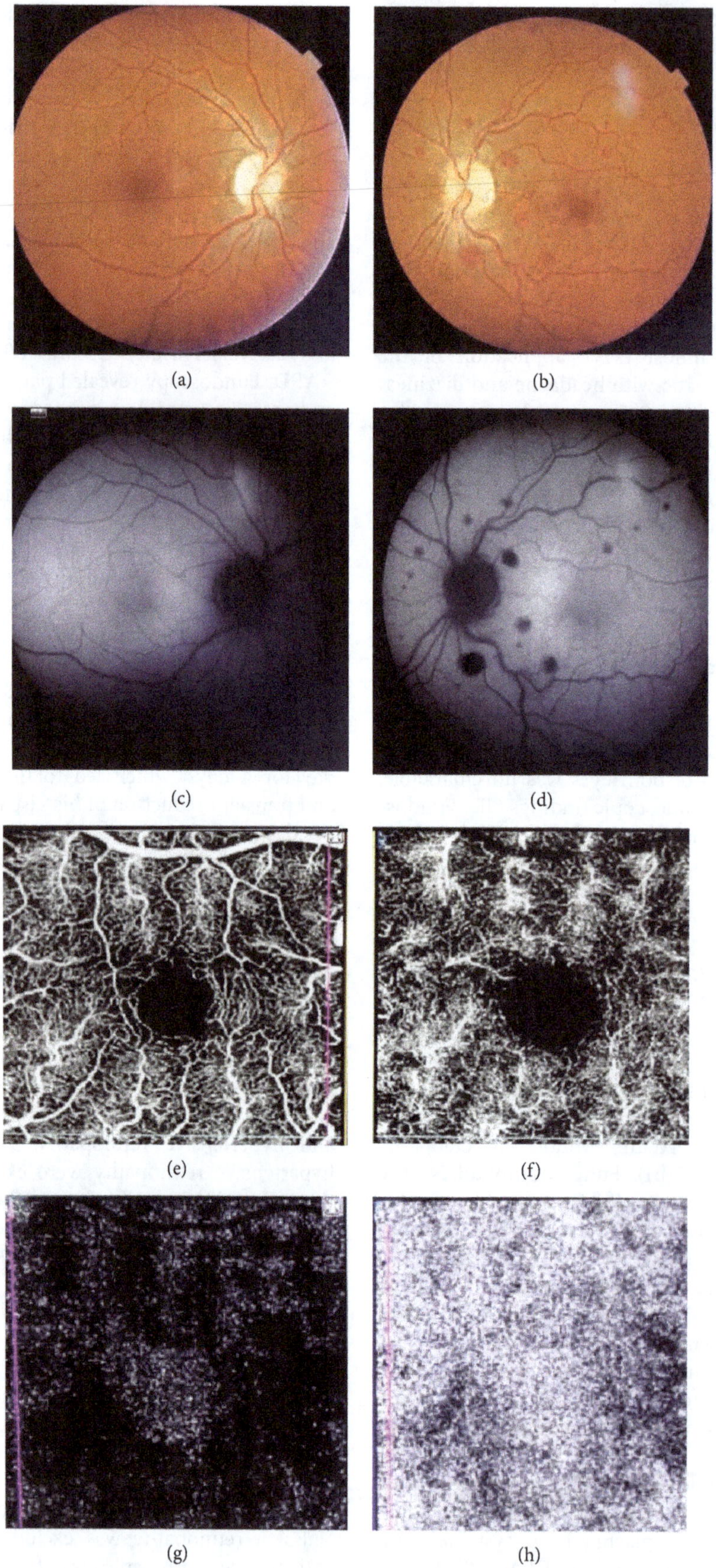

FIGURE 1: Continued.

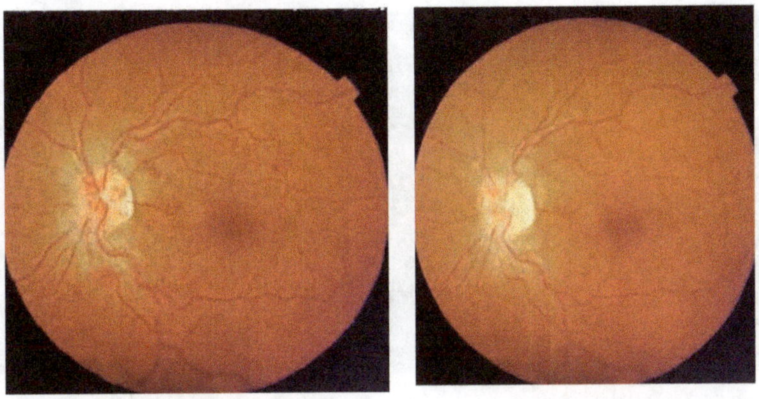

(i) (j)

Figure 1: Fundus photo OD with no evidence of pathology (a). Fundus photo OS with mild retinal venous dilatation and tortuosity with scattered blot hemorrhages (b). Fundus autofluorescence does not reveal hyperfluorescent lesions or RPE changes (c, d) apart from the masking effect from blot hemorrhages OS (d). Optical coherence tomography-angiography demonstrates a focal, small area of capillary dropout in the deep capillary plexus (f). Superficial capillary plexus, outer retina, and choriocapillaris appear normal (e, g, h). Fundus photo OS, 1 month after presentation with fewer blot hemorrhages (i). Fundus photo after 6 months of OS shows complete resolution of the hemorrhages (j).

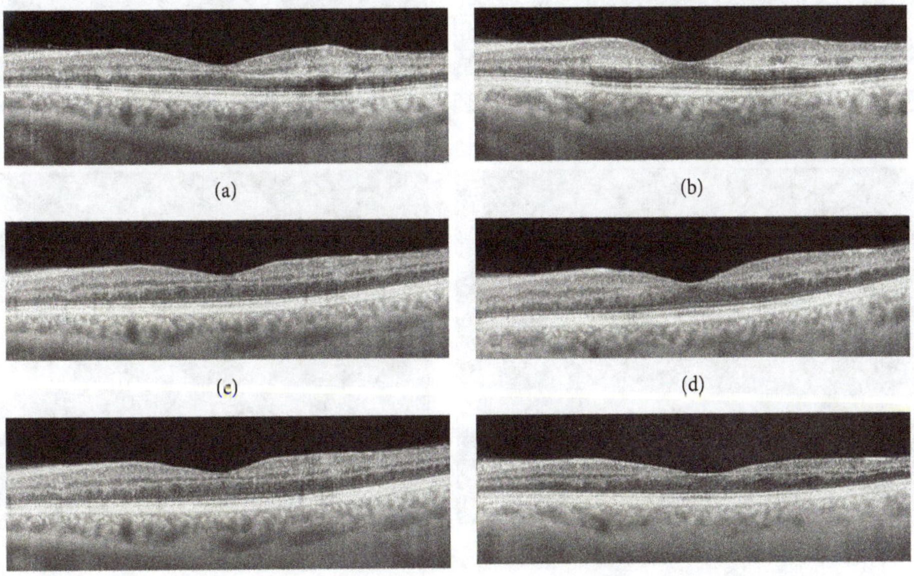

(a) (b) (c) (d) (e) (f)

Figure 2: Swept-source- (SS-) OCT imaging of the left eye. Horizontal scans are presented on the left column and vertical ones on the right one (lines 1 and 6 on DRI OCT Triton, SS-OCT, respectively). OCT scans on presentation demonstrated diffuse, hyperreflective lesions at the level of the inner plexiform layer, inner nuclear layer, and outer plexiform layer (a, b). Partial resolution (one month later) (c, d) and complete resolution (six months later) (e, f) of the lesions are observed along with thinning of the inner retina.

disorder is a result of two possible mechanisms of action, a direct and an indirect one.

The direct mechanism of action involves the nitrate effect on the retinal vessels. As previously stated, nitroglycerin has the ability to cross the blood-ocular barrier and have a vasodilatory effect to the retinal vessels [4], affecting retinal capillaries and veins despite the lack of any elastic or smooth muscle tissue [6]. This effect can explain the retinal vein dilation. It is conceivable that the vasodilatory effect of nitroglycerin in this patient was so potent that it also facilitated dilation of the retinal capillaries of the superior and inferior temporal branches of the central retinal artery to such a degree, causing hypoperfusion. This hypoperfusion led in turn to ischemia at the level of IPL, INL, and OPL, which resulted in PAMM. The fact that the patient had significant symptoms after almost every application of the drug further supports this hypothesis.

The indirect mechanism involves the nitrate effect on the circulatory system. At high doses, nitrates are commonly used for the treatment of acute heart failure by venous and

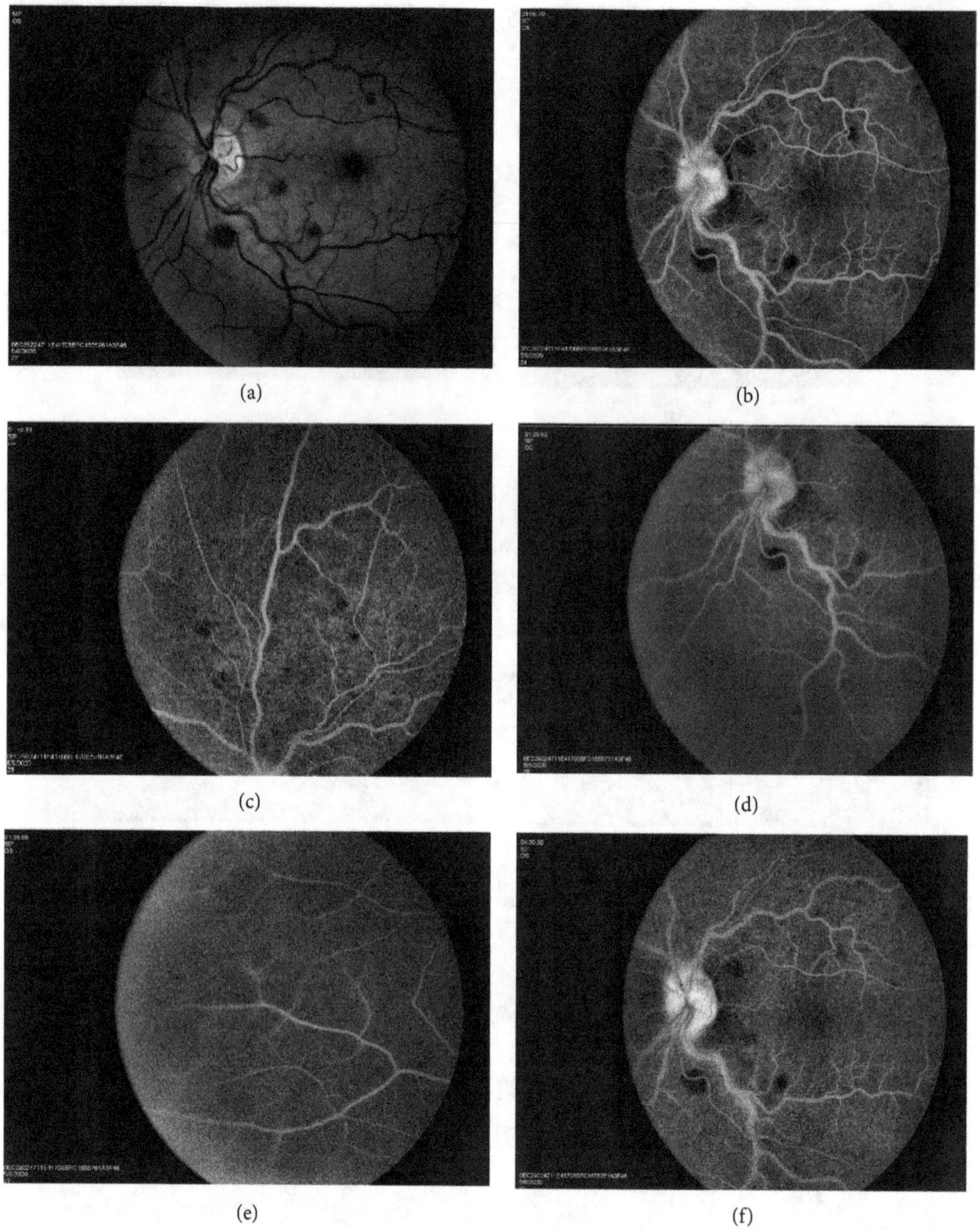

FIGURE 3: Fluorescein angiography (FA) images OS shows a masking effect due to blot hemorrhages and early punctuate leakage in the upper retina: (b) 1.09 min, (c) 1.19 min, (d) 1.29 min, (e) 1.38 min, and (f) 4.30 min.

arterial dilation. Nitrates lower left ventricular filling pressures and reduce systemic resistance. This provides not only preload but also afterload reduction and resolution of symptoms. However, there have been reports of nitroglycerin-induced hypotension and bradycardia [8]. This patient reported episodes of transient postural hypotension. This hypotension may lead to hypoperfusion of the retina at the level of the retinal capillaries leading in turn to macula ischemia and PAMM.

There has been a report of PAMM induced by a different vasodilating drug (PDE5 inhibitor) which further supports our hypothesis [9].

A reasonable counter argument against our diagnosis would be the unilateral presentation of the disease. One could argue that since there is systemic absorption of the drug, both eyes should be roughly equally affected. We believe that since the patient applied the ointment for a relatively short period of time (i.e., two months) and used it excessively for only 15 days; it is justifiable to assume that there was not enough time for the changes to manifest in both eyes. If this type of usage continued, it is possible that both eyes would have similar manifestations.

This is the first report of retinal and vascular abnormalities due to nitrite ointment. Since this type of ointment is widely used for the treatment of anal fissures and hemorrhoids, this case report should raise concerns regarding optimal use of this drug. Patients who have underlying cardiovascular risk factors and/or retinal diseases should be more closely monitored and be advised to seek immediate ophthalmic evaluation, should any visual disturbances occur. Patients who are otherwise healthy should also be advised of potential (albeit rare) visual disturbances especially after overuse. This case report may provide a new insight into an unknown side effect of nitroglycerin ointment. Further studies are needed to confirm a potential correlation between GTN application and vascular abnormalities of the retina.

Consent

The patient in the study has given consent for the clinical study to be published.

References

[1] J. H. Scholefield, J. U. Bock, B. Marla et al., "A dose finding study with 0.1%, 0.2%, and 0.4% glyceryl trinitrate ointment in patients with chronic anal fissures," *Gut*, vol. 52, no. 2, pp. 264–269, 2003.

[2] S. Rattan, A. Sarkar, and S. Chakder, "Nitric oxide pathway in rectoanal inhibitory reflex of opossum internal anal sphincter," *Gastroenterology*, vol. 103, no. 1, pp. 43–50, 1992.

[3] H.-L. Fung, "Clinical pharmacology of organic nitrates," *American Journal of Cardiology*, vol. 72, no. 8, pp. C9–C15, 1993.

[4] G. Weigert, B. Pemp, G. Garhofer et al., "Nitroglycerin-mediated retinal vasodilatation is maintained in patients with diabetes," *Investigative Ophthalmology and Visual Science*, vol. 49, p. 2088, 2008.

[5] M. Hogan and L. Feeney, "The ultrastructure of the retinal blood vessels: I. The large vessels," *Journal of Ultrastructure Research*, vol. 39, pp. 10–28, 1963.

[6] J. Kur, E. A. Newman, and T. Chan-Ling, "Cellular and physiological mechanisms underlying blood flow regulation in the retina and choroid in health and disease," *Progress in Retinal and Eye Research*, vol. 31, no. 5, pp. 377–406, 2012.

[7] D. Sarraf, E. Rahimy, A. Fawzi et al., "Paracentral acute middle maculopathy: a new variant of acute macular neuroretinopathy associated with retinal capillary ischemia," *JAMA Ophthalmology*, vol. 131, no. 10, pp. 1275–1287, 2013.

[8] P. C. Come and B. Pitt, "Nitroglycerin-induced severe hypotension and bradycardia in patients with acute myocardial infarction," *Circulation*, vol. 54, no. 4, pp. 624–628, 1976.

[9] N. Moura-Coelho, T. Gaspar, J. Ferreira, M. Dutra-Medeiros, and J. P. Cunha, "Paracentral acute middle maculopathy—review of the literature," *Graefe's Archive for Clinical and Experimental Ophthalmology*, vol. 258, no. 12, pp. 2583–2596, 2020.

Permissions

All chapters in this book were first published by Hindawi Publishing Corporation; hereby published with permission under the Creative Commons Attribution License or equivalent. Every chapter published in this book has been scrutinized by our experts. Their significance has been extensively debated. The topics covered herein carry significant findings which will fuel the growth of the discipline. They may even be implemented as practical applications or may be referred to as a beginning point for another development.

The contributors of this book come from diverse backgrounds, making this book a truly international effort. This book will bring forth new frontiers with its revolutionizing research information and detailed analysis of the nascent developments around the world.

We would like to thank all the contributing authors for lending their expertise to make the book truly unique. They have played a crucial role in the development of this book. Without their invaluable contributions this book wouldn't have been possible. They have made vital efforts to compile up to date information on the varied aspects of this subject to make this book a valuable addition to the collection of many professionals and students.

This book was conceptualized with the vision of imparting up-to-date information and advanced data in this field. To ensure the same, a matchless editorial board was set up. Every individual on the board went through rigorous rounds of assessment to prove their worth. After which they invested a large part of their time researching and compiling the most relevant data for our readers.

The editorial board has been involved in producing this book since its inception. They have spent rigorous hours researching and exploring the diverse topics which have resulted in the successful publishing of this book. They have passed on their knowledge of decades through this book. To expedite this challenging task, the publisher supported the team at every step. A small team of assistant editors was also appointed to further simplify the editing procedure and attain best results for the readers.

Apart from the editorial board, the designing team has also invested a significant amount of their time in understanding the subject and creating the most relevant covers. They scrutinized every image to scout for the most suitable representation of the subject and create an appropriate cover for the book.

The publishing team has been an ardent support to the editorial, designing and production team. Their endless efforts to recruit the best for this project, has resulted in the accomplishment of this book. They are a veteran in the field of academics and their pool of knowledge is as vast as their experience in printing. Their expertise and guidance has proved useful at every step. Their uncompromising quality standards have made this book an exceptional effort. Their encouragement from time to time has been an inspiration for everyone.

The publisher and the editorial board hope that this book will prove to be a valuable piece of knowledge for researchers, students, practitioners and scholars across the globe.

List of Contributors

Ruchi Goel, Akash Raut, Ayushi Agarwal, Shweta Raghav, Sumit Kumar, Priyanka Golhait and Sushil Kumar
Guru Nanak Eye Centre, Maulana Azad Medical College, New Delhi 110002, India

Simmy Chaudhary
Kallam Anji Reddy Campus, L V Prasad Marg, Banjara Hills, Hyderabad 500034, India

Ravindra Saran
Department of Pathology, Govind Ballabh Pant Post Graduate Institute of Education and Medical Research, New Delhi 110002, India

Beatriz Oliveira Lopes, Margarida Sena Brízido, Margarida Maria Miranda and Susana Morais Pina
Department of Ophthalmology, Beatriz Ângelo Hospital, Loures, Portugal

Ana Isabel Reis
Department of Medicine, Beatriz Ângelo Hospital, Loures, Portugal

Kepa Balparda
Department of Cornea and Refractive Surgery, Black Mammoth Surgical, Medellín, Colombia

Claudia Marcela Vanegas-Ramirez and Johny Márquez-Tróchez
Department of Ophthalmology, Universidad Pontificia Bolivariana, Medellín, Colombia

Tatiana Herrera-Chalarca
Department of Clinical Research, Black Mammoth Surgical, Medellín, Colombia

Mojtaba Abrishami, Seyedeh Maryam Hosseini, Hamid Mohseni, Amir Ghaffarian Mashhadi Nejad, Mohammad Baghi Yazdi, Ghodsieh Zamani, Nasser Shoeibi and Hamid Reza Heidarzadeh
Eye Research Center, Mashhad University of Medical Sciences, Mashhad, Iran

Omar Elghawy and Ryan Duong
University of Virginia School of Medicine, Charlottesville, Virginia, USA

Alice Y. Zhang and Eugene Y. Shildkrot
UVA Health Department of Ophthalmology, Charlottesville, Virginia, USA

William G. Wilson
UVA Health Department of Pediatrics, Charlottesville, Virginia, USA

Andres Gonzalez, Sarina Amin, Stephen Myles Potter and Syed Gibran Khurshid
University of Florida College of Medicine, Department of Ophthalmology, Gainesville, FL, USA

Omar Iqbal
University of Florida College of Medicine, Gainesville, FL, USA

Christopher B. Toomey, Jeffrey Lee and Doran B. Spencer
Viterbi Department of Ophthalmology, Shiley Eye Institute, University of California at San Diego, San Diego, CA, USA

Andrew Gross
McGovern Medical School, University of Texas at Houston Health Science Center, Houston, TX, USA

Kazuhiro Murata, Kenji Ozawa and Kiyofumi Mochizuki
Department of Ophthalmology, Gifu University Graduate School of Medicine, 1-1 Yanagido, Gifu-shi, Gifu 501-1194, Japan

Hideaki Kawakami
Department of Ophthalmology, Gifu Municipal Hospital, 7-1 Kashima-cho, Gifu-shi, Gifu 500-8513, Japan

Kiyofumi Ohkusu
Department of Microbiology, Tokyo Medical University, Japan

Ahgbatouhabeba Ahnoux-Zabsonre, Jérôme Sanou and Gertrude Méda
UFR/SDS University Joseph Ki Zerbo, 03 BP7021, Ouagadougou, Burkina Faso
Yalgado Ouedraogo University Hospital Center, Department of Ophthalmology, 03 BP7022, Captain Sankara Avenue, Ouagadougou, Burkina Faso

Yérénou Ferdinand Lankoandé
Yalgado Ouedraogo University Hospital Center, Department of Ophthalmology, 03 BP7022, Captain Sankara Avenue, Ouagadougou, Burkina Faso

Chantal Bouda
Yalgado Ouedraogo University Hospital Center, Department of Paediatrics, 03 BP7022, Captain Sankara Avenue, Ouagadougou, Burkina Faso

Assita Lamien-Sanou
UFR/SDS University Joseph Ki Zerbo, 03 BP7021, Ouagadougou, Burkina Faso
Yalgado Ouedraogo University Hospital Center, Department of Pathological Anatomy, 03 BP7022, Captain Sankara Avenue, Ouagadougou, Burkina Faso

Mohammad Reza Sedaghat and Mohammad Etezad-Razavi
Eye Research Center, Mashhad University of Medical Sciences, Mashhad, Iran

Hamed Momeni-Moghaddam
Health Promotion Research Center, Zahedan University of Medical Sciences, Zahedan, Iran
Department of Optometry, School of Paramedical Sciences, Mashhad University of Medical Sciences, Mashhad, Iran

Shehzad A. Naroo
Aston University, Ophthalmic Research Group, School of Life and Health Sciences, Aston Triangle, Birmingham B4 7ET, UK
College of Health and Life Sciences, Aston University, Birmingham, UK

Majid Moshirfar
John A. Moran Eye Center, Department of Ophthalmology and Visual Sciences, School of Medicine, University of Utah, USA
Utah Lions Eye Bank, Murray, UT, USA
HDR Research Center, Hoopes Vision, 11820 S. State Street Suite #200, Draper, UT 84020, USA

Elysse S. Tom, K. Matthew McKay and Steven S. Saraf
Department of Ophthalmology, University of Washington, Seattle, WA, USA

Ana Cortesão Costa and Mário Raimundo
Department of Nephrology, Beatriz Ângelo Hospital, Loures, Portugal

Igor Knezović and Sara Djurić
Eye Institute Knezović, Zagreb, Croatia

Majid Razavi
Department of Anesthesiology, School of Medicine, Mashhad University of Medical Sciences, Mashhad, Iran

Charles D. McGuffey, Andrew T. Melson and Kamran M. Riaz
Dean McGee Eye Institute, 608 Stanton L. Young Blvd, Oklahoma City, OK 73104, USA

Asher Khan
Dean McGee Eye Institute, 608 Stanton L. Young Blvd, Oklahoma City, OK 73104, USA
College of Medicine, University of Oklahoma, 800 Stanton L. Young Blvd, Oklahoma City, OK 73117, USA

Harsh Kumar, Mithun Thulasidas and Surbi Taneja
Glaucoma Services, Centre for Sight, B-5/24, Safdarjung Enclave, New Delhi, India

Dinesh Talwar
Vitreoretinal Services, Centre for Sight, B-5/24, Safdarjung Enclave, New Delhi, India

Mohammad-Reza Sedaghat
Eye Research Center, Mashhad University of Medical Sciences, Mashhad, Iran

Michael W. Belin
University of Arizona, Department of Ophthalmology & Vision Science, Tucson, Arizona, USA

Maryam Savardashtaki
Department of Optometry, School of Paramedical Sciences, Mashhad University of Medical Sciences, Mashhad, Iran

Hassan Robabi
Department of Nursing and Midwifery, Zahedan University of Medical Sciences, Zahedan, Iran

William E. Smiddy, Harry W. Flynn and Stephen G. Schwartz
Department of Ophthalmology, Bascom Palmer Eye Institute, University of Miami Miller School of Medicine, 900 NW 17 Street, Miami, FL 33136, USA

Abdelrahman M. Elhusseiny
Department of Ophthalmology, Bascom Palmer Eye Institute, University of Miami Miller School of Medicine, 900 NW 17 Street, Miami, FL 33136, USA
Department of Ophthalmology, Kasr Al Ainy School of Medicine, Cairo University, Egypt

Masaomi Kubota and Takaaki Hayashi
Department of Ophthalmology, Katsushika Medical Center, The Jikei University School of Medicine, 6-41-2, Aoto, Katsushika-ku, Tokyo 125-8506, Japan

Nobumasa Tamura, Haruhiko Yanagisawa and Akira Kojima
Department of Respiratory Medicine, Katsushika Medical Center, The Jikei University School of Medicine, 6-41-2, Aoto, Katsushika-ku, Tokyo 125-8506, Japan

Euido Nishijima and Tadashi Nakano
Department of Ophthalmology, The Jikei University School of Medicine, 3-25-8, Nishi-shimbashi, Minato-ku, Tokyo 105-8461, Japan

Daisuke Nakata
Department of Ophthalmology, Toyokawa City Hospital, Toyokawa, Aichi, Japan
Department of Ophthalmology, Fujita Health University, School of Medicine, Toyoake, Aichi, Japan

Sayaka Kakehi and Hiroshi Okada
Department of Ophthalmology, Toyokawa City Hospital, Toyokawa, Aichi, Japan

Atsuhiro Tanikawa, Yoshiaki Shimada, Masayuki Horiguchi and Yasuki Ito
Department of Ophthalmology, Fujita Health University, School of Medicine, Toyoake, Aichi, Japan

Sunil Ruparelia
Faculty of Medicine, Dalhousie University, Halifax, Nova Scotia, Canada

Nir Shoham-Hazon
Faculty of Medicine, Dalhousie University, Halifax, Nova Scotia, Canada
Miramichi EyeNB Centre of Excellence, Miramichi, NB, Canada

Juliana Wons and Jana Dinges
City Hospital Triemli, Zurich, Switzerland

Matthias D. Becker
City Hospital Triemli, Zurich, Switzerland
University of Heidelberg, Germany

Stephan Michels
City Hospital Triemli, Zurich, Switzerland
University of Zurich, Switzerland

Mariam Raheem, Nimesh A. Patel, Audina M. Berrocal, Alana Grajewski and Mohamed Abou Shousha
Bascom Palmer Eye Institute, Miller School of Medicine, University of Miami, Miami, FL, USA

Taher Eleiwa
Bascom Palmer Eye Institute, Miller School of Medicine, University of Miami, Miami, FL, USA
Department of Ophthalmology, Faculty of Medicine, Benha University, Benha, Egypt

Mustafa Jaffry
Rutgers New Jersey Medical School, Newark NJ, USA

Mark Lister
New York Medical College, Valhalla, New York, USA

Mona Fayad, Richard B. Rosen and Harsha S. Reddy
Department of Ophthalmology, New York Eye and Ear Infirmary of Mount Sinai, 310 E 14th St, New York, NY 10003, USA
Icahn School of Medicine at Mount Sinai, 1 Gustave L. Levy Pl, New York, NY 10029, USA

Hamouda Hamdy Ghoraba
Ophthalmology Department, Faculty of Medicine, Tanta University, Tanta, Egypt
Magrabi Eye Hospital, Tanta, Egypt

Hashem Hamouda Ghoraba
Magrabi Eye Hospital, Tanta, Egypt

Adel Galal Zaky
Ophthalmology Department, Faculty of Medicine, Menoufia University, Shibin el Kom, Egypt

Mladen Bušić, Damir Bosnar and Biljana Kuzmanović Elabjer
Department of Ophthalmology, Reference Center of the Ministry of Health of the Republic of Croatia for Pediatric Ophthalmology and Strabismus, University Hospital "Sveti Duh", Zagreb, Croatia
Faculty of Medicine, Josip Juraj Strossmayer University of Osijek, Osijek, Croatia
Faculty of Dental Medicine and Health Osijek, Josip Juraj Strossmayer University of Osijek, Osijek, Croatia

Mirjana Bjeloš
Department of Ophthalmology, Reference Center of the Ministry of Health of the Republic of Croatia for Pediatric Ophthalmology and Strabismus, University Hospital "Sveti Duh", Zagreb, Croatia
Faculty of Medicine, Josip Juraj Strossmayer University of Osijek, Osijek, Croatia
Faculty of Dental Medicine and Health Osijek, Josip Juraj Strossmayer University of Osijek, Osijek, Croatia
University Eye Clinic, Faculty of Dental Medicine and Health Care Osijek, Faculty of Medicine Osijek, University Josip Juraj Strossmayer in Osijek, University Hospital "Sveti Duh", Zagreb, Croatia

Ana Ćurić and Leon Marković
Department of Ophthalmology, Reference Center of the Ministry of Health of the Republic of Croatia for Pediatric Ophthalmology and Strabismus, University Hospital "Sveti Duh", Zagreb, Croatia
Faculty of Dental Medicine and Health Osijek, Josip Juraj Strossmayer University of Osijek, Osijek, Croatia

Borna Šarić and Benedict Rak
Department of Ophthalmology, Reference Center of the Ministry of Health of the Republic of Croatia for Pediatric Ophthalmology and Strabismus, University Hospital "Sveti Duh", Zagreb, Croatia

Luis Martinez-Velazquez, Kevin K. Ma, Neal S. Patel and Zhonghui Katie Luo
Massachusetts Eye and Ear Infirmary, 243 Charles St, Boston, MA 02114, USA

Roghayeh Dehghan
Department of Genetics and Molecular Biology, School of Medicine, Isfahan University of Medical Science, Isfahan, Iran

Mahdiyeh Behnam
Cellular, Molecular and Genetics Research Center, Isfahan University of Medical Sciences, Isfahan, Iran

Mansoor Salehi
Department of Genetics and Molecular Biology, School of Medicine, Isfahan University of Medical Science, Isfahan, Iran
Pediatric Inherited Diseases Research Center, Research Institute for Primordial Prevention of Non-Communicable Disease, Isfahan University of Medical Sciences, Isfahan, Iran
Child Growth and Development Research Center, Research Institute for Primordial Prevention of Non-Communicable Disease, Isfahan University of Medical Sciences, Isfahan, Iran

Roya Kelishadi
Department of Pediatrics, Child Growth and Development Research Center, Research Institute for Primordial Prevention of Non- Communicable Disease, Isfahan University of Medical Sciences, Isfahan, Iran

Tomas R. Burke
Moorfields Eye Hospital, London, UK

Susan L. Lightman
Moorfields Eye Hospital, London, UK
University College London Institute of Ophthalmology, London, UK

Biljana Kuzmanović Elabjer, Dean Šarić, Mladen Bušić, Mirjana Bjeloš and Andrej Pleše
University Eye Clinic, Faculty of Dental Medicine and Health Care Osijek, Faculty of Medicine Osijek, University Josip Juraj Strossmayer in Osijek, University Hospital "Sveti Duh", Zagreb, Croatia

Alexander R. Bottini, Sean Steinmetz, Kevin J. Blinder and Gaurav K. Shah
The Retina Institute, St. Louis, MO, USA

Kathryn Kelani Braceros, Masumi G. Asahi and Ron P. Gallemore
Retina Macula Institute, Torrance, California, USA

Tahsin Khundkar
Department of Ophthalmology, University of Minnesota, 516 Delaware Street SE, Minneapolis, MN 55455, USA

Syed R. Hasan
AdvantageCare Physicians, 180-05 Hillside Avenue, Queens, NY 11432, USA

Mark P. Breazzano
Department of Ophthalmology, Johns Hopkins University School of Medicine, 87 Thomas Johnson Drive, Frederick, MD 21702, USA

Constance Mei
Department of Ophthalmology, New York Medical College-Jamaica Hospital Medical Center, 134-20 Jamaica Avenue, Richmond Hills, NY 11418, USA

Brandon B. Johnson
New York Retina Center, 161 E 32nd St, New York, NY 10016, USA

Michael J. Schatz, Carl S. Wilkins, Oscar Otero-Marquez, Toco Y. P. Chui, Meenakashi Gupta, Deep Parikh and Alexander Pinhas
Department of Ophthalmology, New York Eye and Ear Infirmary of Mount Sinai, 310 E 14th St, New York, NY 10003, USA

Arjun Shrestha and Rinkal Suwal
BP Eye Foundation, Hospital for Children, Eye, ENT & Rehabilitation Services, Bhaktapur, Nepal

Biju Shrestha
Department of Physiology, Kathmandu Medical College, Kathmandu, Nepal

Justin Torosian and Thomas Mauger
West Virginia University Eye Institute, 1 Medical Center Drive, Morgantown, WV 26506, USA

Winai Chaidaroon, Somsanguan Ausayakhun, Napaporn Tananuvat, Phit Upaphong and Kittipong Thabsuwan
Department of Ophthalmology, Faculty of Medicine, Chiang Mai University, Chiang Mai 50200, Thailand

Tryfon Rotsos, Ioannis Giachos, Konstantinos Tyrlis, Ekaterini Mani and Ilias Georgalas
Department of Ophthalmology, National and Kapodistrian University of Athens, Athens, Greece

Chrysanthos Symeonidis
Department of Ophthalmology, Aristotle University of Thessaloniki, Thessaloniki, Greece

Index

www.ingramcontent.com/pod-product-compliance
Lightning Source LLC
LaVergne TN
LVHW082232200926
848484LV00008B/2341